# HEALTHY GUT, HEALTHY YOU

# HEALTHY GUT, HEALTHY YOU

### The Personalized Plan to Transform
### Your Health from the Inside Out

DR. MICHAEL RUSCIO

Published by The Ruscio Institute, LLC, Las Vegas, NV
www.drruscio.com

Edited and Designed by Girl Friday Productions
www.girlfridayproductions.com

Editorial: Judith Bloch, Katherine Richards, and Carrie Wicks
Interior Design: Paul Barrett
Cover Design: 99 Designs
Image Credits: Cover image © Natalia Aggiato/Shutterstock

ISBN (Paperback): 9780999766804
e-ISBN: 9780999766811

First Edition

Printed in the United States of America

. . . . . . . . . . . . .

Image Credits (Interior) (SS = Shutterstock)

Design elements used throughout: © Marochkina Anastasiia/SS; © Alena Ohneva/SS, © Designnua/SS.

p. 20: © BlueRingMedia/SS (both); p. 28: © Peter Hermes Furian/SS, © Juliann/SS; p. 32: Courtesy Roman Yevseyev Art, romanyevseyev.deviantart.com; p. 33: © Christian Jegou Publiphoto Diffusion/Science Source; p. 34: Reproduced with permission from JAMA. 2007; 297(9): 969–977 Copyright © (2007) American Medical Association. All rights reserved.; p. 40: © paper_Owl/SS; p. 51: Reproduced with permission from Psychoneuroendocrinology Journal. 2015; 53: 233–245. http://dx.doi.org/10.1016/j.psyneuen.2015.01.006. Copyright © (2015) Elsevier; p. 51: Reproduced with permission from Journal of Allergy and Clinical Immunology. 2013; 131(6):1465–1478. http://dx.doi.org/10.1016/j.jaci.2013.04.031. Copyright © (2013) Elsevier; p. 55: © erichon/SS, © Matyas Rehak/SS; p. 75: FODMAPs chart adapted from original BlissfulWriter chart: © Nik Merkulov/SS, © Dan Kosmayer/SS, © Satit Pecharut/SS, © Coprid/SS, © Tim UR/SS, © Grigor Unkovski/SS, © JIANG HONGYAN/SS, © Subject Photo/SS; p. 94: © ekler/SS; p. 106: Reproduced with permission from Autoimmunity Reviews. 2015; 14(6): 479–489. https://doi.org/10.1016/j.autrev.2015.01.009. Copyright © (2015) Elsevier; p. 131: Courtesy Simon Cotterill, with permission from the Kentucky Cancer Registry; p. 134: © ajt/SS; p. 135: © CebotariN/SS, © nui7711/SS; p. 158: © Robert Adrian Hillman/SS, © Alila Medical Media/SS; p. 180: © GraphicsRF/SS, © Teguh Mujiono/SS; p. 187: © Africa Studio/SS; p. 234: © 2003, Center for Biofilm Engineering at Montana State University, P. Dirckx; p. 237: Recreated with permission from Gastroenterol Hepatol (N Y). 2009 Jun; 5(6): 435–442. Copyright © Gastro-Hep Communications, Inc.

# TABLE OF CONTENTS

# INTRODUCTION

I learned the importance of gut health firsthand when I was in my twenties. I had always been a happy, high-energy guy—I played sports and music, dove deep into academics, and had a rich social life. And then a series of events began that would change my entire life.

I noticed that I was always tired. You know those days when you feel like you're dragging? We all have days like that once in a while, but I was feeling it every day. I needed two or three naps a day, had a hard time thinking, and just wanted to put my head down and rest. I was often cold, and I seemed to be wearing more clothes than everyone around me. My hair was thinning.

These symptoms certainly weren't fun, but I wasn't alarmed. I had a lot on my plate (school, work, sports), and I wasn't a kid anymore. I didn't like the way I felt, but I could live with it. What else could I do? I was already eating well, exercising, and getting enough sleep, and I had a happy life.

Then the insomnia started. I would wake up at two in the morning and wouldn't be able to get back to sleep. It was maddening. I also craved sugar. Sometimes I would get in my car and drive to the store at three in the morning to buy a candy bar. When it was time to get up, I was tired. In addition to all this, for the first time in my life, I was having bouts of depression.

I knew this wasn't normal. I thought to myself, *Time to see a doctor. This is what doctors are for, right?* I saw three doctors: a family doctor, an internist, and an endocrinologist. It felt good to take action. I was confident a doctor would find something wrong, we'd fix it, and I'd get on with my life.

Good news and bad news were to follow. The good news was the doctors all said there was nothing wrong with me. The bad news was the doctors all said there was nothing wrong with me! Because the doctors could find nothing wrong with me, they had no recommendations, and apparently there was nothing I could do.

I decided it was time to take matters into my own hands. I was a premed student, working as a personal trainer, and studying holistic nutrition. Because of this training, I already had myself on a healthy diet and exercise program, but obviously I needed to take things to the next level. I started reading and studying everything I could on my symptoms: fatigue, depression, insomnia, feeling cold, thinning hair, and cravings.

Eventually, my studies brought me to a conclusion that took into account all of my symptoms. I had hypothyroidism and adrenal fatigue—essentially hormone imbalances. This had to be the cause of my problems! I started taking a number of supplements that supported the adrenals and thyroid, and I began to feel better, about 30% better. This improvement only lasted a few weeks, though, and then I slowly returned to my unsatisfactory "new normal." I was crushed. I was also irritated because I had spent a few hundred dollars on the supplements.

As if things weren't bad enough, another symptom appeared, this one perhaps the worst of all: brain fog. I experienced episodes where I felt drunk. It was hard for me to speak clearly, I couldn't remember things, and I felt uncoordinated—like my head was in a fog. This would happen after I ate, but what I ate didn't matter; the episodes were completely random. I tried keeping a food journal, but nothing I ate seemed to correlate with the brain-fog episodes.

I continued with my research, trying to get to the root of my problems. Was I feeling this way because of low testosterone? I went on a testosterone-boosting protocol, which, like the last treatment I prescribed for myself, provided about a 30% improvement. And, as before, the improvement was short-lived.

More reading and research followed. Could it be mercury toxicity? I had my urine tested, and the results showed high levels of mercury and lead. *Yes! Finally!* I thought. *This has* got *to be it!* I started on a metal detox program and felt . . . no different. Repeated testing showed that my metal levels had improved, but my symptoms didn't change. I finally tried food-allergy testing. This test showed I was allergic to a whole bunch of foods. I avoided those foods, which was excruciating because it felt like I was on a four-food diet. I did not get better.

At this point, I began to wonder if I was crazy. Clearly something wasn't right, but nothing I'd tried had worked! I went to a weekend workshop that was part of my holistic nutrition training, and there I heard about a doctor who practiced functional medicine, which was apparently the type of

practice everyone in this community went to. I got more information on this doctor, and it seemed like he did exactly what I needed, but he didn't take insurance, and I was a living on a student's budget. I had to save up to afford a haircut, never mind pay $300 for an initial exam. But what did I have to lose? At this point I was desperate; I would have done anything.

This doctor told me he suspected I had a parasitic infection in my intestines. I remember thinking, *Are you kidding me? I don't have diarrhea or other digestive symptoms. Fix my insomnia, depression, and brain fog, please!* However, it turned out he was right. I had an infection in my intestines, and this *one thing* was the underlying cause of *all* my symptoms. As I treated this infection, I experienced slow and steady improvements for all my symptoms. This time, the improvements lasted. Over the course of a few months, I returned to normal. What a relief!

I was so moved by my experience and impressed with that doctor, I decided to follow in his footsteps and practice functional medicine, with a special focus on digestive health. For the past several years, I've helped sick and suffering people determine the cause of their illnesses and not only get better but vastly improve their health. It has truly been an honor and a privilege to do this work. At the same time, I've become increasingly concerned for those who find themselves where I was in my twenties: sick without knowing why, desperately trying to recover their health.

The amount of medical information that people have access to on the Internet is staggering. The downside of this is that people are becoming more and more confused about what to do when they're sick and can't figure out why. So many options, so many opinions . . . you could drown in the possible diagnoses and treatments. You could self-diagnose and try treatments for thirty years and still not exhaust the possibilities. What makes matters worse, this sea of information is polluted by marketing content that's written and designed to look like science to sell you a health-care product. As someone who actually performs and publishes clinical research, I find this appalling. Maybe worst of all, health care is sometimes looked at as a business rather than a healing profession, and there are those who are clearly taking advantage of the fact sick patients are willing to spend lots of money to feel better. All of this has created the perfect storm where health care has become confusing, way too elaborate, and very expensive.

## THE REALIZATION

I have been watching as patients find their way to my office after navigating this increasingly turbulent sea of health-care options. I have often thought to myself, *These patients are going through the same thought process I was, reaching for any possible solution, grasping for straws, self-diagnosing with hypothyroidism, adrenal fatigue, food allergies, toxicity...* I have come to realize what it took to improve *my* health is, in fact, true for the majority of these patients: you must *start* with the gut. This is the most important area to address when starting on your health-care journey. Improving the health of your gut will make most other problems disappear—just like mine did. It's not guaranteed to fix everything, but it's usually the best place to start.

Can this gut-first approach work for you? Let's look at the stories of a few of my patients.

## GETTING RESULTS

The health of your gut has a tremendous impact on the rest of your body. These examples of my patients' stories illustrate how powerful starting with the gut can be. This approach has helped many people regain their health, and it's the same approach contained in the self-help plan in this book—the plan that can now help you.

- **Jen** lost over fifty pounds after treating a fungal overgrowth in her intestines.

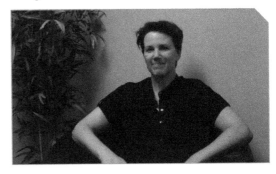

- After healing her gut, **Laura** experienced less joint pain, lost weight, improved her sleep, and was eventually able to decrease her use of thyroid medication.

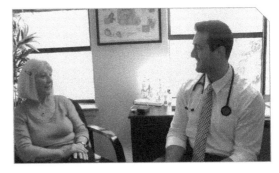

- **Patricia**'s thyroid nodule improved, with reduced swelling and inflammation in her thyroid, after following a diet that heals the gut.
- After clearing a bacterial infection in her gut, **June** saw improved thyroid health. She required less thyroid medication and saw improvement in her energy, sleep, cravings, hot flashes, and joint pain.
- **Bob** was finally able to drink wine and eat certain foods without having unpleasant reactions. He also gained the weight he desperately needed, all after treating a bacterial overgrowth in his intestines.
- **Christine** ended up feeling better at thirty-nine than she did when she was twenty-five. She had better sleep, experienced less bloating, lost over forty pounds, was able to eat more foods, and had

less chemical sensitivity. These health improvements occurred after treating a bacterial overgrowth in her gut.

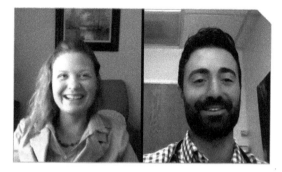

- **Josh** was finally able to overcome a bacterial overgrowth that caused fatigue and brain fog. After seeing every gastrointestinal doc in his area, Josh had nearly given up. But he was able to heal with the same approach we will cover in this book.

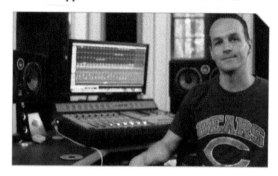

You can achieve results like Jen, Patricia, Josh, and the others. By following the self-help plan you'll find in this book, you can heal your gut and experience the far-reaching benefits that will follow. To learn more about these patients—all from my office—visit my website: http://drruscio.com/patient-conversations/.

As the patient stories above illustrate, improving your gut health can help with a myriad of ailments.

Problems in your digestive tract can manifest as all the symptoms in the above stories. Because fixing gut problems has the potential to remedy these symptoms, all other treatments can become unnecessary if we fix the gut first. It's easy to see why there's so much interest in gut health right now. Laypeople and scientists both want to know why gut health affects things like weight, energy, depression, heart disease, sleep, thyroid, the immune system, and even skin.

After hearing these success stories, it's easy to get excited. However, we must be cautious. It's easy to waste time and money on treatments that are more snake oil than science. This is something I have become increasingly sensitive to after hearing several stories from frustrated patients who wasted enormous amounts of money before coming to me. In this book, I'll focus on the clinically proven steps you can take to improve your health quickly and efficiently, and I'll help you stay clear of what is simply speculation and theory. The more you know, the less likely you are to be taken in by the snake oil.

So, how exactly does the health of your gut affect all these seemingly unrelated symptoms and conditions?

# HOW YOUR GUT AFFECTS EVERY SYSTEM OF YOUR BODY

Here are the main ways your gut affects your entire body.

## INFLAMMATION

The digestive tract is arguably the leading cause of inflammation in your body. When your gut is inflamed, it can cause inflammation throughout your entire body. This inflammation can cause several symptoms:

- Fatigue—inflammation can cause fatigue by creating imbalances in stress hormones; sometimes this is called adrenal fatigue
- Depression or anxiety—when inflammation from the gut gets into the brain, it can alter your neurotransmitters or "happy mood" chemicals

- Brain fog—when inflammation from the gut gets into the brain, it can cause brain fog (cloudy thinking)
- Insomnia—inflammation in the digestive tract has been documented to cause insomnia, as I found out the hard way
- Acne or other skin conditions—it is often said that the skin is a reflection of the gut: a healthy gut equals healthy skin
- Female hormone imbalances—inflammation can directly and indirectly alter the balance of female hormones and cause PMS (fatigue, irritability, bloating), altered cycle length or flow, low libido, and hot flashes
- Male hormone imbalances—inflammation can cause male hormone imbalances, causing fatigue, low libido, erectile dysfunction, muscle loss, and poor memory
- Hypothyroid symptoms—inflammation damages your body's ability to use thyroid hormone, so if your thyroid labs are normal or you are on a thyroid medication but still exhibiting hypothyroid symptoms, inflammation is likely the cause

## IMMUNE DYSREGULATION AND AUTOIMMUNITY

The greatest density of immune cells in your entire body is in your small intestine. When there are problems in the small intestine, like bacterial overgrowths or inflammation, they can cause problems with the immune system. The following are examples of what these immune system problems can look like:

- Hypothyroidism—the leading cause of hypothyroidism is an autoimmune condition known as Hashimoto's disease; treating certain gut infections has been shown to improve thyroid autoimmunity
- Celiac disease and gluten intolerance—both can occur because of immune dysregulation in the small intestine

- IBS (irritable bowel syndrome)—research shows that those with IBS have overactive immune responses in the gut
- Joint pain—rheumatoid arthritis is an autoimmune condition that causes joint damage and pain
- Depression—preliminary evidence shows depression may have an autoimmune component
- Food reactivity—food allergies or intolerances are often because of immune system imbalances in the intestines
- IBD (inflammatory bowel disease)—IBD, such as Crohn's disease and ulcerative colitis, results from an autoimmune response in the intestines

These are just some of the conditions that might be fueled by underlying gut imbalances. There are others.

## NUTRIENT ABSORPTION

Although you might be eating a healthy diet, if you're not absorbing nutrients, it's almost like you're not eating or you're eating junk food. This is known as malabsorption, and it can manifest in the following ways:

- Dry or thinning hair—usually due to protein and fat malabsorption
- Dry or aged skin—usually due to protein and fat malabsorption
- Fatigue—the result of general malnourishment
- Cravings—when people don't absorb nutrients properly, they often crave things like sugar, starch, and fat
- Nutrient deficiencies—the nutrient deficiencies that occur after prolonged malabsorption can cause fatigue, brain fog, depression, hormone imbalances, and other symptoms
- Slowed metabolism—malabsorption can slow metabolism, which causes weight gain, high blood sugar, and even high cholesterol levels

And, of course, let's not forget that problems in the gut can cause digestive symptoms like gas, bloating, constipation, diarrhea, loose stools, reflux, indigestion, and heartburn. Experiencing any of these symptoms is absolute confirmation that a problem in the gut is present.

"Microbiota" and "gut microbiota" are often used interchangeably with the terms "gut health" and "digestive health." What exactly is a microbiota? To put it simply, the microbiota is the world of bacteria that live in your body and have a great impact on your health. The microbiota of your gut contains roughly a thousand different species of bacteria. Almost every surface of your body—your gut, skin, lungs, and urinary tract, for example—has its own microbiota. To make things simpler, in this book we use "microbiota" when we refer specifically to "gut microbiota." If we're discussing a different microbiota, like the skin, we will specify "skin microbiota."

The microbiota we are discussing lives in your digestive tract—your gut. Your digestive tract starts with your mouth and ends at your rectum, with the stomach, small intestine, and large intestine in between. This book will help you better understand your gut and how pivotal it is to optimum health.

We live in symbiosis with this microbiota. A symbiotic relationship is a healthy one because everyone benefits. The opposite, a parasitic relationship, is when only one of the participants benefits. These bacteria help us in different ways, and in exchange we provide them food and shelter.

We've recently discovered that the human body contains more bacterial cells than human cells, and that all these bacteria are important for health and well-being. In fact, we've seen that changes in the microbiota are present in almost every disease state. This is exciting, because if these changes are causing disease, perhaps treating the microbiota will reverse disease. It appears this is true,

although there are some important exceptions that we'll discuss later.

One of the trends we've observed is that a diverse microbiota appears to be healthier than a less diverse one. A hypothetical example of a diverse microbiota is one that contains 1,028 different species of bacteria, whereas a nondiverse microbiota might contain only 859 species. Interestingly, people living in Westernized societies tend to have less diverse microbiotas compared to those living in non-Westernized societies.

Where do these bacteria come from, and why are Westerners' microbiotas less diverse? The environment is a major source of bacteria—think dirt, animals, nature. As Westernized societies have become increasingly sterile and hygienic, they've become disconnected from these major sources of bacteria. In contrast, think about how much dirt a modern-day hunter-gatherer is exposed to compared to someone living in a Westernized society. Hunter-gatherers may go an entire day without washing their hands and will also be in constant contact with animals, dirt—all those sources of bacteria.

People in Western societies have decreased bacterial exposure because of antibiotics, C-section births, less breastfeeding, and antibacterial soaps. Antibiotics and improvements in sanitation unquestionably have benefits, but it appears we are overusing antibiotics and may have become too hygienic and are now suffering the consequences. One consequence of being too clean is the increase in inflammatory and immune-mediated disease that we tend to find in Westernized societies.

Did you know that the occurrence of many conditions associated with Western society is greatly decreased in people who grow up on animal farms? Farm life gives you much greater exposure to a variety of bacteria, bacteria that Westerners are becoming deficient in. We will discuss this more later and provide you with strategies to address this.

Researchers and clinicians have learned how important gut health is for overall health. We have learned that having the right balance of healthy bacteria can vastly improve your health. We have also learned that imbalances in bacteria or the presence of harmful bacteria can detract from your health. The way you eat and live can encourage either a healthy or an unhealthy bacterial balance in your gut. Probiotics, fiber, and certain herbal medicines can also be used to improve the bacterial communities in your gut. This book will help you understand how your gut works and how to optimize your gut health and reap the substantial health benefits.

# HOW TO USE THIS BOOK

Each of the five sections of this book builds upon the previous one, with all the knowledge you've acquired culminating in an action plan. If you work through the sections in order, by the time you're ready to create your action plan, you'll have all the information you need.

Part 1 provides some foundational information: simple gut anatomy and how your gut's work influences many other parts of your body. We also establish a simple framework that will help you understand all the information that follows.

In part 2, we discuss diet and your gut. We'll talk about an anti-inflammatory diet, foods that balance the bacteria in your gut, how many carbs you should eat, and the role of dietary fiber. No one diet is right for everyone, and in part 2 we'll show you the main dietary options and help you identify which diet might be best for you.

Part 3 covers lifestyle factors and your gut. We'll elaborate on the impact sleep, exercise, sunlight, nature, toxins, and stress have on your gut. You'll learn some simple strategies that can substantially improve your health.

Part 4 covers specific treatments for your gut. You'll learn about probiotics, digestive enzymes, antibacterial herbal treatments, special liquid diets, and supplemental fiber.

When you get to part 5, you'll assemble all this information into a personalized action plan—the Great-in-8. You'll determine the diet *you* should eat and the probiotics *you* should take. You'll craft a minimalistic plan that will provide maximal results.

1. Reset—reset your diet and lifestyle
2. Support—support your gut with probiotics and digestive enzymes/acid
3. Remove—remove/reduce unwanted gut bacteria with antimicrobial herbs
4. Rebalance—rebalance gut bacteria after treatment with antimicrobial herbs
5. Reintroduce—reintroduce foods you removed in step 3
6. Feed—feed the good bacteria
7. Wean—wean yourself off the supplements in your plan
8. Maintenance and fun—maintain your improvements, and enjoy your newfound health

We start the action plan with diet and lifestyle because some people will feel better after making only those changes—step 1 is all they need. Others may have imbalances in their intestinal bacteria requiring more than dietary and lifestyle changes. These people may require probiotics or digestive enzymes to fully improve—we address this in step 2.

If you're not feeling better after step 2, you might have a more significant bacterial (or fungal) imbalance in your intestines and require herbal medicines that are specifically antimicrobial. Or you might need a special short-term liquid diet to allow your intestinal tract to heal. You'll find the information you need in step 3. After the herbal antimicrobial treatment or liquid-diet treatment, you'll need a rebalancing period to ensure adequate healing. We address this in step 4.

In steps 5 and 6, you'll broaden your diet through food reintroduction and you'll learn to feed your good gut bacteria.

Finally, in steps 7 and 8, you'll determine the minimum number and doses of supplements you need long term and make sure you have an effective but simple maintenance plan.

We've covered a long list of symptoms and conditions that may be caused by issues in the gut, but is the gut *really* that important? Or is this just another passing fad, like low-fat diets, low-carb diets, the antioxidant craze, or whatever is next? This is a fair question. Let's answer it by going into more detail about why you should consider your gut as the potential root cause of your health problems.

## CONCEPT SUMMARY

- Improving the health of your gut can have tremendous impact on the rest of your body. By improving gut health, you can experience weight loss, improved mood, better blood sugar and cholesterol levels, better energy and sleep, improved thyroid health, balanced hormones, better skin, and less joint pain.

- Your gut's effect on inflammation, immunity/autoimmunity, and nutrient absorption has far-reaching implications for your health.

- It's not uncommon for someone to overlook a problem in the gut as the true cause of his or her health ailments because the symptoms resemble something else, such as hormone imbalance, toxicity, or adrenal fatigue.

# PART 1

---

## THE IMPORTANCE OF YOUR GUT

# CHAPTER 1

# UNDERSTANDING YOUR GUT

## CONDITIONS AND SYMPTOMS THAT CAN BE CAUSED BY PROBLEMS IN THE GUT

The foundational premise here is that the gut has a massively far-reaching impact on your health. We've already discussed how your gut can affect everything from your mood to your skin or even your energy, but let's elaborate on this to give you confidence in this concept.

### THE GUT–DIGESTIVE SYMPTOM CONNECTION

Irritable bowel syndrome (IBS) may affect as much as 30% of the population. Typically, symptoms of IBS include gas, bloating, abdominal pain, and altered bowel function (constipation, diarrhea/loose stools). Did you know that up to 84% of IBS may be caused by an overgrowth of bacteria in the intestines? More importantly, did you know that people can experience relief of these symptoms by following diets that reduce this bacterial overgrowth or by undergoing other treatments that eliminate this bacterial overgrowth?

### THE GUT–BRAIN CONNECTION

It's interesting that when we address these bacterial overgrowths, people often experience mood improvements. Enter the gut-brain connection. Did you know that very high-level science has documented that certain gut treatments (such as certain probiotics) can improve anxiety and depression? There is also evidence showing that brain fog (fuzzy thinking) and impaired memory can improve when healing the gut through diet. Josh, whose case I discussed earlier, illustrates this: after improving his gut health, his digestive symptoms went away and so did his brain fog.

### THE GUT–METABOLISM CONNECTION

Some people have an overgrowth of bad "bugs" (bacteria) in their intestines, which has been correlated to being overweight, having high blood sugar, and having high cholesterol. Preliminary evidence shows improvement in metabolism after treating these bad bugs. There is also data showing that feeding good gut bacteria might be a powerful way to reduce elevated blood sugar, which can be related to diabetes or prediabetes. Remember Jen from earlier? She lost fifty pounds after addressing fungal overgrowth in her intestines.

### THE GUT–THYROID CONNECTION

When we say "metabolism," people often think thyroid. Did you know certain diets that limit inflammatory foods and excess carb intake can improve thyroid autoimmunity and body composition? Thyroid autoimmunity is the most common cause of hypothyroidism. There is preliminary evidence showing that the treatment of a bacteria called H. pylori has been shown to reduce thyroid autoimmunity (Hashimoto's disease). Remember Patricia's, June's, and Laura's stories from earlier? Patricia's thyroid nodules improved dramatically, and June and Laura were able to reduce their thyroid medication after improving their gut health.

### THE GUT–SLEEP CONNECTION

Did you know that inflammation in the intestines has been shown to cause insomnia? Reducing inflammation vastly improves sleep. Of course, if you sleep better, everything else gets better, because sleep is a key pillar to health. I learned this firsthand as my insomnia was almost unbearable and did not improve until I healed my gut.

### THE GUT–SKIN CONNECTION

There is an old saying in naturopathic medicine: "The skin is a reflection of the gut." Certain skin conditions, ones that generally involve pimples, lesions, rashes, and skin inflammation, have been clinically documented to improve after removal of inflammatory foods from the diet or reducing unwanted bacterial overgrowth in the intestines. Many skin conditions originate in your gut and require more than skin creams to be remedied.

### THE GUT–HORMONE CONNECTION

The gut bacteria play an important role in the breakdown of hormones and their removal from the blood. This is especially important for women because problems in this area can easily cause imbalances in estrogen. What can this look like? PMS, irritability, depression, weight gain, and accelerated aging are a few symptoms. We also discussed how the gut can be a source of inflammation. High levels of inflammation can cause higher testosterone in women (not a good thing) and higher estrogen levels in men (also not a good thing). This is why it's not unusual for hormone-related symptoms to improve after improving your gut health. This might look like improved libido, mood, PMS, energy, or stamina. Remember June, who eliminated her hot flashes after improving the health of her gut?

## GETTING TO KNOW YOUR GUT

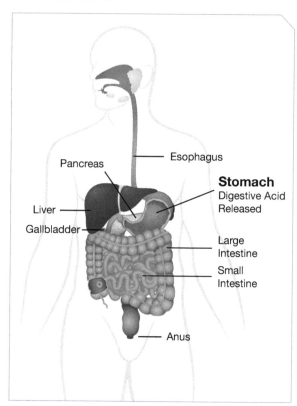

I hope you are starting to appreciate the impact of your gut health. Let's now briefly acquaint you with your gut (more formally known as your digestive system). This diagram helps us visualize the key features of your digestive system, which include the

- mouth and esophagus
- stomach
- small intestine
- liver, gallbladder, and pancreas
- large intestine (the colon)
- rectum

The digestive process begins in the mouth, where food is chewed and digestive enzymes are released. When you swallow food, it travels down your esophagus and into your stomach, where things start to get interesting. In the stomach, we see the digestive process ramp up. Your stomach releases acid to help break down your food. This acid helps kill any unwanted bacteria, fungus, or parasites that may be present in your food. If you have too little acid or if you're taking acid-lowering medications, your risk for bacterial and fungal overgrowths or even parasitic infections increases.

On the other hand, if you have stomach-acid levels that are too high, you can be at risk for ulcers and irritation of the stomach (gastritis). Acid imbalance in the stomach can contribute to indigestion, reflux, and heartburn. As we discussed earlier, certain bacteria in the stomach (namely H. pylori) may cause or worsen the autoimmunity associated with hypothyroidism. Inflammation in the stomach can cause an inability to absorb key minerals like iron and B vitamins, which can then lead to anemia, which causes fatigue.

Food then moves from your stomach into your small intestine, which might be the most important of all the sections of your digestive system. Most nutrient absorption occurs here, but this section is the most sensitive and prone to damage and inflammation. To complicate things further, the small intestine is a common source of bacterial and fungal imbalance. The liver, gallbladder, and the pancreas release important digestive secretions

into the small intestine to assist with digestion. These include bile from the liver and gallbladder and pancreatic enzymes from the pancreas.

There is a lot happening here. The stomach has to do a good job prepping food for the small intestine. The liver, gallbladder, and pancreas also have to do their jobs and release their respective secretions into the small intestine. The small intestine itself releases digestive enzymes to aid in digestion. Additionally, the small intestine has to make sure to absorb nutrients—the good stuff—but keep out bacteria and parasites, the bad stuff. We will mention the small intestine many times throughout this book because it's a key part of your digestive tract.

As we pass the midway point of the digestive process, food moves into the large intestine (the colon). Some digestion and absorption of nutrients occurs here, but not as much as in the small intestine. Here in the large intestine, bacteria assist with digestion and detoxification, among other things. More specifically, in the large intestine bacteria help us digest dense fibers, just as bacteria in a cow's digestive tract break down tough grasses. This is a key point for later.

The large intestine is an area where bacterial and fungal overgrowth, as well as infection, can occur. Inflammation can also negatively affect the large intestine. The large intestine is less prone to problems than the small intestine, but it's still important to maintain a healthy environment here to prevent inflammation, polyps, and cancer.

By the time food nears the end of our digestive tract, we have extracted much of the nutrition from it and packaged some toxins that need to be excreted. What once was food has now become stool, ready for expulsion from the body via the rectum.

# INFLAMMATORY FOODS AND FOOD AND COMPOUNDS THAT FEED GUT BACTERIA

We've discussed the symptoms and conditions caused by inflammation and problems with gut bacteria, but we need to look at the foods and compounds that cause those issues in the first place.

## INFLAMMATORY FOODS

You've probably heard this admittedly vague term before. We'll cover it in more detail when we get into our specific dietary plan. For now, we'll cover just a few basics.

The term "inflammatory food" typically refers to foods that your body doesn't do well on because they cause your immune system to react and attack. For people who are allergic to nuts, this is often a very obvious reaction. People with celiac disease have a noticeably adverse reaction to foods containing wheat and gluten. However, there are other foods that produce a less obvious inflammatory response. Some people become inflamed when eating gluten, but the reaction is not as noticeable as it is for those with celiac disease. Others may not do well with dairy, eggs, or soy.

What's tricky is that each of us has a different set of foods our body treats as inflammatory. A large part of determining the ideal diet for you involves figuring out which foods are inflammatory for your body and which ones are not. We'll work through this process later in the book.

## FOODS AND COMPOUNDS THAT FEED GUT BACTERIA

Because our Western environment leaves us deficient in bacterial exposure, it's sometimes recommended that we feed our gut bacteria by eating

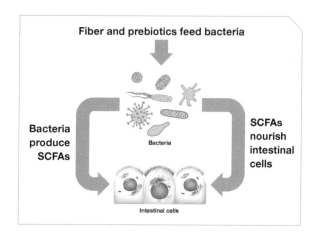

fiber and prebiotics, which are often found in carbohydrate-rich foods. However, this overlooks the fact that many people have *too much* bacteria (bacterial overgrowth) and should *not* be feeding their gut bacteria and encouraging even more growth.

Another reason it's sometimes recommended that we feed gut bacteria with prebiotics and fiber is that if we feed them, our gut bacteria will then produce short-chain fatty acids (SCFAs). SCFAs nourish our intestinal cells and may help prevent intestinal inflammation and intestinal damage (often called "leaky gut"). This sounds like a good idea, right? Not always. In a recent review paper, it was shown that obese people often produce excessive levels of SCFAs, which might contribute to weight gain.[1] This has been found in other studies as well.[2] The reason overweight and obese people have high levels of SCFAs is because they have too much bacteria in the small intestine. Yes, increased levels of small-intestinal bacteria have been found in those who are overweight.[3] If you have ever felt bloated or gassy, you might have been feeling the effects of too much bacteria in your small intestine. This is likely why diets that feed gut bacteria have been shown to be the least effective for weight loss—because many who are overweight already have too much bacteria to begin with.

Now that we have a lay of the land that is your digestive system, let's establish a simple framework to help you understand all the gut information we will discuss. This framework will help you understand why no one diet works for everyone. It will also help you appreciate the individualized plan we'll work through a little later.

## YOUR GUT IS AN ECOSYSTEM

As we delve deeper into our discussion of the gut and gut microbiota, it's important to provide an overview to help organize and understand the concepts we'll be covering. You already know that the gut is important and can affect many aspects of your health. Now you'll learn the concepts related to gut healing. The fundamental principle is this:

> *Your gut and gut microbiota are an ecosystem.*

Think of your gut and microbiota as a life system just as complex as a rain forest. This ecosystem lives in the environment that is your body, just like some rain forests live in the environment of South America. It is the health of the environment that dictates the health of the ecosystem. If the rain forest has an environment with plenty of rain, it will thrive; if there is a prolonged drought, the rain forest can die. When it comes to your gut (the ecosystem) and body (the environment),

> *a healthy body equals healthy bacteria.*

By providing your gut bacteria the healthiest environment possible, we'll allow the healthiest bacteria to grow, and you'll then reap all the health benefits that follow. Think of it like this: If you were a gardener and your plants were dying, what would you do? In medicine, we often focus on the problem (the symptoms), not the cause. But in gardening, a more *holistic* view is required. With the holistic-gardener view, we ask the question, why is this plant dying? We examine the environment the plant is in and then work to provide the plant with the environment it needs to grow and thrive. We may find there is not enough sun exposure and too much moisture, and, as a result, the soil is infected with fungus. We trim some overgrowth brush that is blocking the sun, which helps to reduce moisture, and use agents to aid in removing the fungus. This is the same approach we must take to repair your gut and microbiota ecosystem. Yes, sometimes a branch must be cut off, but this is what we will work to avoid.

In addition to being holistic, we need an *individualized* approach. It's interesting that in nutrition we seem to fall into the trap of recommending one diet for all. For example, researchers have observed that African hunter-gatherers have very healthy guts and gut microbiotas. This has led many to make the oversimplified recommendation of replicating the Africans' diet, thinking this would then cause our microbiotas to look like theirs. But the ecosystem of your gut is far too complex to micromanage.

> *You can't micromanage an ecosystem.*

And, as we'll discuss later, what's good for someone else, like an African hunter-gatherer, might be harmful to you. We need to create the *optimum environment* for *your ecosystem* through an individualized approach.

Think of it this way, life on the outside affects life on the inside. If you abuse the "outside" (your body) with stress, lack of sleep and exercise, and by eating poison, what do you think the world of bacteria on the inside will look like?

We've established that your gut is like an ecosystem. It probably won't surprise you to learn that just as there are different types of ecosystems, there are ***different types of guts***. What will help one ecosystem may severely damage another. To accommodate this fact, our recommendations for healing your gut ecosystem are individualized. To return to our rain-forest metaphor, some ecosystems need lots of rain and sun, while others need more shade and less rain. If the amount of rainfall that occurs in a rain forest suddenly fell in an arid region like Southern California, it would create problems. A sudden burst of rain in Southern California can create mudslides that decimate communities and cause fatalities. If we see something working in one ecosystem, it doesn't mean it's going to be good for another system. Some gut ecosystems will need little fiber and carbs. Others will need more carbs and fiber. Although it's true that you can't micromanage your gut ecosystem, you *can* listen to it, learn from it, and tend to it like a good gardener attends a garden.

## CONCEPT SUMMARY

- The somewhat sterile environments many Westerners live in deprive us of the bacterial exposure needed to train our immune systems and prevent inflammatory and autoimmune conditions.

- The gut microbiota is like an ecosystem. It requires the appropriate environment to flourish.

- Just like different ecosystems require different amounts of rain, different guts require different amounts of carbs, prebiotics, and fiber.

- By creating a healthy internal environment, you will allow healthy bacteria to grow.

1    Rosa Krajmalnik-Brown et al., "Effects of Gut Microbes on Nutrient Absorption and Energy Regulation," *Nutrition in Clinical Practice* 27, no. 2 (April 24, 2012): 201–14, doi:10.1177/0884533611436116.

2    Alexandra L. McOrist et al., "Fecal Butyrate Levels Vary Widely among Individuals but Are Usually Increased by a Diet High in Resistant Starch," *Journal of Nutrition* 141, no. 5 (May 1, 2011): 883–89, doi:10.3945/jn.110.128504.

3    Enzo Ierardi et al., "Macronutrient Intakes in Obese Subjects with or without Small Intestinal Bacterial Overgrowth: An Alimentary Survey," *Scandinavian Journal of Gastroenterology* 51, no. 3 (March 3, 2016): 277–80, doi:10.3109/00365521.2015.1086020.

# CHAPTER 2

# THE SMALL INTESTINE

## A FEW THINGS YOU SHOULD KNOW

### BACTERIAL OVERGROWTHS IN THE SMALL INTESTINE MAY CONTRIBUTE TO HYPOTHYROIDISM, CELIAC DISEASE, AND IBS.

We briefly touched on the small intestine as a key area of your digestive tract. In fact, the small intestine has much relevance to hypothyroidism, celiac disease (gluten allergy), and IBS (gas, bloating, abdominal pain, constipation, and diarrhea). Although Westerners tend to be deficient in exposure to environmental bacteria because of our overly hygienic environment, we tend to have overgrowths of bacteria in the small intestine. *"SIBO" (small-intestinal bacterial overgrowth)* is a term we'll be talking about more later. As we will detail in this book, this overgrowth of bacteria explains why approaches that feed bacteria may not work well for conditions like hypothyroidism, celiac disease, and IBS. If you have a bacterial overgrowth, feeding bacteria can make you worse. Let's cover some of the basics regarding your small intestine and then talk more about its bacteria.

*The small intestine accounts for over 56% of our intestinal tract.*

By comparison, the colon or large intestine represents roughly 20%. Key changes early in human evolution allowed us to rely more on the small intestine for digestion and less on the colon. This is why *the small intestine is responsible for 90% of caloric absorption*. Yes, 90% of the food you eat is absorbed through your small intestine—so it's a big deal.

It is very important to mention *the small intestine has a profound impact on your immune system. The largest mass of immune cells in your entire body is seen in the small intestine.*[1]

This is why small-intestinal health is so impactful on immune and autoimmune conditions—as we discussed earlier. The small intestine has a thin, protective mucous membrane and is much more prone to damage (which results in leaky gut) than the large intestine. This damage underlies many immune and autoimmune conditions, food reactivity, and the malabsorption of nutrients.

The small intestine harbors a relatively small number of bacteria compared to the large intestine. This is important because it explains why the small and large intestines have different needs.

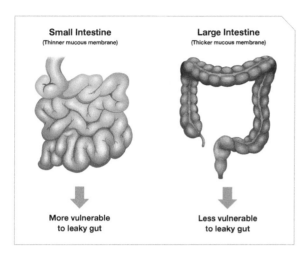

| Small Intestine | Large Intestine |
|---|---|
| (Thinner mucous membrane) | (Thicker mucous membrane) |
| More vulnerable to leaky gut | Less vulnerable to leaky gut |

Current recommendations seem to favor the large intestine—feed your gut bacteria by eating lots of fiber, carbs, and prebiotics. However, following this advice often creates problems for the small intestine.

I hope it's clear that the small intestine is the most important section of your gut and your entire digestive tract. When we look at the entire gut ecosystem and the methods for creating a healthy internal environment in your gut ecosystem, it's usually the interventions that work best for the small intestine that have the most overall benefit. We'll continue to think about your digestive tract holistically, but it's important to understand much of what we do will be driven by the needs of the small intestine. For example, sometimes it's best to reduce bacteria rather than feed them, because reducing bacteria is often what the small intestine needs. If there's already overgrowth in the small intestine, feeding bacteria can cause gas, bloating, diarrhea, constipation, high blood sugar, high cholesterol, and weight gain. Because the small intestine is so important, when it becomes imbalanced it can cause a wide range of negative health effects. Why are these issues more common in the small intestine? Again, because the small intestine is fragile and more prone to dysfunction.

## IS THERE MORE TO LIFE THAN BACTERIA?

Yes! Fungi are an important part of your gut ecosystem. This fungal world, known as your mycome or mycobiota, includes 355 species of fungus!

We will discuss fungal overgrowths and their cousin, candida, a little later, but did you know one of the most successful probiotics is a fungus? Saccharomyces boulardii is a healthy fungus that has been studied in clinical trials in humans and has shown very positive results.[2]

Not only can the small intestine experience bacterial overgrowth, it can also experience fungal overgrowth, called SIFO (small-intestinal fungal overgrowth).[3]

There is also a collection of viruses that inhabit your gut, known as the virome. There are other organisms like worms and protozoa that can have a strong impact on your gut and whole-body health. Fungi, viruses, worms, and protozoa *are not* part of current microbiota testing, which is likely another reason why the tests have limited clinical usefulness. However, gut tests *do* include these other organisms. In part 5, we will cover testing and treatment recommendations to make sure you have all this covered.

How do bacteria and the small intestine tie in with celiac disease and hypothyroidism? Many with celiac disease and hypothyroidism have too much bacteria in their small intestine and thus do better with approaches that reduce or rebalance bacterial levels. Let's expand on how this pertains to celiac disease.

### CELIAC DISEASE AND THE SMALL INTESTINE

Celiac disease is the most severe form of gluten intolerance—it causes inflammation and autoimmune damage to your intestines. Several human studies have shown that there is increased bacterial count and diversity in the small intestine of those with celiac disease—essentially, they have bacterial overgrowths.[4]

An increased diversity in the healthy bacterial species of bifidobacteria has been shown in children with celiac disease when compared to healthy controls.[5] This same increased diversity in bifidobacteria has been shown in adults with celiac disease.[6] Although all studies don't agree on this,[7] there is certainly enough evidence to suggest bacterial overgrowth is an issue for many with celiac disease. It's also important to point out that celiac disease predominantly affects the small intestine, not the large.[8]

We talked earlier about the short-chain fatty acids produced by bacteria. Children and adults with celiac disease often have increased short-chain fatty acids in their stools.[9]

### GUT GEEKS
*Butyrate is the short-chain fatty acid that appears in stool of people with celiac disease.*

This suggests that ***those with celiac disease may have bacterial overgrowth—that is, too much bacteria in their small intestines***. So, although short-chain fatty acids in the appropriate levels can be beneficial, high levels have been documented in those with celiac disease and in those who are obese. In summary, the reason those with celiac disease have high levels of short-chain fatty acids is likely because of the bacterial overgrowth. Too much bacteria equals too many short-chain fatty acids. The good news is that levels of short-chain fatty acids appear to normalize after treatment with a gluten-free diet![10]

### GUT GEEKS
*It's possible that those with celiac disease aren't absorbing nutrients, thus making available more substrate for bacterial feeding. This feeding causes bacterial overgrowth and subsequent elevated production of short-chain fatty acids.*

Why else might bacterial overgrowth be common in those with celiac disease? People with celiac disease may have impaired motility, which causes bacterial overgrowth. Motility is the ability of your intestines to keep food moving through them at an appropriate pace. Inflammation, which is often elevated in those with celiac disease, impairs this motility.[11] When food doesn't move through your intestines quickly enough, it can cause bacterial overgrowth. It's similar to water: stagnant pond water isn't safe to drink because of high bacteria levels. Running river water is safer to drink because it contains less bacteria. Running water doesn't encourage bacterial overgrowth; stagnant water does. Stagnant food in your intestine fosters bacterial overgrowth, while moving food does not.

### GUT GEEKS
*Inflammation may decrease the repair rate of the interstitial cells of Cajal.*

It has been shown that inflammation causes an unfavorable balance of bacteria in the gut. Why? Because inflammation is a major factor in the health of your internal environment! Inflammation can kill good bacteria and encourage growth of bad bacteria.[12]

This introduces an important concept:

> *eating to reduce inflammation is more important than eating to feed gut bacteria.*

We will expand on this concept later, but again this ties back to our holistic view of creating a healthy environment that will foster healthy bacterial growth. An inflamed environment is unhealthy; therefore, an inflamed environment equals unhealthy bacteria.

The bottom line is those with celiac disease might need an approach that reduces excessive bacteria in the small intestine. Accordingly, it has been documented that SIBO (small-intestinal bacterial overgrowth) is a common reason why people's symptoms don't improve on a gluten-free diet.[13] And, more importantly, after treating their SIBO properly, these patients become symptom-free.[14] SIBO can be assessed with a simple breath test. However, you do not need to do this test now, even if this sounds like you, because working through the steps in part 5 will address SIBO, as well as other gut imbalances.

If people with celiac disease can have too much bacteria, as in SIBO, does this mean they should avoid probiotics? No, it does not. This is a common and understandable misconception. The logic is, why take a bacterial supplement (probiotic) if you already have too much bacteria? But probiotics can actually kill the unwanted bacteria of bacterial overgrowths and have been shown to be a viable treatment, as we will discuss in part 4.

## HYPOTHYROIDISM AND THE SMALL INTESTINE

What about hypothyroidism? This same issue of having too much bacteria in the small intestine seems to be true for hypothyroidism as well. Research has shown that hypothyroidism is associated with small-intestinal bacterial overgrowth.[15]

You might be wondering if this overgrowth occurs because of the hypothyroidism itself. We don't know for sure, but bacterial overgrowth has been seen in both hypothyroidism and hyperthyroidism.[16] In hypothyroidism, your intestinal motility can slow down, which can then cause

bacterial overgrowth, like SIBO. However, we also see bacterial overgrowth in hyperthyroid disease, where motility speeds up.

So, what does this mean? It suggests the bacterial overgrowth is not being caused by thyroid disease but rather that the overgrowth is causing the thyroid disease. This makes sense when considering most thyroid disease is autoimmune in nature. Remember the largest density of immune cells are contained in your small intestine and the small intestine has a large impact on autoimmunity.

Perhaps this is why we see that when people with thyroid autoimmunity follow a lower-carb diet, their thyroid autoimmunity improves.[17] Remember, a lower-carb diet tends to starve bacteria, which can reduce bacterial overgrowth. Starving the bacteria helps heal the small intestine, and since the small intestine is tightly tied to your immune system, the autoimmune condition of hypothyroidism then improves. Again, this does not mean everyone should be on a lower-carb diet, but this is important information to consider.

## IBS AND THE SMALL INTESTINE

How does the small intestine connect to IBS? SIBO is known to cause gas, bloating, constipation, diarrhea, and abdominal pain—in other words, the symptoms of IBS. Current treatment guidelines state those with SIBO shouldn't feed their gut bacteria,[18] or at least should do so very cautiously. There are herbs that have been shown effective in treating SIBO and IBS and even an FDA-approved antibiotic that has been shown helpful for IBS because of its anti-SIBO properties.[19]

## THE FAR-REACHING EFFECTS OF THE GUT

We're learning that problems in the gut, such as small-intestinal bacterial overgrowth, can cause or contribute to problems in other parts of the body. These problems include but are not limited to brain fog, depression, fatigue, skin conditions, joint pain, hypothyroidism, and other autoimmune conditions. It's so important for you to achieve optimal gut health because there's a good chance a gut imbalance underlies your current symptoms. I can't guarantee that this is the case, but an examination of your gut health is a very smart place to start. Remember, you can have a problem in the gut that is manifesting *only* as non-digestive symptoms, like fatigue or depression.[20]

We're beginning to develop a context for understanding your gut and your gut microbiota. The small intestine is a crucial aspect of your digestive tract and holds much potential for improving your overall health. But what about the microbiotas of other cultures? Earlier we mentioned that hunter-gatherers in Africa have healthier guts. Let's now look at what we can learn from the guts and microbiotas of other cultures and our prehistoric ancestors.

## CONCEPT SUMMARY

- The small intestine is an often-overlooked but crucially important area of your digestive tract.

- The small intestine makes up the majority—56%—of our intestinal tract.

- The small intestine is responsible for 90% of caloric absorption.

- The small intestine has a profound impact on your immune system. The largest mass of immune cells is seen in the small intestine.

- The small intestine has a thin, protective mucous membrane and is much more prone to damage (leaky gut) than the large intestine is.

- The small intestine harbors a relatively small number of bacteria compared to the large intestine.

- Bacterial overgrowth commonly occurs in the small intestine and can cause gas, bloating, diarrhea, constipation, high blood sugar, high cholesterol, and weight gain.

- People with celiac disease, IBS, or hypothyroidism might have bacterial overgrowth, often in the small intestine. These people may want to avoid recommendations that they feed their gut bacteria.

- People who have trouble regulating bacteria and fungus in their guts should avoid too much feeding via fiber and carbs.

- Eating to reduce inflammation is more important than eating to feed gut bacteria.

1   Sahar El Aidy et al., "The Small Intestine Microbiota, Nutritional Modulation and Relevance for Health," *Current Opinion in Biotechnology* 32 (April 2015): 14–20, doi:10.1016/j.copbio.2014.09.005.

2   Margret Irmgard Moré and Alexander Swidsinski, "Saccharomyces Boulardii CNCM I-745 Supports Regeneration of the Intestinal Microbiota after Diarrheic Dysbiosis—A Review," *Clinical and Experimental Gastroenterology*, August 2015, doi:10.2147/CEG.S85574; H. Szajewska et al., "Systematic Review with Meta-Analysis: *Saccharomyces Boulardii* Supplementation and Eradication of *Helicobacter Pylori* Infection," *Alimentary Pharmacology & Therapeutics* 41, no. 12 (June 2015): 1237–45, doi:10.1111/apt.13214.

3   Askin Erdogan and Satish S. C. Rao, "Small Intestinal Fungal Overgrowth," *Current Gastroenterology Reports* 17, no. 4 (April 19, 2015): 16, doi:10.1007/s11894-015-0436-2.

4    Esther Nistal et al., "Differences of Small Intestinal Bacteria Populations in Adults and Children with/without Celiac Disease: Effect of Age, Gluten Diet, and Disease," *Inflammatory Bowel Diseases* 18, no. 4 (April 2012): 649–56, doi:10.1002/ibd.21830; Yolanda Sanz et al., "Differences in Faecal Bacterial Communities in Coeliac and Healthy Children as Detected by PCR and Denaturing Gradient Gel Electrophoresis," *FEMS Immunology & Medical Microbiology* 51, no. 3 (December 2007): 562–68, doi:10.1111/j.1574 -695X.2007.00337.x; Maria Carmen Collado et al., "Specific Duodenal and Faecal Bacterial Groups Associated with Paediatric Coeliac Disease," *Journal of Clinical Pathology* 62, no. 3 (March 1, 2009): 264–69, doi:10.1136/jcp.2008.061366; Serena Schippa et al., "A Distinctive 'Microbial Signature' in Celiac Pediatric Patients," *BMC Microbiology* 10, no. 1 (June 17, 2010): 175, doi:10.1186/1471-2180 -10-175; Raffaella Di Cagno et al., "Duodenal and Faecal Microbiota of Celiac Children: Molecular, Phenotype and Metabolome Characterization," *BMC Microbiology* 11, no. 1 (October 4, 2011): 219, doi:10.1186/1471-2180-11-219.

5    Ester Sanchez et al., "Intestinal Bacteroides Species Associated with Coeliac Disease," *Journal of Clinical Pathology* 63, no. 12 (December 1, 2010): 1105–11, doi:10.1136/jcp.2010.076950.

6    Esther Nistal et al., "Differences in Faecal Bacteria Populations and Faecal Bacteria Metabolism in Healthy Adults and Celiac Disease Patients," *Biochimie* 94, no. 8 (August 2012): 1724–29, doi:10.1016/j.biochi.2012.03.025.

7    Esther Nistal et al., "Differences of Small Intestinal Bacteria Populations in Adults and Children with/without Celiac Disease: Effect of Age, Gluten Diet, and Disease," *Inflammatory Bowel Diseases* 18, no. 4 (April 2012): 649–56, doi:10.1002/ibd.21830; Yolanda Sanz et al., "Differences in Faecal Bacterial Communities in Coeliac and Healthy Children as Detected by PCR and Denaturing Gradient Gel Electrophoresis," *FEMS Immunology & Medical Microbiology* 51, no. 3 (December 2007): 562–68, doi:10.1111/j.1574 -695X.2007.00337.x; Jing Cheng et al., "Duodenal Microbiota Composition and Mucosal Homeostasis in Pediatric Celiac Disease," *BMC Gastroenterology* 13, no. 1 (December 11, 2013): 113, doi:10.1186/1471-230X-13-113; Tim G. J. de Meij et al., "Composition and Diversity of the Duodenal Mucosa-Associated Microbiome in Children with Untreated Celiac Disease," *Scandinavian Journal of Gastroenterology* 48, no. 5 (May 27, 2013): 530–36, doi:10.3109/00365521.2013.775666.

8    MUSC Health Digestive Disease Center, "Celiac Disease (Celiac Sprue)," accessed October 9, 2017, http://ddc.musc.edu/public /diseases/small-intestine/celiac-disease.html.

9    Esther Nistal et al., "Differences in Faecal Bacteria Populations and Faecal Bacteria Metabolism in Healthy Adults and Celiac Disease Patients," *Biochimie* 94, no. 8 (August 2012): 1724–29, doi:10.1016/j.biochi.2012.03.025; Bo Tjellstrom et al., "Gut Microflora Associated Characteristics in Children with Celiac Disease," *American Journal of Gastroenterology* 100, no. 12 (December 1, 2005): 2784–88, doi:10.1111/j.1572-0241.2005.00313.x.

10   Bo Tjellström et al., "Faecal Short-Chain Fatty Acid Pattern in Childhood Coeliac Disease Is Normalised after More Than One Year's Gluten-Free Diet," *Microbial Ecology in Health & Disease* 24, no. 0 (September 25, 2013), doi:10.3402/mehd.v24i0.20905.

11   Kenton M. Sanders, "Interstitial Cells of Cajal at the Clinical and Scientific Interface," *Journal of Physiology* 576, no. 3 (November 1, 2006): 683–87, doi:10.1113/jphysiol.2006.116814.

12   Claudia Lupp et al., "Host-Mediated Inflammation Disrupts the Intestinal Microbiota and Promotes the Overgrowth of Enterobacteriaceae," *Cell Host & Microbe* 2, no. 2 (August 16, 2007): 119–29, doi:10.1016/j.chom.2007.06.010; Bärbel Stecher et al., "Salmonella Enterica Serovar Typhimurium Exploits Inflammation to Compete with the Intestinal Microbiota," ed. Matt Waldor, *PLoS Biology* 5, no. 10 (August 28, 2007): e244, doi:10.1371/journal.pbio.0050244; Laura G. Patwa et al., "Chronic Intestinal Inflammation Induces Stress-Response Genes in Commensal Escherichia Coli," *Gastroenterology* 141, no. 5 (November 1, 2011): 1842 -51-10, doi:10.1053/j.gastro.2011.06.064; Frederic A. Carvalho et al., "Transient Inability to Manage Proteobacteria Promotes Chronic Gut Inflammation in TLR5-Deficient Mice," *Cell Host & Microbe* 12, no. 2 (August 16, 2012): 139–52, doi:10.1016/j.chom.2012.07.004.

13   Antonio Tursi et al., "High Prevalence of Small Intestinal Bacterial Overgrowth in Celiac Patients with Persistence of Gastrointestinal Symptoms after Gluten Withdrawal," *American Journal of Gastroenterology* 98, no. 4 (April 1, 2003): 839–43, doi:10.1111/j.1572-0241.2003.07379.x.

14   Ibid.

15   Camilla Virili and Marco Centanni, "Does Microbiota Composition Affect Thyroid Homeostasis?," *Endocrine* 49, no. 3 (August 17, 2015): 583–87, doi:10.1007/s12020-014-0509-2.

16   Lei Zhou et al., "Gut Microbe Analysis between Hyperthyroid and Healthy Individuals," *Current Microbiology* 69, no. 5 (November 27, 2014): 675–80, doi:10.1007/s00284-014-0640-6; Mairi H. McLean et al., "Does the Microbiota Play a Role in the Pathogenesis of Autoimmune Diseases?," *Gut* 64, no. 2 (February 1, 2015): 332–41, doi:10.1136/gutjnl-2014-308514.

17   Teresa Esposito et al., "Effects of Low-Carbohydrate Diet Therapy in Overweight Subject with Autoimmune Thyroiditis: Possible Synergism with ChREBP," *Drug Design, Development and Therapy* 1 (September 14, 2016): 2939–946. doi:10.2147/dddt.s106440.

18    Mark Pimentel, "An Evidence-Based Treatment Algorithm for IBS Based on a Bacterial/SIBO Hypothesis: Part 2," *American Journal of Gastroenterology*, no. 105 (June 2010): 1227–230, doi:10.1038/ajg.2010.125.

19    US Food & Drug Administration, "FDA Approves Two Therapies to Treat IBS-D," news release, May 27, 2015, www.fda.gov /NewsEvents/Newsroom/PressAnnouncements/ucm448328.htm.

20    Carlos Isasi et al., "Non-Celiac Gluten Sensitivity and Rheumatic Diseases," *Reumatología Clínica* 12, no. 1 (December 11, 2015): 4–10 . doi:10.1016/j.reuma.2015.03.001.

# CHAPTER 3

# ALL GUTS ARE NOT THE SAME

## GUT EVOLUTION AND THE MICROBIOTAS OF OTHER CULTURES

Those in nonindustrialized parts of the world, like rural Africa, have healthier guts, microbiotas, and immune systems than people in the Westernized world. This is predominantly because of less antibiotic use, more exposure to environmental bacteria (having a less hygienic environment), the consumption of virtually no processed food, and vastly different lifestyles. Why does this matter? It matters because we see much less inflammatory and immune-related illness, like hypothyroidism, celiac disease, obesity, IBS, depression, and heart disease, in these populations, which might tell us how we can reduce the incidence of these conditions in Westerners.

This has led many to insist that a woman from California, for example, should try to have a microbiota like a woman of the Hadza tribe in Africa. Is this true? Should you strive to have the microbiota of someone from such circumstances? In some ways, yes, and in some ways, no. It comes down to one of our fundamental concepts: you cannot micromanage an ecosystem. You cannot

force your microbiota to match that of a hunter-gatherer (in fact, you may hurt yourself if you try to). But you can try to improve the health of *your* environment and by doing so create an environment that supports healthy bacteria. We can provide the stage for change, and then the body can find its own healthy equilibrium. What we cannot do is force the specific change we think is best. When we do the former, we experience healing; when we do the latter, things often don't end well.

## BORROWING THE DIETS OF OTHER CULTURES

"I've heard studies show those with healthier microbiotas, like some Africans, eat more carbs, especially grains. Should I do this?" This is a question people often ask after hearing about some of the research coming out of Africa. Think about this from the perspective of our environmental analogy: different environments require different amounts of rain. If your ecosystem is not African, would it make sense for you to suddenly expose your ecosystem to the rainfall level of Africa? Western ecosystems are quite different from systems. In fact, eating like an African hunter-gatherer could cause harm, just like sudden downpours can cause flash flooding and mudslides in arid climates. This leads to an important point:

## *Do not replicate another culture's or population's diet or microbiota if you are not in that culture or population.*

There are a number of reasons for this. It has been well established that the closer to the equator a population is, the higher in carbohydrates and lower in protein and fat the diet tends to be.[1]

Why does this matter? As researchers have been attempting to identify what a healthier microbiota is, they've studied non-Westernized groups, like the African hunter-gatherer Hadza. We've learned a lot from this research; however, there is one major problem here. Most of the groups studied live in equatorial regions. Why is this a problem? Differences in climate mean that the available foods differ and, therefore, diet differs. If you are of European descent, you might not do well with a dietary balance like that consumed by those of Central African descent. Historically, Europeans in general come from a history of relatively lower carbohydrate intake, while Africans historically have a relatively higher carbohydrate intake. The world map above highlights the narrow equatorial zone where most of our current microbiota research comes from. Compare this to the entire globe, and you see most of Europe, Asia, and North America are left out of the sample. The red star and yellow star show where much of the African research is performed—in fact any research in Africa can be considered equatorial because of Africa's equatorial location. If your heritage is of European or Asian descent, your gut ecosystem has different needs than the gut ecosystem of someone of African descent. Later, we will discuss a study that drives this point home

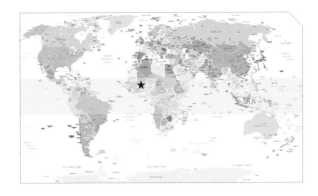

and can help you determine your ideal carbohydrate consumption—again, because carb intake is the main dietary factor that changes at different latitudes. Before we do, though, there are a few other important reasons for being cautious about replicating another culture's diet.

In 2010, a study was performed comparing a group of urban Italians to a group of rural Africans from Burkina Faso (see black star on map).[2] This study received quite a bit of attention because the Africans had significantly different microbiotas from the Italians. The Africans had better overall bacterial diversity and had more of the Bacteroidetes bacteria group and less Firmicutes bacteria. Correspondingly, the Africans had healthier body weights than the Italians. The Africans also ate lots of carbohydrates and grains.

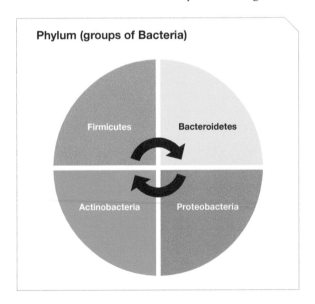

**Phylum (groups of Bacteria)**

Firmicutes | Bacteroidetes
Actinobacteria | Proteobacteria

This caused many health-care professionals to recommend that Westerners consume more carbs and grains in order to make our guts more like the guts of the Africans. In other words, the observation that Africans had healthier weights, better bacterial diversity, and less Firmicutes, plus the observation that they consumed high amounts of grains and carbs, led many to conclude (mistakenly) that everyone should now eat more grains and carbs to improve diversity, decrease Firmicutes, and be skinny, like the Africans.

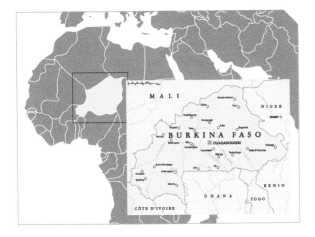

Does this overly assumptive logic smell funny? It should. It's this type of wishful thinking that accompanies many dietary fads. Some important factors are left out of this assumption. The Africans

- consumed about half the calories the Italians did;
- consumed virtually no processed foods and ate minimally processed grain;
- presumably were far more active (having to hand grind their grains before eating them, for example);
- had an incredible amount of contact with their less hygienic environment and all the bacteria it contained;
- presumably had far less stress and far more sun exposure than most Westerners.

The importance of the Africans' less hygienic living conditions cannot be overstated. The bacterial exposure in these types of environments has been repeatedly shown to have a tremendously positive impact on the development of a healthy immune system. This then helps prevent inflammatory and autoimmune conditions like celiac disease, thyroid disease, inflammatory bowel disease, allergies, asthma, IBS, and obesity or being overweight. The Africans are saturated in bacteria all day long, which is a major reason for their increased microbiota bacterial diversity and healthy immune systems.

So, the environment has a large impact on your bacterial diversity and immune system. Did you know that children who grow up in households that use a sponge to clean dishes have fewer allergic diseases than those growing up in households that use a dishwasher?[3]

This is likely because using a sponge leaves more bacteria on the dishes, giving the children contact with more bacteria, which then tones their immune systems and helps prevent allergic diseases. Even the frequency of how often you vacuum has been shown to influence your microbiota.[4] In part 3, we will detail these environmental factors and how you can use them in your favor.

Can we extract just the diet of an entire culture, apply it to a Westernized population, and expect the same results? Can we force our microbiotas to look like Africans' even though we are completely different, with different genes, different lifestyles, and different immune systems? It is extremely, extremely unlikely. In fact, we have performed clinical studies to answer this question, and we already know the answer: for many people, taking the approach of copying the diet of another—very different—population is a bad idea.

I would estimate that the Africans would be very healthy *regardless* of their diet, due to their substantially lower caloric intake and, more importantly, their environment and lifestyle!

Much of this book illustrates this important message—environment has a tremendous impact on your microbiota and your health. Findings from China help illustrate this point. When comparing those in urban versus rural China, the urban Chinese were more inflamed than rural Chinese, even after taking diet into account![5] This shows us that environment might be more important than diet in causing inflammation. Perhaps this is why we see Africans thriving on a diet that might make many Westerners sick—it's their healthier environment.

Another important fact to mention is that the Africans in this study were technically farmers, not hunter-gatherers. The negative health implications of humans abandoning a more hunter-gatherer diet/lifestyle and adopting a farming/grain-based diet/lifestyle have been well documented. Additionally, a number of people notice they feel better on gluten-free/grain-free diets. Remember, if the African-like high-carbohydrate and grain-based diet worked so well for everyone, we would have seen much better results with the old food-pyramid-diet model where grains and other carb-rich foods were the foundation. So while these African rural farmers might not have had an ideal diet, they were living in a very healthy environment (contact with dirt and germs, more activity, less stress), and this environment likely contributed to their gut health.

Does this mean all grains and carbs are bad? Absolutely not. I simply want you to understand why we cannot excise the diet from an entire culture and force it upon another.

One final point to consider regarding observations from non-Westernized societies: for the most part, the cultures and populations that have been studied are fairly poor and are only able to afford cheap-to-produce carbohydrate products, like grains and potatoes, rather than animals, which are significantly more expensive to raise. This is important to keep in mind, because these cultures may not be eating this way because they think it's healthier but because it's all they can afford.

It sounds like we can't replicate the diet of rural Africans, but what about Asians? Aren't they healthier than Americans? This question brings up a key point:

> *A population's diet is often accompanied by unique changes in their microbiota, changes that allow them to thrive on that diet.*

Asians provide two examples of this point. Traditional Asian diets typically include soy and seaweed, and the microbiotas of Asians have adapted accordingly. Most Asians' gut microbiotas contain unique bacteria that can break down soy to produce a compound known as (S)-equol. However, gut microbiotas of only 25%–30% of Westerners are able to do this.[6] The Japanese have also been shown to harbor intestinal bacteria that break down seaweed, bacteria that are undetected in North Americans' gut microbiota.[7]

We see another example of this in the Hadza, the African hunter-gatherers we discussed earlier. They consume a high amount of dense dietary fiber, and they harbor bacteria rarely found in Westerners. Those bacteria help to break down the dense fiber.[8] Even more interesting is that the Hadza have no Bifidobacterium![9] Bifidobacterium is one of the most beneficial probiotics for digestive health in Westerners and is used in many probiotic formulas.[10]

## BORROWING THE DIET OF OUR ANCESTORS

Are you sure you want an African or hunter-gatherer-like microbiota? Many people would probably answer *"Yes, because I'm Paleo!"* What does that have to do with anything? Paleo-diet enthusiasts often strive to replicate our hunter-gatherer ancestors. I understand the desire to learn from and replicate the environment of our Paleolithic predecessors or our non-Westernized counterparts, but we shouldn't do this blindly.

Allow me to introduce you to a member of your gut microbiota known as Methanobrevibacter smithii or M. smithii for short. Human studies have repeatedly shown that when this bug over-grows, it causes constipation, gas, and bloating. It has also been suggested M. smithii may cause high cholesterol and blood sugar levels and even weight gain when it overgrows in Westerners.[11]

Correspondingly, treatment of this bug may help improve cholesterol and blood sugar levels and has been shown to relieve constipation, gas, and bloating.

So, high levels of M. smithii are not good if you're a Westerner. However, the *highest* levels of M. smithii are seen in African hunter-gatherer-like populations![12] Does this mean Africans are constipated and overweight? No. For Africans, having high levels of M. smithii is likely a survival advantage. This is because M. smithii slows the movement of food through the intestinal tract, allowing more breakdown and absorption of food and calories. For Africans who eat a diet high in hard-to-digest fibrous plant foods, one that's often low in calories, this is beneficial.[13]

However, as we mentioned, for someone in a Westernized society, this could cause constipation, weight gain, higher cholesterol, and higher blood sugar levels (which are linked to diabetes). So, this is a case where we may want to rethink the ancestral replication paradigm. This all reinforces the notion that we can't treat every ecosystem the same. *Your* gut ecosystem is different from an *African hunter-gatherer or your Paleolithic ancestors.* To improve *your* health, we have to create the environment that is ideal for *your ecosystem.*

## AN EVOLUTIONARY OR ANCESTRAL PERSPECTIVE

As the human gastrointestinal tract evolved, the large intestine became shorter and we became less dependent upon it. The large intestine harbors lots of bacteria, and these bacteria help to break down hard-to-digest foods. This process is known as fermentation. Think of a cow's long intestinal tract, which helps break down the rigid grasses that it eats. As our early ancestors started eating a higher-quality diet, they enjoyed easy-to-digest, nutrient-dense, calorie-rich foods. It might seem that calorie-rich foods are a bad thing, but for our hunter-gatherer ancestors, it was a constant strug-gle to obtain enough calories to survive. As our ancestors became better hunters, they could obtain these easy-to-digest, nutrient-dense, calorie-rich foods—such as animals, with their high amounts of fat and protein, and ripe fruits—instead of hard-to-digest leaves and grasses. As the quality of their diet improved, their intestines changed. They didn't need as much large intestine to break down leaves and grasses, so they relied more heavily on their small intestine. The improvements in their diets and availability of more calories enabled brain growth. It all really comes down to energy. When our early ancestors ate foods that did not supply a lot of calories (energy), foods like grasses and leaves, they could barely meet their energy requirements. Because they could barely meet their energy requirements, there wasn't much extra energy for growth. But when they started eating easy-to-digest, calorie-rich foods, they had extra energy for growth, in this case, brain growth.

But why did the large intestine shorten? Again, because when our ancestors started eating food that they could digest more easily, they didn't need a lengthy digestive tract anymore. The specific area that was no longer needed was the large intestine, where hard-to-digest, fibrous material is broken down with the assistance of bacteria. This shift is reflected in our current intestinal anatomy. The small intestine represents over 56% of the intestinal tract, with the large intestine representing about 20%.[14] As we have been discussing, to optimize gut health, we need to pay particular attention to the small intestine.

Easy-to-digest, nutrient-dense, calorie-rich foods are often assumed to be ones that are high in protein and fat, such as animal foods. However, it's important to mention that access to carbohydrates that were easy to digest, like ripe fruits and cooked starches, also fueled the shortening of the large intestine.[16]

These are carbohydrates that require minimal bacterial digestion (fermentation) in the large intestine and instead utilize the small intestine for digestion. This again reinforces the importance of the small intestine. To put this simply, as we have evolved, our digestion has become more dependent upon the small intestine and less dependent upon the large intestine.

An evolutionary face-off between two of our most ancient ancestors illustrates this concept. The face-off was between Paranthropus boisei ("nut cracker" man, top image) versus Homo habilis (bottom image). Boisei was like a modern-day gorilla. He had extremely powerful jaws, which allowed him to chew his highly fibrous diet of tough roots and other fibrous plant foods. He also likely had a digestive tract that was highly fermentative, like a cow's, with a long intestinal tract, a long large intestine, and lots of bacteria to help break down food. Habilis was more of a scavenger, eating carcasses and foraging for honey but unable to digest the tough foodstuffs of the boisei's diet.

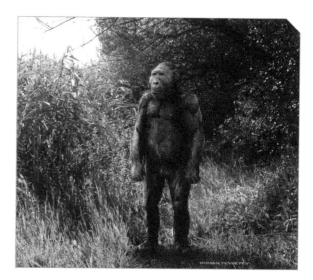

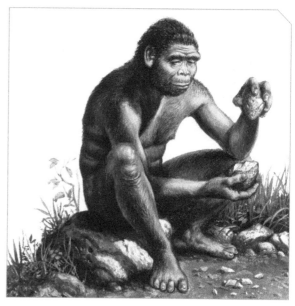

Initially, life was easy for the boisei. He ate the plant matter that was all around him. Life for the habilis, however, was difficult. He had to work hard to find a meal—scavenging from carcasses or climbing trees for honey. Sometime later, the climate changed. Africa became more arid, and plant life dwindled. This made things hard for the boisei, as his food supply was dwindling, and he soon became extinct because he could only eat his highly fibrous plant-food diet. The habilis, on the other hand, was able to survive due to his variable omnivorous diet—he wasn't dependent upon one type of food. Also, because the habilis was eating meat and fat, his brain was able to grow, thus improving his intellect. This was likely a key turning point in our evolution, setting us on a path away from a boisei-like large-intestine and fermentation-dependent digestion and toward habilis-like small-intestinal-dominated digestion.

Returning to the modern age, we see research showing Africans have different microbiotas from Westerners. But this does not mean that by replicating their microbiotas we will become healthier. If everyone ate an African-like diet that was high in carbs and prebiotics, people with celiac disease, thyroid disease, IBS, SIBO, and even diabetes, obesity, and fungal overgrowths wouldn't feel better, they'd feel worse.

This is likely because while these diets are good for the large intestine, they are often not good for the small intestine. I would like to reiterate that I am not saying a higher-carb and prebiotic diet is bad for everyone. There are clearly those it will help, but there are some it will make worse. With the current microbiota craze, everyone seems to be jumping on the bandwagon of more carbs and prebiotics because carbs and prebiotics feed gut bacteria. We know that optimizing your gut and microbiota requires an approach that creates the optimum environment for *your ecosystem* and not a one-size-fits-all approach. This is exactly what we will work toward in this book. Thank you for hanging in there as we cover these details, the details that are *behind* the recommendations we'll be making.

# DIFFERENT CULTURES REQUIRE DIFFERENT CARB INTAKES

## CARBS, WEIGHT, DIABETES, AND HEART DISEASE

We have established that different guts require different carb intake, just like different ecosystems require differing amounts of rain. We have already discussed how those with obesity, celiac disease, and thyroid disease may have preexisting bacterial overgrowths and that a higher carbohydrate and prebiotic diet might be a bad idea for these people. We have established that for many a lower-carb dietary approach that can reduce bacterial overgrowth might be the best strategy. There is even more data suggesting the ideal dietary approach may be a lower-carb one that actually helps prune back these bacterial overgrowths and, by doing so, improves the environment in and the health of the small intestine.

Dr. Christopher Gardner from Stanford conducted a study comparing popular diets that ranged from high fat/low carb through high carb/low fat. Remember, carbs and fat usually share an inverse relationship in diet: when one goes up, the other goes down. In his "A to Z Weight Loss Study,"[17] Dr. Gardner compared the following diets:

- Atkins (low carb)
- LEARN and Ornish (high carb)
- Zone (moderate carb/Mediterranean-like)

Gardner's study showed **the most improvement in overall cardiovascular risk profiles, blood sugar, and weight occurred on a low-carb diet**. He also showed this was the diet participants found easiest to stick with. Remember that a low-carb diet doesn't feed your gut bacteria to the extent of a higher-carb diet (such as the Ornish diet). In fact,

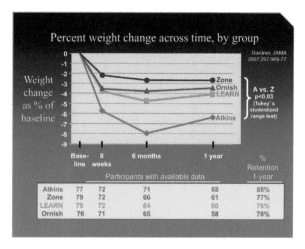

Percent weight change across time, by group

Gardner, JAMA 2007;297:969-77

A vs. Z
p<0.03
(Tukey's studentized range test)

| | Base-line | 8 weeks | 6 months | 1 year | % Retention 1-year |
|---|---|---|---|---|---|
| | | | Participants with available data | | |
| Atkins | 77 | 72 | 71 | 68 | 88% |
| Zone | 79 | 72 | 66 | 61 | 77% |
| LEARN | 79 | 72 | 64 | 60 | 76% |
| Ornish | 76 | 71 | 65 | 58 | 78% |

a lower-carb diet can help reduce bacterial and fungal overgrowths. What this tells us is that it's more important to eat the appropriate amount of carbohydrates than it is to feed your gut bacteria. This brings us to another principle:

## *eating to control blood sugar is more important than eating to feed gut bacteria.*

This is likely because eating to control blood sugar is also good for your small intestine. Now, the appropriate level of carb intake is not the same for everyone. It's important to mention that *all* the diets evaluated in this study were helpful; however, the lower-carb diet was the most helpful. We will help you find your ideal level of carb intake in part 5.

## CARBS AND IBS

What about SIBO (small-intestinal bacterial overgrowth) and SIFO (small-intestinal fungal overgrowth)? It has been shown that bacterial and fungal overgrowths may underlie IBS. In fact, it has been shown that those with IBS (gas, bloating, loose stools, constipation, abdominal pain) can have a heightened inflammatory response to their normal intestinal bacteria (their microbiotas)

when compared to healthy controls.[18] This is likely why a well-established, published treatment algorithm for SIBO calls for *restriction* of foods that encourage bacterial growth—or, said another way, recommends a diet that prunes back or reduces intestinal bacteria. Specifically, this diet restricts high-FODMAP foods. High-FODMAP foods are foods that are high in prebiotics (remember, prebiotics feed gut bacteria).[19] Numerous studies have shown that those with digestive problems do much better when avoiding these prebiotic-rich high-FODMAP foods. In other words, these people do better with a dietary approach that reduces bacterial overgrowth.[20]

So, a carb- and prebiotic-*rich* diet works for Africans, but if you are a Westerner, and especially if you are a Westerner with some gut issues, a high-carb and prebiotic diet might be the exact opposite of what you need. It may feed bacteria that your immune system is attacking. If you feed these bacteria, it can cause your intestines to be inflamed and contribute to the whole host of gut-related problems that we discussed earlier. Does this mean everyone should follow a low-carb diet? Again, no. In the recommendations sections that come later, I will provide you with a strategy to personalize your carb and prebiotic intake.

You've probably heard something about fungus (sometimes referred to as candida). Maybe you have a friend who treated fungus/candida and felt much better. Or perhaps someone you know did a candida diet and improved. You may have also heard people mention that they can't eat many carbs because if they do, their candida will flare up. Is this legitimate? To some extent, yes. Why does this group of people feel better when they avoid excess dietary carbs? Generally speaking, carbs feed fungus similarly to how they feed bacteria. Some people have genetic variations that make them susceptible to fungal overgrowths. These gene variations, two of which are known as Dectin-1 and CARD9, result in enhanced susceptibility to fungal infections and overgrowths because they cause alterations in the immune system's ability to control fungal growth.[21] People with these gene variations need to eat in a way that prevents fungal overgrowth.

It's even been suggested that this inability of the immune system to regulate fungus may lead to fungal overgrowth that then causes the autoimmune attack seen in inflammatory bowel disease, specifically Crohn's disease.[22] Similarly, increased bacterial diversity has been observed in diverticulitis, an inflammatory condition of the intestines. It has been suggested that increased diversity on microbiota testing could be used as a test for diverticulitis.[23] Again, we see that some people need help rebalancing or even reducing bacteria and fungus in their guts and should not blindly attempt to increase their bacteria.

"But I have a friend that lost weight and feels great on a moderate/higher-carb diet; aren't carbs good?" This is a great question. The answer again comes from Gardner's work. While Gardner clearly noted that the lower-carb diet seemed to work best, there were *some* subjects that responded equally well to the higher-carb diets. Gardner wanted to know why, so he analyzed his results further. He discovered that

- those who were more prone to diabetes (those who were most insulin *resistant*) seemed to only respond to the lower-carb diet;
- those who were the most insulin *sensitive* appeared to be able to lose weight on any diet, high carb or low carb.

His results have been replicated by others.[24]

*Insulin sensitive* means you process carbs well, and *insulin resistant* means you don't. This tells us that not everyone has to follow one diet! This is an important point to keep in mind, and it should encourage a dietary approach that helps individuals determine where they fit on the spectrum of carbohydrate intake.

## CONCEPT SUMMARY

- Westerners who attempt to replicate another culture's microbiota might get sick.

- A population's diet is often accompanied by unique changes in their microbiota, which allows them to thrive on that diet.

- Evolution has shortened our intestines and caused us to rely more on the small intestine and less on the bacterial fermentation of the large intestine.

- Eating to control your blood sugar is more important than eating to feed your gut bacteria.

- Carbohydrate intake is not a one-size-fits-all matter. Some will do better on more carbs, and some will do better on less. The goal is to find where you fall on the carb/prebiotic spectrum.

- You can't "custom manipulate" your microbiota, but you can optimize your gut environment/ecosystem to allow the healthiest microbiota. A healthy environment equals healthy bacteria.

1   Alexander Ströhle et al., "Latitude, Local Ecology, and Hunter-Gatherer Dietary Acid Load: Implications from Evolutionary Ecology," *American Journal of Clinical Nutrition* 92, no. 4 (October 1, 2010): 940–45, doi:10.3945/ajcn.2010.29815; Loren Cordain et al., "The Paradoxical Nature of Hunter-Gatherer Diets: Meat-Based, yet Non-Atherogenic," supplement, *European Journal of Clinical Nutrition* 56, no. S1 (March 2002): S42–S52, doi:10.1038/sj/ejcn/1601353; Alexander Ströhle and Andreas Hahn, "Diets of Modern Hunter-Gatherers Vary Substantially in Their Carbohydrate Content Depending on Ecoenvironments: Results from an Ethnographic Analysis," *Nutrition Research* 31, no. 6 (June 1, 2011): 429–35, doi:10.1016/J.NUTRES.2011.05.003; Alexander Ströhle et al., "Estimation of the Diet-Dependent Net Acid Load in 229 Worldwide Historically Studied Hunter-Gatherer Societies," *American Journal of Clinical Nutrition* 91, no. 2 (February 1, 2010): 406–12, doi:10.3945/ajcn.2009.28637.

2   Carlotta de Filippo et al., "Impact of Diet in Shaping Gut Microbiota Revealed by a Comparative Study in Children from Europe and Rural Africa," *Proceedings of the National Academy of Sciences of the United States of America* 107, no. 33 (August 17, 2010): 14691–96, doi:10.1073/pnas.1005963107.

3   Bill Hesselmar et al., "Allergy in Children in Hand versus Machine Dishwashing," *Pediatrics* 135, no. 3 (March 1, 2015): e590–7, doi:10.1542/peds.2014-2968.

4   Ekaterina Avershina et al., "Potential Association of Vacuum Cleaning Frequency with an Altered Gut Microbiota in Pregnant Women and Their 2-Year-Old Children," *Microbiome* 3, no. 1 (December 21, 2015): 65, doi:10.1186/s40168-015-0125-2.

5   Amanda L. Thompson et al., "Multilevel Examination of the Association of Urbanization with Inflammation in Chinese Adults," *Health & Place* 28 (July 1, 2014): 177–86, doi:10.1016/J.HEALTHPLACE.2014.05.003.

6   Catherine A. Lozupone et al., "Diversity, Stability and Resilience of the Human Gut Microbiota," *Nature* 489, no. 7415 (September 12, 2012): 220–30, doi:10.1038/nature11550; Jan-Hendrik Hehemann et al., "Transfer of Carbohydrate-Active Enzymes from Marine Bacteria to Japanese Gut Microbiota," *Nature* 464, no. 7290 (April 8, 2010): 908–12, doi:10.1038/nature08937.

7   Ibid.

8   Stephanie L. Schnorr et al., "Gut Microbiome of the Hadza Hunter-Gatherers," *Nature Communications* 5 (April 15, 2014): ncomms4654, doi:10.1038/ncomms4654.

9   Ibid.

10   Robin Spiller, "Review Article: Probiotics and Prebiotics in Irritable Bowel Syndrome," *Alimentary Pharmacology & Therapeutics* 28, no. 4 (August 1, 2008): 385–96, doi:10.1111/j.1365-2036.2008.03750.x; Magnus Simrén et al., "Intestinal Microbiota in Functional Bowel Disorders: A Rome Foundation Report," *Gut* 62, no. 1 (January 2013): 159–76, doi:10.1136/gutjnl-2012-302167.

11   Robert J. Basseri et al., "Intestinal Methane Production in Obese Individuals Is Associated with a Higher Body Mass Index," *Gastroenterology & Hepatology* 8, no. 1 (January 2012): 22–28, www.ncbi.nlm.nih.gov/pubmed/22347829; Ruchi Mathur et al., "Methane and Hydrogen Positivity on Breath Test Is Associated with Greater Body Mass Index and Body Fat," *Journal of Clinical Endocrinology & Metabolism* 98, no. 4 (April 2013): E698–702, doi:10.1210/jc.2012-3144; Catherine A. Mbakwa et al., "Gut Colonization with *Methanobrevibacter Smithii* Is Associated with Childhood Weight Development," *Obesity* 23, no. 12 (December 2015): 2508–16, doi:10.1002/oby.21266; Andrew Curry, "Certain Bacteria Might Make Type 2 More Likely," *Diabetes Forecast*, November 2012, accessed October 9, 2017, www.diabetesforecast.org/2012/nov/certain-bacteria-might-make-type-2-more-likely.html.

12   Nadia Gaci et al., "Archaea and the Human Gut: New Beginning of an Old Story," *World Journal of Gastroenterology* 20, no. 43 (November 21, 2014): 16062–78, doi:10.3748/wjg.v20.i43.16062.

13   Ibid.

14   Katherine Milton, "A Hypothesis to Explain the Role of Meat-Eating in Human Evolution," *Evolutionary Anthropology: Issues, News, and Reviews* 8, no. 1 (January 1, 1999): 11–21, doi:10.1002/(SICI)1520-6505(1999)8:1<11::AID-EVAN6>3.0.CO;2-M.

15   Jens Walter and Ruth Ley, "The Human Gut Microbiome: Ecology and Recent Evolutionary Changes," *Annual Review of Microbiology* 65, no. 1 (October 13, 2011): 411–29, doi:10.1146/annurev-micro-090110-102830.

16   Anna Revedin et al., "Thirty Thousand-Year-Old Evidence of Plant Food Processing," *Proceedings of the National Academy of Sciences of the United States of America* 107, no. 44 (November 2, 2010): 18815–19, doi:10.1073/pnas.1006993107; Katherine Milton, "A Hypothesis to Explain the Role of Meat-Eating in Human Evolution," *Evolutionary Anthropology: Issues, News, and Reviews* 8, no. 1 (January 1, 1999): 11–21, doi:10.1002/(SICI)1520-6505(1999)8:1<11::AID-EVAN6>3.0.CO;2-M; Karen Hardy et al., "The Importance of Dietary Carbohydrate in Human Evolution," *Quarterly Review of Biology* 90, no. 3 (September 26, 2015): 251–68, doi:10.1086/682587.

17    Christopher D. Gardner et al., "Comparison of the Atkins, Zone, Ornish, and LEARN Diets for Change in Weight and Related Risk Factors among Overweight Premenopausal Women," *JAMA* 297, no. 9 (March 7, 2007): 969, doi:10.1001/jama.297.9.969.

18    Ohanna Sundin et al., "Cytokine Response after Stimulation with Key Commensal Bacteria Differ in Post-Infectious Irritable Bowel Syndrome (PI-IBS) Patients Compared to Healthy Controls," *PLOS ONE* 10, no. 9 (September 14, 2015): e0134836, doi:10.1371/journal.pone.0134836.

19    Mark Pimentel, "An Evidence-Based Treatment Algorithm for IBS Based on a Bacterial/SIBO Hypothesis: Part 2," *American Journal of Gastroenterology* 105, no. 6 (June 1, 2010): 1227–30, doi:10.1038/ajg.2010.125.

20    Abigail Marsh et al., "Does a Diet Low in FODMAPs Reduce Symptoms Associated with Functional Gastrointestinal Disorders? A Comprehensive Systematic Review and Meta-Analysis," *European Journal of Nutrition* 55, no. 3 (April 17, 2016): 897–906, doi:10.1007/s00394-015-0922-1; Richard B. Gearry et al., "Reduction of Dietary Poorly Absorbed Short-Chain Carbohydrates (FODMAPs) Improves Abdominal Symptoms in Patients with Inflammatory Bowel Disease—a Pilot Study," *Journal of Crohn's and Colitis* 3, no. 1 (February 1, 2009): 8–14, doi:10.1016/j.crohns.2008.09.004; Ashley Charlebois et al., "The Impact of Dietary Interventions on the Symptoms of Inflammatory Bowel Disease: A Systematic Review," *Critical Reviews in Food Science and Nutrition* 56, no. 8 (June 10, 2016): 1370–78, doi:10.1080/10408398.2012.760515.

21    Scott G. Filler, "Insights from Human Studies into the Host Defense against Candidiasis," *Cytokine* 58, no. 1 (April 1, 2012): 129–32, doi:10.1016/J.CYTO.2011.09.018; Andre Franke et al., "Genome-Wide Association Study for Ulcerative Colitis Identifies Risk Loci at 7q22 and 22q13 (IL17REL)," *Nature Genetics* 42, no. 4 (April 14, 2010): 292–94, doi:10.1038/ng.553; Erik Glocker and Bodo Grimbacher, "Chronic Mucocutaneous Candidiasis and Congenital Susceptibility to Candida," *Current Opinion in Allergy and Clinical Immunology* 10, no. 6 (December 2010): 542–50, doi:10.1097/ACI.0b013e32833fd74f; Bart Ferwerda et al., "Human Dectin-1 Deficiency and Mucocutaneous Fungal Infections," *New England Journal of Medicine* 361, no. 18 (October 29, 2009): 1760–67, doi:10.1056/NEJMoa0901053; Erik-Oliver Glocker et al., "A Homozygous *CARD9* Mutation in a Family with Susceptibility to Fungal Infections," *New England Journal of Medicine* 361, no. 18 (October 29, 2009): 1727–35, doi:10.1056/NEJMoa0810719; Philip R. Taylor et al., "Dectin-1 Is Required for -Glucan Recognition and Control of Fungal Infection," *Nature Immunology* 8, no. 1 (January 10, 2007): 31–38, doi:10.1038/ni1408; Dermot P. B. McGovern et al., "Genome-Wide Association Identifies Multiple Ulcerative Colitis Susceptibility Loci," *Nature Genetics* 42, no. 4 (April 14, 2010): 332–37, doi:10.1038/ng.549.

22    Stephan J. Ott et al., "Fungi and Inflammatory Bowel Diseases: Alterations of Composition and Diversity," *Scandinavian Journal of Gastroenterology* 43, no. 7 (January 8, 2008): 831–41, doi:10.1080/00365520801935434; Annie Standaert-Vitse et al., "Candida Albicans Colonization and ASCA in Familial Crohn's Disease," *American Journal of Gastroenterology* 104, no. 7 (July 26, 2009): 1745–53, doi:10.1038/ajg.2009.225.

23    L. Daniels et al., "Fecal Microbiome Analysis as a Diagnostic Test for Diverticulitis," *European Journal of Clinical Microbiology & Infectious Diseases* 33, no. 11 (November 4, 2014): 1927–36, doi:10.1007/s10096-014-2162-3.

24    Cara B. Ebbeling et al., "Effects of a Low–Glycemic Load vs Low-Fat Diet in Obese Young Adults," *JAMA* 297, no. 19 (May 16, 2007): 2092, doi:10.1001/jama.297.19.2092.

# CHAPTER 4

# HOW TO EVALUATE HEALTH RECOMMENDATIONS

## THREE WAYS TO AVOID CONFUSION IN THE DIETARY-HEALTH CONTROVERSY

Do you ever feel confused about what you should and shouldn't eat? For example, maybe somewhere you read we should all follow a low-carb diet, and then somewhere else you read that fat and meat are unhealthy for you and we should eat a high-carb plant-based diet. Or maybe you've read we should eat high-fiber diets because fiber is good for us. But you've also read that if you have gas, bloating, and diarrhea, high-fiber diets can make you worse. Maybe you've read that probiotics are good for SIBO but heard others say probiotics are bad for it. What do you do? This book will answer all these questions, but I would like to share with you how you can use the same screening process we use to cut through the confusion with health claims.

## 1. DON'T THINK SMALL

You may hear or read something along the lines of "those who are diabetic have low levels of [insert bacteria name here], while those who are healthy have high levels of it. So, we need to increase our levels of this bacteria to become healthier."

This is a very alluring concept. It's reminiscent of the magic-pill idea that we so easily fall in love with. However, as I am sure you know, there are no magic pills. This type of thinking is highly reductive, and your gut doesn't play by these rules. Your gut is an ecosystem brimming with life, and it can't simply be reduced to a few bacteria. Let's look at an example.

Faecalibacterium prausnitzii is a bacterium said to have antiobesity and antidiabetes effects. You can't take F. prausnitzii as a probiotic, but you can take prebiotics or eat more carb/prebiotic-rich foods that will help increase your levels of this bacteria. Great, right? Well, this is where speculation gets us in trouble.

Some studies show that a low-carb diet increases F. prausnitzii.[1] Other studies show a high-carb diet increases F. prausnitzii.[2] Some studies show diabetics and obese people have lower levels of F. prausnitzii.[3] But other studies show diabetics and the obese people have higher levels of F. prausnitzii.[4] Along these same lines, a placebo control study was recently performed where obese women were given prebiotics. The prebiotics caused an increase in F. prausnitzii levels but did not cause any change in weight![5]

When it comes to the gut, thinking too small will get us into trouble. Here is another example, this one from mice studies regarding a bacterium called Prevotella copri DSM 18205.[6] I don't like citing animal data, but this study helps illustrate the point. When Prevotella copri DSM 18205 was transplanted into one group of mice, it showed the ability to improve glucose levels. This suggests it may help with conditions like diabetes. However, when transplanted into a different group of mice, the bacteria caused arthritis.[7] Also, when these same bacteria were transferred into mice that had been previously given antibiotics, they formed colitis or inflammation in the intestines. The same bacteria act in very different ways in different contexts because your gut is a complex ecosystem.

This is also why the small intestine has been overlooked by many of the gut gurus; everyone is looking at your gut health through the narrow lens of the large intestine.

Making health-care decisions based upon what happens to one bacteria is a "zoomed-in" approach; it's like navigating from Massachusetts to California by looking through a magnifying glass.

OK, so don't think small. How, then, do we think big? Looking at clinical trials in humans is how we think big, and transitions us to our second point.

## 2. DEMAND HUMAN-OUTCOME STUDIES (CLINICAL TRIALS). DON'T GET SWEPT UP IN ANIMAL-MODEL STUDIES, CELL STUDIES, OR OBSERVATIONAL STUDIES

The reason you've been told feeding your gut bacteria is the next "cure" for obesity might be because of a mistake that is repeated with almost every health-care fad: overextrapolation. When a rat study shows an interesting finding in five rats, or a clump of cells in a petri dish produces a novel result, fad enthusiasts shout from the rooftops and the media searches for a sound bite that will grab your attention. However, before we jump for joy, these results must be confirmed in human trials. These human trials should show favorable outcomes like weight loss, improved mood, less inflammation, or dampened autoimmunity. Failing to do this is the source of confusion surrounding most topics in health care. These confirming human trials are called *clinical trials* or *randomized clinical trials*, RCT for short.

You should demand human-outcome data before trying a new test or treatment. If you don't have that data, *you're* the guinea pig. Doctors rely heavily on clinical trials before adopting new treatments for their patients. This will help you cut through much confusion, debate, and speculation. Yes, there are occasional exceptions to this rule, but for the most part, following this principle is an excellent strategy.

We touched on animal studies and cell studies, but what about observational studies—what are those? Observational studies are simply when we observe other people, like the Africans we talked about earlier. We observe that the Africans eat lots of fiber, carbs, and grains and also have healthy weights and immune systems. But, as we have already discussed, this doesn't mean that if we do what the Africans do, we'll become healthy. In fact, doing so ends up making many people sick. Just because we observe another group of people doing something doesn't mean we will see our health improve when we do the same thing. Try drinking the Africans' water for example, and see how that goes. Also, remember the reason why the Africans do well with *their* diet might be because of the high levels of the M. smithii in their guts—the same M. smithii that makes Westerners sick. Their gut ecosystem is different, and, therefore, they have different needs.

## 3. AVOID MAKING DECISIONS BASED UPON ONE STUDY

One study does not prove anything. You can find one study to support almost anything. Using one study to generate a recommendation is not good practice. Rather, what we should do is examine *all* the available studies to establish what the body of evidence as a whole suggests.

This might sound complicated, but you do this every day. Thirty people have been to Café Triste, the new Italian café in town. Would asking one person what he or she thought give a true representation of this café? Isn't it possible that one person could have an unusually good or bad experience? Yes, of course. We would want to ask all thirty people what they thought to get an accurate gauge. The same thing applies to studies. The results of one study could be misleading, but if we consider what *all* the studies show, we will have a much more accurate opinion on an issue.

Here is another example: What if one study showed that supplementing with prebiotics improved diarrhea, but another eighteen studies showed that supplementing with prebiotics worsened diarrhea? If you only knew about the one study, you would be in trouble.

The three points we just covered can be rolled into one simple ideal: use high-quality scientific evidence rather than low-quality evidence.

Here is what you should look for to determine the quality of the evidence you're considering:

- RCTs—randomized clinical trials (also known as randomized control trials) are human studies that control for the placebo effect and usually look at health outcomes like prolonged life, weight loss, improved blood sugar, less inflammation, and less bloating. These studies are arguably the highest level of scientific evidence.
- Systematic reviews—these review many RCTs and other data. It's like a summary of what thirty people had to say about the café. Just remember it's a review *of* all the data, hence a systematic review.
- Meta-analyses—these are like taking the reviews of the thirty people eating at the café and then using math to give the café a numeric score. For example, when asking people what they think about the café, you ask them to rate it on a scale of one to one hundred. Then, you take the average of all the scores. The average score of this café might have been twenty-five out of one hundred. Or if you asked just one person, he or she might have rated the café as a ninety-five. If the average score was a twenty-five out of one hundred, the chance of you having a ninety-five-out-of-one-hundred experience is very slim. Simple, right? Meta means "big picture." So, a meta-analysis is just a big-picture analysis or summary.

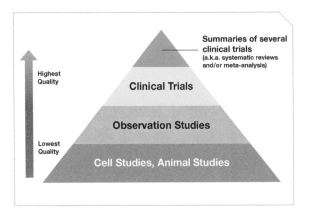

Again, you likely use systematic reviews and meta-analyses in your day-to-day life without even realizing it. Think about an important financial decision you need to make—let's say the best way to save for your retirement. Would you follow the plan of the first financial adviser you spoke to? Or would you speak with several financial advisers and feel most comfortable with the strategies that were agreed upon by most of them? You would likely look for the trends or commonalities recommended by a majority of top financial advisers. This is what we will do throughout this book with health-care information.

The terms "systematic review" and "meta-analysis" sound intimidating, but when we break them down, they are merely big words that essentially mean "to summarize." This is what you want, a summary of all the data.

## WHY LEVELS OF EVIDENCE ARE SO IMPORTANT

Let's take the example of trying to increase your income to become wealthy to illustrate this.

- A *mechanism* or *cell study* is like saying people become wealthy because they have more money going into their accounts than out of their accounts. OK, great. Does this tell you how to become wealthy? No. Does this tell you how you can change your situation to always have more money going into your bank account than out? No.
- An *observational study* might report that you have a greater chance of becoming rich if you grew up in a certain town. For example, it might observe that a high percentage of people from this town end up becoming wealthy. But this still doesn't tell you how to become wealthy now. The people from this town could simply have been born into wealthy families.
- A *clinical trial/outcome study/RCT* would be akin to discovering that 80% of people who followed a particular investing strategy became wealthy within five years. This tells you how you can become wealthy—by following this investment strategy. It

tells you what action you can take to improve your situation. Levels of evidence are important and should matter to you.

You can waste huge amounts of time and money by investing in health-care theories. Instead, invest your time and energy into health-care recommendations that have been proved by high-quality science, such as the recommendations we're making in this book. Clinical trials answer the question: What happens to someone when they do X, Y or Z? This is what you need to know. You don't benefit from knowing what happened to a rat, a cell, or a group of people from a different culture and environment whose gut microbiota are nothing like yours. Make sense?

Sometimes we have little scientific evidence to work with and have to make the best decision we can based on the limited data we have. However, what happens all too often is the science to inform us is out there, but an author, doctor, or another "authority" has already made up his or her mind on an issue and merely cherry-picks studies to support a preconceived belief. This is not good. We should use science to learn and update our opinion and improve our recommendations, not to footnote an erroneous or preexisting belief. When science is used incorrectly like this, it's you the consumer who suffers; when it's used correctly, you benefit.

Throughout this book we'll review the effectiveness of available microbiota and gut treatments in order to craft a plan to improve your health. Nearly every study we will examine will be the high-quality type listed above. We will predominantly look at clinical trials (RCTs) or summaries of clinical trials (systematic reviews or meta-analyses). This ensures you will be provided with the most effective plan for improving your gut health and overall health.

## CONCEPT SUMMARY

There are three simple ways to avoid being misled
by microbiota and health claims:

- Don't focus on one bacteria but rather think more
broadly about your gut health and gut ecosystem.

- Rely on randomized clinical studies (RCTs) in
humans rather than animal or cell-culture studies.

- Look to the aggregate findings of numerous
studies—systematic reviews and meta-analyses—
instead of basing decisions upon one study.

1    Harry J. Flint et al., "The Role of the Gut Microbiota in Nutrition and Health," *Nature Reviews Gastroenterology & Hepatology* 9, no. 10
      (September 4, 2012): 577–89, doi:10.1038/nrgastro.2012.156.

2    F. Fava et al., "The Type and Quantity of Dietary Fat and Carbohydrate Alter Faecal Microbiome and Short-Chain Fatty Acid
      Excretion in a Metabolic Syndrome 'at-Risk' Population," *International Journal of Obesity* 37, no. 2 (February 13, 2013): 216–23,
      doi:10.1038/ijo.2012.33.

3    Herbert Tilg and Alexander R. Moschen, "Microbiota and Diabetes: An Evolving Relationship," *Gut* 63, no. 9 (September 1,
      2014): 1513–21, doi:10.1136/gutjnl-2014-306928; Marlene Remely et al., "Effects of Short-Chain Fatty Acid Producing Bacteria on
      Epigenetic Regulation of FFAR3 in Type 2 Diabetes and Obesity," *Gene* 537, no. 1 (March 2014): 85–92, doi:10.1016/j.gene.2013.11.081.

4    Ramadass Balamurugan et al., "Quantitative Differences in Intestinal Faecalibacterium Prausnitzii in Obese Indian Children,"
      *British Journal of Nutrition* 103, no. 3 (February 23, 2010): 335, doi:10.1017/S0007114509992182; J. Graessler et al., "Metagenomic
      Sequencing of the Human Gut Microbiome Before and After Bariatric Surgery in Obese Patients with Type 2 Diabetes: Correlation
      with Inflammatory and Metabolic Parameters," *Pharmacogenomics Journal* 13, no. 6 (December 2, 2013): 514–22, doi:10.1038
      /tpj.2012.43.

5    Evelyne M. Dewulf et al., "Insight into the Prebiotic Concept: Lessons from an Exploratory, Double Blind Intervention Study with
      Inulin-Type Fructans in Obese Women," *Gut* 62, no. 8 (August 1, 2013): 1112–21, doi:10.1136/gutjnl-2012-303304.

6    Ruth E. Ley, "Gut Microbiota in 2015: Prevotella in the Gut: Choose Carefully," *Nature Reviews Gastroenterology & Hepatology* 13, no. 2
      (February 1, 2016): 69–70, doi:10.1038/nrgastro.2016.4.

7    Jose U. Scher et al., "Expansion of Intestinal *Prevotella Copri* Correlates with Enhanced Susceptibility to Arthritis," *eLife* 2 (Novem-
      ber 5, 2013): e01202, doi:10.7554/eLife.01202.

# CHAPTER 5

# HOW EARLY LIFE AND ENVIRONMENT IMPACT YOUR GUT AND IMMUNE SYSTEM

## EARLY LIFE'S IMPACT ON YOUR MICROBIOTA AND IMMUNE SYSTEM

As we've discussed, environment has a major influence on your microbiota. Beginning in utero and continuing through the first few years of life, environment appears to have a particularly powerful impact. This is because the world of bacteria that will be with you the rest of your life (your gut microbiota) develops to a large extent by the second to third year of life.[1] The colonization starts while a mother is pregnant and seems to be mostly complete by age two or three. It also appears that your immune system develops in tandem with this, because your early microbiota is crucial in developing a healthy immune system.

The importance of early life on development of the immune system cannot be overemphasized. It has been well documented that early life exposure to dirt, germs, and bugs aids in the development of your immune system, and if you have robust exposure, you'll be less inflamed and have a healthier immune system later in life.

It has been theorized that problems with this early life development is one of the major reasons industrialized countries have higher levels of inflammatory and autoimmune/immune diseases.[2] We'll discuss some of the most common autoimmune diseases a little later in this chapter.

I find it fascinating that as we have transitioned from hunter-gatherer bands to living in modern Westernized societies, we have lost exposure to a lot of the dirt, bacteria, and other environmental microbes that have been essential for proper microbiota and immune system development.

It's important to remember there is a trade-off here. We greatly reduced infectious diseases and infant mortality because of our improved sanitation. However, we may have gone too far in the hygienic direction and damaged our immune systems, which has led to a rise in allergic and autoimmune diseases. Entire books have been written about this topic. (One of my favorites is *An Epidemic of Absence,* by Moises Velasquez-Manoff.)

# UNDERSTANDING THE ENVIRONMENT, HYGIENE, IMMUNE SYSTEM, AND AUTOIMMUNE DISEASE

It's not unreasonable for parents to want to protect their children, and this certainly includes protecting them from infections. However, too much protection can have unintended side effects of inflammatory, autoimmune, and allergic disorders. But how does all this work? Your body has its own army (your immune system) to defend against invasion (infection). Like any army, your immune system needs practice and training to operate effectively.

We evolved under circumstances of constant exposure to dirt, bacteria, animals, and germs— great training for your immune system. Picture our prehistoric ancestors. They would likely be covered in dirt most of the day. They would work all day, making tools, repairing their shelters, gathering foods, and butchering animals—all without washing their hands. Infants and children of these ancestors would be in contact with the environment and with their "dirty" moms and dads.

Whether you're the infant, child, or adult in this scenario, you're getting lots of exposure to dirt, bacteria, and animals. All this exposure was fantastic training for the army that is your immune system. Because of this, your immune system would have been well trained and well behaved—meaning no allergies, inflammation, or autoimmune disease.

Fast-forward to today: many children are lathered with antibacterial soaps daily, hardly ever touch dirt, are given antibiotics, and, compared to how we used to live, exist in a germ-free bubble.

Their armies are poorly trained. An untrained army—immune system—might attack the wrong target or attack at the wrong time, and this is what causes inflammatory, autoimmune, and allergic disorders. Autoimmunity occurs when your immune system inappropriately attacks your body's healthy tissue. Allergies are when your immune system mistakenly reacts to things that aren't threats, things like grasses, pollens, or foods. Both autoimmunity and allergies cause an increase in inflammation.

## SOME COMMON AUTOIMMUNE DISEASES AND THEIR TARGETS

- celiac disease—intestinal tissue
- inflammatory bowel disease (Crohn's and ulcerative colitis)—intestinal tissue
- hypo- and hyperthyroidism (Hashimoto's disease and Graves' disease)—thyroid gland
- rheumatoid arthritis—joint tissue
- depression—brain tissue[3]
- psoriasis, eczema—skin tissue
- anemia (pernicious anemia)—stomach cells
- MS (multiple sclerosis)—nervous system cells
- myasthenia gravis—nervous system receptors

There is even some research suggesting heart disease may have an autoimmune component.

> *If autoimmune diseases were measured as one group, they would be as common as heart disease.*

Heart disease is the most common disease in the United States—more common than cancer. Cancer is the second most prevalent disease. For cancer, we add up *all* cancer types to measure how many people have the disease. However, we do not do this for autoimmune diseases. Autoimmune diseases aren't measured as one large group but rather as many smaller subgroups. Because of this, the statistics regarding autoimmune conditions may be misleading.

Here is a statement from the National Institutes of Health's Autoimmune Diseases Coordinating Committee regarding autoimmune disease:

> *collectively [autoimmune diseases] are thought to affect approximately 5 to 8 percent of the United States population—14 to 22 million persons. To provide a context to evaluate the impact of autoimmune diseases, cancer affected approximately 9 million people in the United States in 1997 and heart disease affected approximately 22 million people in the United States in 1996.[4]*

It has been repeatedly observed that those living in less sterile, non-Westernized societies have far less inflammatory, autoimmune, and allergic diseases.[5] Again, this is likely because the immune systems of people in those societies get the training they need to function properly. Is this the *only* reason for this? Probably not, but it appears to be a major factor. This supports the assertion that it's the environment that makes some societies—such as the Africans we discussed earlier—healthy, not their diet.

This hints at an interesting question. If I have an autoimmune disease, is there something wrong with *me* or something wrong with the *environment*? I certainly think we can say the environment. This is important to keep in mind, because some of my patients with autoimmune conditions are very hard on themselves. While I understand how frustrating a health ailment can be, some self-love and self-appreciation may also be in order.

*Those with a tendency toward autoimmune and allergic conditions today may have been most protected from infection when the environment wasn't as clean.*

This is because those with autoimmune and allergic conditions tend to have a strong immune system (I'm using the term "strong" loosely, to mean "quick to react"). This was very helpful when we didn't have modern medicine and you could be killed by an infection. However, today things are a little different. We don't have the constant exposure to dirt and germs to train our immune system army. If you combine a strong army with poor training, you can get reckless behavior—like your immune system attacking tissues of your own body as in autoimmune conditions.

This is not speculative. We have modern-day examples of how this plays out. Sardinia is a beautiful Italian island that has one of the highest populations of centenarians (those who live to a hundred or longer) in the world. Sardinia used to have a high infection rate of malaria. But despite the high malarial infection rate, Sardinians appeared generally healthy, likely because they had strong immune systems that could hold malaria in check.

In the 1950s, Sardinia underwent a malaria-eradication program that virtually eliminated this infection from the population.[6] Since then, Sardinia's rate of the autoimmune disease multiple sclerosis (MS) has skyrocketed.[7] Here's what we think happened: The Sardinian immune system evolved to be strong under the constant pressure from malaria. Once malaria was gone, the strong immune system didn't know what to do. It was so used to being in a constant battle with malaria that once malaria was gone, it started attacking the Sardinian nervous system tissue, causing MS.

We have discussed the concept that those with autoimmune conditions may in fact have strong immune systems and how these strong immune systems may protect from infection. In support of this reasoning is this: It has been observed that those with autoimmunity against their stomach tissue are protected from H. pylori bacteria infecting their stomachs—possibly because of this strong immune system we have been discussing.[8] Other studies have confirmed that those with this stomach autoimmunity appear to be protected from H. pylori infection in the stomach.[9] So, those with a strong immune system that causes autoimmunity to stomach tissue are actually protected against infection in that same stomach tissue. Additionally, the genes associated with celiac disease (which is autoimmune reactivity to intestinal tissue triggered by dietary gluten) have also been shown to offer protection against bacterial infection.[10]

When we look at all this evidence, a picture emerges: as our environment has changed, a strong immune system may have become a liability.[11] Remember, though, this same immune system may have been a major asset in a different environment. If *you* have an autoimmune condition, don't be too hard on yourself. Now that we have a better understanding of the immune system and how autoimmunity develops, let's discuss some crucial early life factors that impact the development of your immune system.

# EFFECTS OF ANTIBIOTIC USE AND ENVIRONMENTAL EXPOSURES IN EARLY LIFE

Antibiotics should be used on babies and young children only when absolutely necessary. This is because antibiotics kill bacteria, the good along with the bad. If an antibiotic is used before the colonization of your microbiota is complete, around age two or three, you risk losing some bacteria forever. And, unfortunately, this can cause lifelong problems. I understand this is a powerful statement. This is not to say you should *never* use antibiotics on young children, but you should do so only when absolutely necessary. Let's discuss why.

## EARLY LIFE ANTIBIOTICS AND ECZEMA, ASTHMA, AND ALLERGY

The trend in medical literature strongly suggests that early life antibiotic use increases the risk of eczema, asthma, and allergies. Of the eleven available high-quality studies I reviewed, nine show an increased risk,[12] while two do not.[13] Of the nine studies showing increased risk, two were systematic reviews and one was a meta-analysis. They showed antibiotics increased risk of eczema and asthma, respectively.[14] Remember, this is powerful information because both of these study types are reviews that examine the available studies to see what the trend is. In these two studies, "early" life is defined as within a child's first year.

Does this mean that using antibiotics after a child's first year is OK? Interestingly, another asthma study found that antibiotics were still a problem when used *after* one year of age but were significantly less problematic (over 50% less).[15] It was also shown that the more antibiotic the child used, the higher the child's risk of asthma. This certainly seems logical. This hints at our concept of timing, meaning antibiotics do the most harm while your microbiota is forming (earlier in life) and are less harmful once your microbiota is more formed (later in life). In other words,

> *the earlier in life antibiotics are used, the more damaging they are.*

Again, the microbiota predominantly forms by age two or three.

## EARLY LIFE ANTIBIOTICS, WEIGHT GAIN, AND OBESITY

Can using antibiotics early in life put a child at risk for being overweight later in life? The general trend seen in the medical literature suggests yes. Some reoccurring themes are seen here also. It appears the earlier the use, the more times used, and the broader the spectrum (broad-spectrum antibiotics target more types of bacteria compared to narrow-spectrum antibiotics), the greater the risk of weight gain or obesity later in life.[16]

In the case of antibiotics affecting weight gain and obesity, how early is early? Most of the studies used here define this as between six months and two years of life. But even within this time frame, it appears antibiotic use at six months may be more damaging than at two years.[17] Again, the earlier the more damaging.

How much weight is usually gained? This is harder to define due to variations in the studies. But we do know there is an increased risk of being classified as overweight and even obese. So, clearly the weight gain is more than just a few pounds.

Could something else in the child's life be what caused the weight gain? Were there other factors that could have affected the accuracy of these studies? People may say things like "Maybe heavier kids are less healthy and, therefore, more often have infections and need antibiotics," or "Did breastfeeding affect the results?" or "Did the mom gain excessive weight while pregnant?" The researchers cited here have controlled for other factors, which means that even after attempting to *isolate for the effect of antibiotics alone*, the relationship between antibiotics and weight gain still remains.

## EARLY LIFE ANTIBIOTICS AND INFLAMMATORY BOWEL DISEASE (IBD)

It does appear that early life exposure to antibiotics increases the risk of inflammatory bowel disease.[18] One meta-analysis, again very high-quality data, found that "All antibiotics were associated with IBD, with the exception of penicillin." And two antibiotics in particular, metronidazole and fluoroquinolone, were most strongly associated with IBD.

Another study found a 2.9 times increased risk of IBD after using antibiotics in children.[19] It also appears that the risk of developing Crohn's disease is greater than that of developing ulcerative colitis after using antibiotics early in life.[20]

Before we leave the topic of antibiotics, let's consider this question: Are antibiotics the *only* reason for the changes Westerners see in their microbiotas? Likely not. Looking at a nonindustrialized tribe in Papua New Guinea, we see something interesting. This group still lives a largely non-Westernized tribal life but *also* regularly uses antibiotics.[21] The members of this tribe have much greater diversity in their gut bacteria than what is seen in the United States and a much lower incidence of allergies and autoimmune diseases.[22] Even though they use antibiotics, they still have better gut diversity and immune system health. This suggests the environment may be more important than antibiotics.

So, should we be like the New Guineans? Well, if we were to *only* look at this question through a narrowed window of bacterial diversity, maybe. However, it's important to realize that the New Guineans have a lower life expectancy and higher rate of infant mortality. What does all this mean? It means there are pros and cons for *every* environment—from the "dirty" hunter-gatherer at the one end to the "sterile" Westerner at the other. We trade one thing for another. In this case, it appears we trade life expectancy and infant mortality for allergy and autoimmune conditions.

- Westerners experience increased life expectancy and survival rate of children but also experience increased autoimmune conditions and allergies.
- Hunter-gatherers experience decreased life expectancy and survival rate of children but also experience decreased autoimmune conditions and allergies.

We have established antibiotic use early in life can have negative impacts later in life, likely by killing off some of the good bacteria in your gut. We've talked about how important the environment is in shaping the microbiota and immune system. So, does having more exposure to bacteria (and, therefore, more bacteria in your gut) early in life lead to positive health impacts later in life? In short, yes.

There are several important ways in which infants and children become exposed to these bacteria, bacteria that help colonize their guts to form their microbiota and train their immune systems. Some of the most important exposures are through the birthing process, breastfeeding, and early life environmental exposure.

## THE BIRTHING PROCESS

When children are born, they are exposed to a massive dose of bacteria as they pass through their mothers' vaginal canals. In fact, some researchers now think that the stress of labor causes temporary leaky gut in the mother, which then allows the mom's gut bacteria to colonize the child.[23] It has been clearly documented that children who are born vaginally have different bacterial colonization than those born by C-section. Those birthed vaginally have bacteria that resemble their moms' bacteria; those born by C-section have bacteria that reflect the delivery room.

I hope you're asking, "Well, OK, but what does this really mean in terms of real-world effects?"

Fortunately, we have some good data here. In 2008, researchers published a meta-analysis of observational studies. This is high-level scientific data because it analyzed the twenty available studies to see what the consensus of the data was. They also attempted to control for other variables that could confound the findings. For example, maybe older mothers were more prone to having C-sections, and, therefore, the study findings could have been due to increased maternal age and *not* because of the C-sections. After attempting to isolate for other variables like this, it was found the C-section babies have a more than 20% increased risk of developing type 1 diabetes.[24]

One additional paper found birth by C-section increases risk of chronic inflammatory conditions—celiac disease, type 1 diabetes, asthma, and obesity—compared to vaginal birth.[25] In yet another study, ulcerative colitis, celiac disease, lower respiratory tract infection, juvenile arthritis, and asthma were more common in C-section babies compared to vaginal birth after following over 750,000 children for fourteen years.[26]

Does this mean you or your child is doomed if you have been born by or have had a child by C-section? Of course not. But it's important for you to understand what it might mean and for you to try even harder in the other health-promoting areas you *can* control. Let's discuss those areas.

## BREASTFEEDING AND FARM LIFE

In 2013, a paper titled "Reshaping the Gut Microbiota at an Early Age: Functional Impact on Obesity Risk?" was published. The title gives away what this study was about, but let's discuss the association of early life factors, the microbiota, obesity, and some other interesting stuff.

When breastfed infants were compared to bottle-fed infants, breastfed infants had[27]

- reduced risk of infection;
- improved cognitive development;

- decreased occurrence of celiac disease, asthma, and high cholesterol later in life;
- decreased occurrence of type 2 diabetes and obesity later in life.

Absence of or short-term breastfeeding was found to be a risk factor for obesity in another study. Additionally, this study found short sleep duration to be a risk factor for obesity. We will discuss the importance of sleep later.

Interestingly, this paper also noted that calorie consumption doesn't appear to fully account for changes in obesity rates.[28] This means there must be something else going on. One factor might be calorie quality, whether your calories are coming from junk foods or healthy foods. Another factor might be how the microbiota affects metabolism. The microbiota can affect how efficiently you extract calories from your food. Perhaps this is one of the underappreciated reasons why some gain weight and others do not.

There is more to the development of the microbiota and immune system than access to breast milk and mode of delivery. The environments of the mom while pregnant and of the child early in life also have an impact. As we discussed earlier, our increasingly sterile environments may be contributing to increasing rates of autoimmune and allergic diseases. Conversely, it has been noted that children growing up on farms have fewer allergies, and, in 2006, researchers wanted to have a closer look at this. The researchers monitored over eight thousand children and performed additional blood testing on over three hundred. They tracked how much exposure the mom and the child had to things like farm animals and how this exposure correlated with immune system markers and later development of skin allergy and asthma. The researchers found that if the mom had exposure to farm animals while pregnant, the child was protected from developing these immune disorders later in life. In fact, they found that for every additional animal the mom had exposure to, there was a corresponding increased benefit. They noted a benefit if the *child* was exposed to animals, but the impact was much greater if the exposure started when the mom was pregnant.[29] This suggests a child's immune system, and maybe even microbiota, start developing before birth. So, the earlier the exposure the better—exposure while pregnant might be better than exposure at one year of age, for example.

Has this association been verified by other research? Yes. Other studies have found similar results,[30] and even our highly revered review papers have found this trend to be consistent across the body of evidence as a whole.[31]

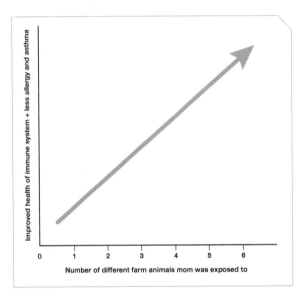

Let's come back to this 2006 study. In it, the researchers discussed protective factors for asthma and immune disorders.

Protective factors included

- farm (raw) milk consumption;
- regular contact with farm animals;
- frequent stable or barn work;
- maternal stable work during pregnancy (this was the factor that gave the most protection).[32]

So, all this asks the question: Are dirt and bacteria bad? While the answer may not be a simple yes or no, this information certainly makes us rethink cleanliness trends such as obsessive dirt avoidance and sterilization. One observation that really jolted me into rethinking my feelings about dirt involved bedbugs. Essentially, a study found that the more endotoxin (bacteria fragments) found in a child's mattress, the lower the child's rate of allergies and asthma.[33] Sounds a bit gross but again reinforces the concept we have been discussing—

## early life bacterial exposure helps train our immune system.

## LOCAL PLANT LIFE

You might not have to move to a farm to obtain exposure to healthy microbes. It has been shown that if you have a diverse array of **naturally occurring** plant life around your home, you will have more diverse bacteria on your skin, a.k.a. a more diverse skin microbiota.[35] In fact, teenagers with more diverse plant life surrounding their homes had higher diversity of skin bacteria, which then correlated with a lower level of skin allergies (such as rashes and eczema).[36] So, proximity to natural environments appears to be good for your skin and immune system.

## MORE DIRT, LESS PROBLEMS

It's natural for parents to want to protect their children, but sometimes the best thing we can do for children is let them learn on their own and to avoid overprotecting them. The same logic applies to the immune system. Remember that "training" we discussed earlier? Let's look at a few examples of how childhood infection—which might seem like a bad thing—might be valuable training for a child's immune system.

One example involves Crohn's disease, an autoimmune disease of the intestines. Roughly two thousand children were monitored to assess the association between early life infection and later risk of Crohn's disease. You guessed it. It was found that early life infection was protective against developing Crohn's disease later in life.[37] Immune system training, anyone?

Remember H. pylori, the bacteria that inhabits the stomach? You may have heard of it in the context of causing ulcers, which it can. However, H. pylori has been shown to be protective against issues like reflux and esophageal cancer.[38] Although the association between H. pylori and health is complex, timing is a noteworthy aspect. In alignment with our recurring theme, early exposure to H. pylori may be protective. Children colonized with H. pylori appear to be protected against stomach and intestinal autoimmunity. More specifically, these children are protected against Crohn's disease, ulcerative colitis, and stomach autoimmunity.[39] It has been shown that as H. pylori colonization increases, allergic diseases decrease.[40] Even food allergies decreased.[41] However, it's possible that those with H. pylori are living in a "dirtier" environment and it's the environment that is protective, not specifically the H. pylori. In either case, this still reinforces the theme of early exposure to "dirt" as protective. This same "early exposure is protective" association may also hold true for certain viruses, like Epstein Barr, which can cause mononucleosis.[42]

Campylobacter is a bacterium that can cause acute diarrhea. Unlike H. pylori, campylobacter seems to have no benefit in adults. However, it has been shown that infants infected with campylobacter are greatly protected against allergic conditions later in life.[43] So, while it may be distressing to watch an infant suffer with a bout of diarrhea, fever, vomiting, and abdominal pain, as the infant's immune system cleans out this bug, it receives some valuable training. This campylobacter infection is usually self-limiting, meaning the body will clear it on its own. Antibiotics have been shown to only reduce the length of illness by 1.3 days.[44] This is a great example of when it might be a good idea to pass on the antibiotics. This doesn't mean you should ignore modern medicine. You should work with your doctor to use antibiotics only when there is no other option. If you have a child and notice symptoms like those described, please check in with your doctor.

When should you use antibiotics? Here is a general rule: if your child acquires an infection for which the worst outcome is a few days of diarrhea, antibiotics may not be needed. If your child acquires an infection that could potentially cause long-term damage or even death, of course an antibiotic makes sense. This is the type of logic and practicality you should be looking for from your doctor.

The relationship between bacteria, infections, dirt, and the immune system is a complicated one, and not all the data show early infection is protective. Some data do show early life infection to be detrimental to immune system development.[45]

It's likely not as simple as colonizing an infant with one missing bacteria or having early exposure to one pathogen to achieve a desired outcome. But hopefully understanding how important environment is in shaping the immune system will spark more research and changes in policy to allow us to regain some of the valuable exposures we are now deficient in.

## LIFESTYLE INTERVENTIONS TO IMPROVE MICROBIOTA AND IMMUNE HEALTH IN EARLY LIFE

As you can see, early life is a crucial time for the development of the microbiota and immune system. This includes the time while the child is in the womb through the first few years of life.

### THESE EXPOSURES MAY HAVE A BENEFICIAL IMPACT ON YOUR MICROBIOTA AND IMMUNE SYSTEM:

- Natural birth is protective compared to C-section birth
- Breastfeeding is protective compared to formula feeding
- Farm life (working in barns and stables, access to raw milk, for example) is protective
- Diverse wild plant life growing around your home is protective
- Early life exposure to infection and exposure to bacteria like H. pylori and campylobacter and viruses like Epstein Barr *may* be protective

In addition to the early life exposures we discussed, there are some lifestyle factors that can help develop the immune system and microbiota. One of my favorite strategies comes from researchers in Sweden. After over a thousand Swedish children were surveyed, it was noted that in families that hand wash their dishes (instead of using a dishwasher), there was significantly less allergic disease. There was even less allergic disease if those families served their children fermented foods and if they purchased foods directly from farms.[46] If you can hand wash your dishes, buy from a farm or maybe a farmers' market, and serve fermented foods, you may feed your microbiota and see some nice immune system benefits. The common thread here is that all of these behaviors—hand washing dishes, buying your food from a farmer, and eating fermented foods—will increase your exposure to bacteria.

---

**SOME COMMON FERMENTED FOODS**

- sauerkraut
- kimchi
- yogurt/kefir
- kombucha
- pickled foods, like cucumbers, garlic, beets, radishes, corn relish
- natto, miso, tempeh
- soy sauce, fermented tofu
- naturally fermented and unpasteurized beers

---

Fermented foods are rich in healthy probiotic bacteria. Bacteria feed off and break down sugars in foods. This means the bacteria are alive, which is great for your immune system. These bacteria also produce important vitamins, like vitamin $K_2$. Vitamin $K_2$ is important for bone and artery health. Fermented foods can be bought from a grocery store or made at home. In my opinion, at least a few servings a week of fermented foods should be incorporated into your diet.

You may have heard of other lifestyle factors that contribute to healthy immune system development, factors like day care or having pets. There is some evidence that attending day care, having siblings, and having pets may all help prevent allergic and immune diseases. The findings here are somewhat inconsistent however. Some studies show day care attendance decreases allergic diseases, and other studies show it increases allergic

diseases.[47] One study found if a child attended day care before the age of two and was breastfed, the risk of type 1 diabetes decreased.[48] However, if the child attended day care before the age of two and was *not* breastfed, there was an *increased* risk of type 1 diabetes. Perhaps a child needs the immune-developing breast milk to successfully handle the immune system training provided by the bombardment of bacteria from day care.

Studies with pets show the same inconsistent findings—sometimes pets help, and sometimes they make immune conditions worse.[49] What may be happening here comes back to our theme of timing. One systemic review suggested that if pet exposure occurs in early childhood (before age six), it may be protective; whereas if exposure occurs in later childhood (after six), it may be detrimental.[50] Again, the picture that starts to emerge from the research is that timing is a key factor. As we just discussed, the same exposure might be protective for a young child but detrimental for an older child or an adult. Do you recall our bedbugs from earlier, where the increased bacterial fragments in children's mattresses seemed to protect them from allergic and autoimmune diseases? Well, for adults, this increased bacteria between the sheets may *increase* allergic diseases.[51]

Could there be a downside to increased exposure, even from seemingly healthy farm exposure? Maybe. Some studies have shown early life exposure to farms and farm animals may increase allergic diseases.[52] Confused? This violates our theory of early exposure being good. In a recent conversation with Moises Velasquez-Manoff, author of *An Epidemic of Absence*, he theorized an excellent explanation. The immune system may require *continuous* exposure to environmental bacteria, or dirt, if it is to have a healthy impact. If the exposures are *occasional*, the immune system may look at each exposure as an attempted invasion. I should clarify that in studies where early life farm exposure was "bad" for the immune system,

the children were not *living* on a farm but periodically *visiting* one. What may be happening here is
the beneficial effect of farming may occur if your
immune system develops/lives in the dirtier, bac-
terially rich environment—in other words, if it is
receiving constant training. But if the exposure is
just once and a while, your immune system may go
to war, because it's trying to protect you from this
unusual influx of bacteria.

Think of it like playing a game of basketball.
If you have a regular routine of playing basketball, playing an all-out game would likely be very
healthy. But if you're sedentary except for one
Saturday every month, when you go all out and
play a strenuous game, you have a much higher
risk of injury. Constant stimulus is good; occasional stimulus is bad. Remember to listen to your
body. Something that works great for someone
else may not work great for you. A friend or
friend's child might feel great eating lots of fermented foods (every day or even multiple servings
a day), but you or your child may not. Even though
pets can help, you may notice you or your child's
allergies become worse with a pet. You may read
a magazine article with a catchy title about the
benefit of farm life, but remember this may not be
helpful for everyone. Through experimenting and
listening to your body, you will find what works
best for you or your child. You have more power
than you may think; just be confident, observant,
and patient in applying these principles.

## ALL DIRT IS NOT CREATED EQUAL

Please remember just because we are learning the
importance of increased bacterial exposure does
not mean you should participate in indiscriminate
exposure to dirt. There is a common-sense principle here—I like to think of this as "old dirt" versus
"new dirt."

Old dirt is the type of dirt you would be
exposed to as a hunter-gatherer: soil, animals,
or plants, for example. New dirt is the type of

dirt you would be exposed to in more man-made
environments, such as sewage, slums, and trash.
Why is old dirt healthier than new dirt? Part of
the reason is that different environments allow
different types of bacteria to flourish. When we
lived in hunter-gatherer bands, we lived in small
groups. One group would be separated from
another group by a large distance. It was therefore
in the best interest of a bacteria not to kill its host
but rather be able to live in harmony with it. If a
bacterium were deadly to it host, it could quickly
wipe out a tribe, thereby running out of hosts.
Without a host, the bacteria would die. So, again,
the bacteria we saw in hunter-gatherer environments were less likely to kill you and more likely
to live with you because it was not in the bacteria's
best interest to kill you, its host. But today, with so
many hosts (people) in such close contact, even a
bacterium that killed its host would have no short-
age of places to live. It could just go from person
to person and have billions of available hosts. This

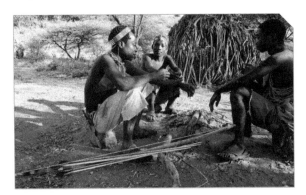

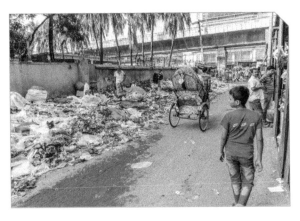

is likely why we see more examples of deadly and epidemic bacteria occurring in modern living situations but not in more primitive living situations.

An illustrative example of old dirt versus new dirt can be seen when we compare children from the slums of Bangladesh, US children, and Hadza hunter-gatherers. Children growing up in slums in Bangladesh live in more of a new-dirt type of environment. This exposure to dirt does give them a more diverse microbiota compared to US children, but the children in Bangladesh also have high rates of diarrheal conditions.[53] Conversely, the Hadza hunter-gatherers have exposure to old dirt, which gives them more microbiota diversity than US children, but not the increase in diarrheal diseases of the Bangladeshi children.[54] These types of findings have been replicated in other cross-cultural comparisons.[55] What this ultimately boils down to is that not all dirt, germs, or bacteria are good for you. If you go to the bathroom, you should wash your hands. If you are in a dirty city area, you should wash your hands. If you have just returned from a hike in the woods, it might be a good time *not* to wash your hands.

# EARLY LIFE PREBIOTICS AND PROBIOTICS TO IMPROVE MICROBIOTAL AND IMMUNE HEALTH

Now that we have discussed environment and lifestyle strategies for optimal microbiotal and immune health, what about probiotics and prebiotics? As a quick refresher, probiotics are healthy bacteria and prebiotics are foods that feed these bacteria. Feel free to skip to the end of this section if you just want a quick summary of the effectiveness of probiotics and prebiotics for common conditions.

We have discussed that the earlier in life antibiotics are used, the more harmful they can be on a child's microbiota and immune system. If we kill bacteria early, it's bad, but what if we support bacteria early? Could early bacterial support be good? Yes. It appears the earlier a child takes a probiotic, the more helpful it can be. This has been reinforced by one study, which found early probiotic supplementation (at the ages of zero to twenty-seven days) was associated with a decreased risk of type 1 diabetes (pancreatic autoimmunity) when compared with probiotic supplementation *after* twenty-seven days or compared to no probiotic supplementation at all.[56] This reinforces our concept of how influential early life factors are on the microbiota and immune system. Let's now discuss this further.

## EARLY LIFE PROBIOTICS, PREBIOTICS, AND ENVIRONMENTAL ALLERGIES, ASTHMA, AND ECZEMA

The effect of early life probiotics and prebiotics on allergies, atopic disorders (an umbrella term for skin allergies and rashes), and eczema is the most well studied relative to other areas like weight gain and food allergies.

A systematic review with meta-analysis recently examined the effect of probiotics and prebiotics on eczema. Again, this is extremely high-level scientific data that examines most/ all of the available research to establish what the overall trend in the science is. This study found that a mixture of traditional lactobacillus- and bifidobacterium-type probiotics reduced the incidence of eczema when given to children under two. Interestingly, the benefit only occurred if a mixture (meaning many strains as opposed to a one-strain probiotic) was used.[57] Two other systematic reviews with meta-analysis reinforced these findings,[58] as did other randomized control trials (RCTs).[59]

Probiotics have been shown to be helpful in treating seasonal/environmental allergies (allergic rhinitis). A systematic review concluded that the majority of clinical trials showed symptomatic improvement in seasonal allergies when taking probiotics.[60] Another RCT showed reduced symptoms and reduced allergy medication use in children taking a probiotic.[61] These findings have been reinforced in other RCTs.[62] Probiotics have also been shown to make antihistamine drugs work better.

Does this mean probiotics can help every childhood immune disorder? Well, since probiotics are extremely safe and fairly inexpensive, it certainly seems reasonable to give them a try. However, the answer to the question is no. Probiotics have not been shown to help with every childhood immune disorder.

Probiotics have not been shown to benefit asthma. Three high-level reviews (systematic reviews with meta-analyses) have shown probiotics did not help with asthma.[63] One of these review papers even attempted to assess if probiotic use during pregnancy helped with asthma. Unfortunately, there was no benefit.[64] This does not mean you should avoid probiotics if your child has asthma—remember, they have other benefits. While the majority of the data is not encouraging for asthma, one study found that using probiotics and prebiotics together helped with asthma symptoms.[65]

We have discussed probiotics, but what about prebiotics? Prebiotics might be especially important for young children because breast milk is high in oligosaccharides and other prebiotics.[66] For infants especially, prebiotics likely play an important role in establishing a healthy microbiota. The studies of prebiotics used in infants show promising results. In one study, either a placebo or prebiotic was given to infants during their first six months of life. The infants were then tracked to see if there was a difference in allergic diseases diagnosed within the first two years of life. Less wheezing, hives, and upper respiratory tract infections were seen in the prebiotic group.[67]

A similar study used the same prebiotic in the first six months of life. The children receiving the prebiotic experienced less seasonal/environmental allergies, and the effect lasted up till five years of age.[68] Again, not all the data agree on this, but it certainly seems reasonable to use prebiotics with your child or infant because they are safe and inexpensive.[69]

Another example of how early life is an important time for immune system development is illustrated by a study on infants and intestinal inflammation. Intestinal inflammation at two months of age predicted skin allergy and asthma at six years of age.[70] We know probiotics have anti-inflammatory effects, so perhaps this is part of the reason probiotics benefit skin allergy.

## EARLY LIFE PROBIOTICS AND FOOD ALLERGY

There are not many studies examining the effect of probiotics on food allergy. Because of this, I look more to the robust studies on environmental allergy, asthma, and skin disorders to infer what type of effect might be seen on food allergy. Based upon the fact that probiotics and prebiotics have been shown to help with these other problems, it seems reasonable to try a probiotic/prebiotic to aid in your child's food allergy. Although there are few studies, let's look at what we do know about probiotics and food allergy.

Two studies have shown probiotics benefit food allergy in children. One RCT showed that probiotics allowed children with a cow's milk allergy to overcome their allergy more quickly than kids not taking a probiotic.[71] Another study also looked at children with a cow's milk allergy. This study found that the constipation caused by consuming milk was decreased after taking a probiotic.[72] However, another RCT showed that probiotics did *not* allow children with a cow's milk allergy to overcome their allergy more quickly.[73] Overall, it seems prudent to try a probiotic if your child has food allergies, especially in light of the other benefits obtained from probiotics.

## EARLY LIFE PROBIOTICS, PREBIOTICS, AND WEIGHT

One RCT study has shown probiotics taken by moms while pregnant and breastfeeding can prevent excessive weight gain in children. In this study, half of the moms took probiotics, the other half received a placebo, and their children's weight was tracked for about five years. The favorable effects on weight were only present until the child was about four years old. After reaching age four, there was no longer any difference in the placebo versus control group.[74] However, two other RCTs showed no effect. One study looked at a probiotic/prebiotic mixture.[75] The other looked at probiotics alone.[76] In this case, probiotics might help, but the evidence is not strong.

Can probiotics cause weight gain? No. I mention this because one researcher did publish a paper stating that probiotics may cause weight gain and that we should be careful with them because we might be harming our children.[77] After fact-checking the paper, it was clear the author had used poor-quality references and the claims lacked scientific support. A rebuttal paper that stated probiotics are safe and may even help fight obesity was published by two other researchers.[78]

## EARLY LIFE PROBIOTICS, PREBIOTICS, INFECTION, AND SAFETY

Probiotics appear to be safe, even for infants[79] and preterm infants.[80] Probiotics have been shown to protect against intestinal fungus (candida) overgrowth[81] and to reduce risk of ear and respiratory infection.[82]

Bear in mind, though, that probiotics are not always protective. If a child is very ill, they may not be helpful or may even be detrimental. This was demonstrated in a study that showed babies in pediatric intensive care units had slightly more infections when given a probiotic.[83] Probiotics appear to be safe, as long as your child is not in intensive care.

My overall recommendation is to use a multiple-strain probiotic along with a prebiotic in infants and children. For most childhood immune ailments, prebiotics/probiotics have been shown helpful. If your child is critically ill, you should not use probiotics/prebiotics until your child has recovered.

**GUT GEEKS**

*Summary of early life probiotic/prebiotic recommendations*

- **Eczema**—*Multiple-strain probiotics with or without prebiotics are helpful, according to very high-level evidence.*

- **Seasonal allergy**—*Probiotics are helpful, can reduce symptoms, and/or help allergy drugs work better, according to very high-level evidence.*

- **Asthma**—*The majority of the evidence suggests probiotics do not help with asthma, but trying a probiotic might be worthwhile due to their other health benefits.*

- **Prebiotics**—*When used early in life (before six months of age), prebiotics have been shown to reduce wheezing, hives, and upper respiratory tract infections. Prebiotics have also been shown to reduce seasonal and environmental allergies. This is supported by moderate-level evidence.*

- **Food allergy**—*Probiotics may or may not be helpful. Again, a trial of probiotics/prebiotics might be worthwhile.*

- **Weight gain**—*Probiotics may or may not be helpful in preventing weight gain. Again, a trial of probiotics/prebiotics might be worthwhile.*

- **Safety**—*Probiotics and prebiotics appear safe for infants and young children. Probiotics have been shown to protect against multiple types of infection. However, if your child is critically ill (in the intensive care unit), probiotics may increase likelihood of infection.*

We have discussed the importance of the early life factors in developing the microbiota and immune system, including early life environment/hygiene, early life antibiotics use, birthing method, breastfeeding, and using probiotics/prebiotics in children and infants. Let's next discuss how we can use diet for a favorable impact on the guts, micro-biotas, and immune systems of children *and adults.*

## CONCEPT SUMMARY

- The world of bacteria that will be with you the rest of your life (your microbiota) begins forming while in utero and is mostly developed by the second to third year of life.

- It has been well documented that consistent early life exposure to dirt, bacteria, and animals aids in the development of a healthier immune system later in life.

- If autoimmune diseases were measured as one group, they would rival the number of Americans with heart disease.

- Individuals with a tendency toward autoimmune and allergic conditions today may have been the most protected from infection when their environment wasn't so "clean."

- Today, we don't have the constant exposure to dirt and germs to train our immune systems; in some individuals, the immune system starts attacking body tissues (autoimmune disease).

- The earlier in life antibiotics are used, the more damaging they are.

- Antibiotics should be used at a young age only when absolutely necessary. Antibiotics kill good and bad bacteria, and if you use them before the colonization of your microbiota is complete, you risk losing some bacteria forever.

- Early life bacterial exposure helps train our immune system. The birthing process, breastfeeding, and environmental exposures such as farm life and diverse wild plant life all help to form a child's microbiota.

- It has been clearly documented that children who are born vaginally have different bacterial colonization than those born by C-section.

- Birth by C-section increases the risk of inflammatory, autoimmune, and immune disorders.

- Fermented foods are rich in healthy probiotic bacteria; however, overconsumption can be problematic for some.

- Not all dirt is created equal. Not all dirt is good for you. Old dirt (soil, animals, plants) is better for you than new dirt (man-made dirt such as sewage, trash, and slums).

- Probiotics are healthy bacteria, and prebiotics are foods that feed these bacteria.

- The earlier a child takes a probiotic supplement, the more helpful it could be.

- Certain probiotics have been shown to reduce the incidence of eczema and to be effective in treating seasonal allergies.

- Prebiotics likely play an important role in establishing a healthy microbiota in infants.

- Use a multiple-strain probiotic along with a prebiotic in infants and children. For most childhood immune ailments, prebiotics/probiotics have been shown helpful. If your child is critically ill, you should not use them until your child has recovered.

1    Akihito Endo et al., "Long-Term Monitoring of the Human Intestinal Microbiota from the 2nd Week to 13 Years of Age," *Anaerobe* 28 (August 1, 2014): 149–56, doi:10.1016/J.ANAEROBE.2014.06.006.

2    Scott T. Weiss, "Eat Dirt—The Hygiene Hypothesis and Allergic Diseases," *New England Journal of Medicine* 347, no. 12 (September 19, 2002): 930–31, doi:10.1056/NEJMe020092.

3    Michael Maes et al., "Increased Autoimmune Activity against 5-HT: A Key Component of Depression That Is Associated with Inflammation and Activation of Cell-Mediated Immunity, and with Severity and Staging of Depression," *Journal of Affective Disorders* 136, no. 3 (February 1, 2012): 386–92, doi:10.1016/j.jad.2011.11.016.

4    "Autoimmune Diseases | NIH: National Institute of Allergy and Infectious Diseases," *National Institute of Allergy and Infectious Diseases*, accessed October 9, 2017, www.niaid.nih.gov/diseases-conditions/autoimmune-diseases.

5    H. Okada et al., "The 'Hygiene Hypothesis' for Autoimmune and Allergic Diseases: An Update," *Clinical & Experimental Immunology* 160, no. 1 (March 11, 2010): 1–9, doi:10.1111/j.1365-2249.2010.04139.x.

6    Eugenia Tognotti, "Program to Eradicate Malaria in Sardinia, 1946–1950," *Emerging Infectious Diseases* 15, no. 9 (September 2009): 1460–66, doi:10.3201/eid1509.081317.

7    Stefano Sotgiu et al., "Hygiene Hypothesis: Innate Immunity, Malaria and Multiple Sclerosis," *Medical Hypotheses* 70, no. 4 (January 1, 2008): 819–25, doi:10.1016/j.mehy.2006.10.069.

8    Tse-Ling Fong et al., "Helicobacter Pylori Infection in Pernicious Anemia: A Prospective Controlled Study," *Gastroenterology* 100 (1991): 328–32, www.gastrojournal.org/article/0016-5085(91)90199-U/pdf.

9    V. G. Djurkov et al., "A Study of Helicobacter Pylori Infection in Patients with Pernicious Anemia," *Folia Medica* 42, no. 2 (2000): 23–27, www.ncbi.nlm.nih.gov/pubmed/11217279.

10   Alexandra Zhernakova et al., "Evolutionary and Functional Analysis of Celiac Risk Loci Reveals SH2B3 as a Protective Factor against Bacterial Infection," *American Journal of Human Genetics* 86, no. 6 (June 11, 2010): 970–77, doi:10.1016/j.ajhg.2010.05.004.

11   Elinor K. Karlsson et al., "Natural Selection and Infectious Disease in Human Populations," *Nature Reviews Genetics* 15, no. 6 (April 29, 2014): 379–93, doi:10.1038/nrg3734.

12   T. Tsakok et al., "Does Early Life Exposure to Antibiotics Increase the Risk of Eczema? A Systematic Review," *British Journal of Dermatology* 169, no. 5 (November 1, 2013): 983–91, doi:10.1111/bjd.12476; Debra L. Wohl et al., "Intrapartum Antibiotics and Childhood Atopic Dermatitis," *Journal of the American Board of Family Medicine : JABFM* 28, no. 1 (January 1, 2015): 82–89, doi:10.3122 /jabfm.2015.01.140017; Fawziah Marra et al., "Does Antibiotic Exposure during Infancy Lead to Development of Asthma?," *Chest* 129, no. 3 (March 1, 2006): 610–18, doi:10.1378/chest.129.3.610; Kristen Wickens et al., "Antibiotic Use in Early Childhood and the Development of Asthma," *Clinical and Experimental Allergy* 29, no. 6 (June 1, 1999): 766–71, doi:10.1046/j.1365-2222.1999.00536.x; Sunia Foliaki et al., "Antibiotic Use in Infancy and Symptoms of Asthma, Rhinoconjunctivitis, and Eczema in Children 6 and 7 Years Old: International Study of Asthma and Allergies in Childhood Phase III," *Journal of Allergy and Clinical Immunology* 124, no. 5 (November 1, 2009): 982–89, doi:10.1016/j.jaci.2009.08.017; Chang-Hung Kuo et al., "Early Life Exposure to Antibiotics and the Risk of Childhood Allergic Diseases: An Update from the Perspective of the Hygiene Hypothesis," *Journal of Microbiology, Immunology and Infection* 46, no. 5 (October 1, 2013): 320–29, doi:10.1016/j.jmii.2013.04.005; William Murk et al., "Prenatal or Early-Life Exposure to Antibiotics and Risk of Childhood Asthma: A Systematic Review," *Pediatrics* 127, no. 6 (June 1, 2011): 1125–38, doi:10.1542/peds.2010-2092; Carsten Flohr and Lindsey Yeo, "Atopic Dermatitis and the Hygiene Hypothesis Revisited,"

Pathogenesis and Management of Atopic Dermatitis, 1–34, Basel: KARGER, 2011, doi:10.1159/000323290; Ischa Kummeling et al., "Early Life Exposure to Antibiotics and the Subsequent Development of Eczema, Wheeze, and Allergic Sensitization in the First 2 Years of Life: The KOALA Birth Cohort Study," *Pediatrics* 119, no. 1 (January 1, 2007): e225–31, doi:10.1542/peds.2006-0896.

13  J. C. Celedon et al., "Antibiotic Use in the First Year of Life and Asthma in Early Childhood," *Clinical Experimental Allergy* 34, no. 7 (July 1, 2004): 1011–16, doi:10.1111/j.1365-2222.2004.01994.x; M. Kusel, "Antibiotic Use in the First Year of Life and Risk of Atopic Disease in Early Childhood," *Clinical & Experimental Allergy* 38, no. 12 (December 1, 2008): 1921–28, doi:10.1111/j.1365-2222.2008.03138.x.

14  T. Tsakok et al., "Does Early Life Exposure to Antibiotics Increase the Risk of Eczema? A Systematic Review," *British Journal of Dermatology* 169, no. 5 (November 1, 2013): 983–91, doi:10.1111/bjd.12476; William Murk et al., "Prenatal or Early-Life Exposure to Antibiotics and Risk of Childhood Asthma: A Systematic Review," *Pediatrics* 127, no. 6 (June 1, 2011): 1125–38, doi:10.1542/peds.2010 -2092; Fawziah Marra et al., "Does Antibiotic Exposure during Infancy Lead to Development of Asthma?," *Chest* 129, no. 3 (March 1, 2006): 610–18, doi:10.1378/chest.129.3.610.

15  Kristen Wickens et al., "Antibiotic Use in Early Childhood and the Development of Asthma," *Clinical and Experimental Allergy* 29, no. 6 (June 1, 1999): 766–71, doi:10.1046/j.1365-2222.1999.00536.x.

16  M. B. Azad et al., "Infant Antibiotic Exposure and the Development of Childhood Overweight and Central Adiposity," *International Journal of Obesity* 38, no. 10 (October 11, 2014): 1290–98, doi:10.1038/ijo.2014.119; L. Charles Bailey et al., "Association of Antibiotics in Infancy with Early Childhood Obesity," *JAMA Pediatrics* 168, no. 11 (November 1, 2014): 1063, doi:10.1001/jamapediatrics .2014.1539; Antti Saari et al., "Antibiotic Exposure in Infancy and Risk of Being Overweight in the First 24 Months of Life," *Pediatrics* 135, no. 4 (April 1, 2015): 617–26, doi:10.1542/peds.2014-3407; R. Murphy et al., "Antibiotic Treatment during Infancy and Increased Body Mass Index in Boys: An International Cross-Sectional Study," *International Journal of Obesity* 38, no. 8 (August 21, 2014): 1115–19, doi:10.1038/ijo.2013.218; L. Trasande et al., "Infant Antibiotic Exposures and Early-Life Body Mass," *International Journal of Obesity* 37, no. 1 (January 21, 2013): 16–23, doi:10.1038/ijo.2012.132.

17  Saari et al., "Antibiotic Exposure in Infancy and Risk of Being Overweight in the First 24 Months of Life," *Pediatrics* 135, no. 4 (April 1, 2015): 617–26, doi:10.1542/peds.2014-3407; L. Trasande et al., "Infant Antibiotic Exposures and Early-Life Body Mass," *International Journal of Obesity* 37, no. 1 (January 21, 2013): 16–23, doi:10.1038/ijo.2012.132.

18  Ryan Ungaro et al., "Antibiotics Associated with Increased Risk of New-Onset Crohn's Disease but Not Ulcerative Colitis: A Meta-Analysis," *American Journal of Gastroenterology* 109, no. 11 (November 16, 2014): 1728–38, doi:10.1038/ajg.2014.246; Souradet Y. Shaw et al., "Association Between the Use of Antibiotics in the First Year of Life and Pediatric Inflammatory Bowel Disease," *American Journal of Gastroenterology* 105, no. 12 (December 12, 2010): 2687–92, doi:10.1038/ajg.2010.398; L. Virta et al., "Association of Repeated Exposure to Antibiotics with the Development of Pediatric Crohn's Disease—A Nationwide, Register-Based Finnish Case-Control Study," *American Journal of Epidemiology* 175, no. 8 (April 15, 2012): 775–84, doi:10.1093/aje/kwr400.

19  Souradet Y. Shaw et al., "Association between the Use of Antibiotics in the First Year of Life and Pediatric Inflammatory Bowel Disease," *American Journal of Gastroenterology* 105, no. 12 (December 12, 2010): 2687–92, doi:10.1038/ajg.2010.398.

20  L. Virta et al., "Association of Repeated Exposure to Antibiotics with the Development of Pediatric Crohn's Disease—A Nationwide, Register-Based Finnish Case-Control Study," *American Journal of Epidemiology* 175, no. 8 (April 15, 2012): 775–84, doi:10.1093/aje /kwr400.

21  Michaeleen Doucleff, "How Modern Life Depletes Our Gut Microbes," *Goats and Soda*, National Public Radio, April 21, 2015, accessed October 9, 2017, www.npr.org/sections/goatsandsoda/2015/04/21/400393756/how-modern-life-depletes-our-gut-microbes.

22  Inés Martínez et al., "The Gut Microbiota of Rural Papua New Guineans: Composition, Diversity Patterns, and Ecological Processes," *Cell Reports* 11, no. 4 (April 28, 2015): 527–38, doi:10.1016/j.celrep.2015.03.049.

23  Raakel Luoto et al., "Reshaping the Gut Microbiota at an Early Age: Functional Impact on Obesity Risk?," *Annals of Nutrition & Metabolism* 63 Suppl 2 (2013): 17–26, doi:10.1159/000354896.

24  C. R. Cardwell et al., "Caesarean Section Is Associated with an Increased Risk of Childhood-Onset Type 1 Diabetes Mellitus: A Meta-Analysis of Observational Studies," *Diabetologia* 51, no. 5 (May 22, 2008): 726–35, doi:10.1007/s00125-008-0941-z.

25  Ibid.

26  Kim Kristensen and Lonny Henriksen, "Cesarean Section and Disease Associated with Immune Function," *Journal of Allergy and Clinical Immunology* 137, no. 2 (February 1, 2016): 587–90, doi:10.1016/j.jaci.2015.07.040.

27  C. R. Cardwell et al., "Caesarean Section Is Associated with an Increased Risk of Childhood-Onset Type 1 Diabetes Mellitus: A Meta-Analysis of Observational Studies," *Diabetologia* 51, no. 5 (May 22, 2008): 726–35, doi:10.1007/s00125-008-0941-z.

28   L. Monasta et al., "Early-Life Determinants of Overweight and Obesity: A Review of Systematic Reviews," *Obesity Reviews* 11, no. 10 (March 16, 2010): 695–708, doi:10.1111/j.1467-789X.2010.00735.x.

29   Markus Johannes Ege et al., "Prenatal Farm Exposure Is Related to the Expression of Receptors of the Innate Immunity and to Atopic Sensitization in School-Age Children," *Journal of Allergy and Clinical Immunology* 117, no. 4 (April 1, 2006): 817–23, doi:10.1016/j.jaci.2005.12.1307.

30   Josef Riedler et al., "Exposure to Farming in Early Life and Development of Asthma and Allergy: A Cross-Sectional Survey," *Lancet* 358, no. 9288 (2001): 1129–33, doi:10.1016/S0140-6736(01)06252-3.

31   Erika von Mutius and Katja Radon, "Living on a Farm: Impact on Asthma Induction and Clinical Course," *Immunology and Allergy Clinics of North America*, 2008, doi:10.1016/j.iac.2008.03.010.

32   Josef Riedler et al., "Exposure to Farming in Early Life and Development of Asthma and Allergy: A Cross-Sectional Survey," *Lancet* 358, no. 9288 (2001): 1129–33, doi:10.1016/S0140-6736(01)06252-3.

33   Charlotte Braun-Fahrländer et al., "Environmental Exposure to Endotoxin and Its Relation to Asthma in School-Age Children," *New England Journal of Medicine* 347, no. 12 (September 19, 2002): 869–77, doi:10.1056/NEJMoa020057.

34   Maartje A. C. Zijlmans et al., "Maternal Prenatal Stress Is Associated with the Infant Intestinal Microbiota," *Psychoneuroendocrinology* 53 (March 1, 2015): 233–45, doi:10.1016/j.psyneuen.2015.01.006.

35   Ilkka Hanski et al., "Environmental Biodiversity, Human Microbiota, and Allergy Are Interrelated," *Proceedings of the National Academy of Sciences of the United States of America* 109, no. 21 (May 22, 2012): 8334–39, doi:10.1073/pnas.1205624109.

36   L. Ruokolainen et al., "Green Areas around Homes Reduce Atopic Sensitization in Children," *Allergy* 70, no. 2 (February 1, 2015): 195–202, doi:10.1111/all.12545.

37   Vicky Springmann et al., "Timing, Frequency and Type of Physician-Diagnosed Infections in Childhood and Risk for Crohn's Disease in Children and Young Adults," *Inflammatory Bowel Diseases* 20, no. 8 (August 2014): 1346–52, doi:10.1097/MIB.0000000000000098.

38   Derek Lin and Britt Koskella, "Friend and Foe: Factors Influencing the Movement of the Bacterium *Helicobacter Pylori* along the Parasitism-Mutualism Continuum," *Evolutionary Applications* 8, no. 1 (January 1, 2015): 9–22, doi:10.1111/eva.12231.

39   Jay Luther et al., "Association between Helicobacter Pylori Infection and Inflammatory Bowel Disease," *Inflammatory Bowel Diseases* 16, no. 6 (June 2010): 1077–84, doi:10.1002/ibd.21116; Alexandra Frolkis et al., "Environment and the Inflammatory Bowel Diseases," *Canadian Journal of Gastroenterology* 27, no. 3 (2013): e18–24, doi:10.1155/2013/102859; K. L. Kolho et al., "Parietal Cell Antibodies and Helicobacter Pylori in Children," *Journal of Pediatric Gastroenterology and Nutrition* 30, no. 3 (2000): 265–68, http://pesquisa.bvsalud.org/ghl/resource/en/mdl-10749409.

40   Elena Lionetti et al., "Helicobacter Pylori Infection and Atopic Diseases: Is There a Relationship? A Systematic Review and Meta-Analysis," *World Journal of Gastroenterology* 20, no. 46 (2014): 17635–47, doi:10.3748/wjg.v20.i46.17635.

41   Sang Pyo Lee et al., "Correlation between Helicobacter Pylori Infection, IgE Hypersensity, and Allergic Disease in Korean Adults," *Helicobacter* 20, no. 1 (2015): 49–55, doi:10.1111/hel.12173.

42   Michael P. Pender, "CD8+ T-Cell Deficiency, Epstein-Barr Virus Infection, Vitamin D Deficiency, and Steps to Autoimmunity: A Unifying Hypothesis," *Autoimmune Diseases*, 2012, doi:10.1155/2012/189096.

43   Dara Jovanovic et al., "Campylobacter Jejuni Infection and IgE Sensitization in up to 2-Year-Old Infants," *Vojnosanitetski Pregled* 72, no. 2 (2015): 140–47, doi:10.2298/VSP1502140J.

44   A. Ternhag et al., "A Meta-Analysis on the Effects of Antibiotic Treatment on Duration of Symptoms Caused by Infection with Campylobacter Species," *Clinical Infectious Diseases* 44, no. 5 (2007): 696–700, doi:10.1086/509924.

45   C. J. Edwards et al., "Infections in Infancy and the Presence of Antinuclear Antibodies in Adult Life," *Lupus* 15, no. 4 (2006): 213–17, doi:10.1191/0961203306lu2286oa; C. Carlens et al., "Perinatal Characteristics, Early Life Infections and Later Risk of Rheumatoid Arthritis and Juvenile Idiopathic Arthritis," *Annals of the Rheumatic Diseases* 68, no. 7 (2009): 1159–64, doi:10.1136/ard.2008.089342; C. J. Edwards et al., "The Presence of Anticardiolipin Antibodies in Adults May Be Influenced by Infections in Infancy," *QJM* 101, no. 1 (2008): 41–47, doi:10.1093/qjmed/hcm119.

46   Bill Hesselmar et al., "Allergy in Children in Hand versus Machine Dishwashing," *Pediatrics* 135, no. 3 (2015): e590–7, doi:10.1542/peds.2014-2968.

47   C. Svanes et al., "Early Exposure to Children in Family and Day Care as Related to Adult Asthma and Hay Fever: Results from the European Community Respiratory Health Survey," *Thorax* 57, no. 11 (2002): 945–50, doi:10.1136/thorax.57.11.945.

48   Katelyn Hall et al., "Daycare Attendance, Breastfeeding, and the Development of Type 1 Diabetes: The Diabetes Autoimmunity Study in the Young," *BioMed Research International* (2015): doi:10.1155/2015/203947.

49   A. Simpson and A. Custovic, "Early Pet Exposure: Friend or Foe?," *Current Opinion in Allergy and Clinical Immunology* 3, no. 1 (2003): 7–14, doi:10.1097/01.all.0000053261.39029.7a; Marco Waser et al., "Exposure to Pets, and the Association with Hay Fever, Asthma, and Atopic Sensitization in Rural Children," *Allergy: European Journal of Allergy and Clinical Immunology* 60, no. 2 (2005): 177–84, doi:10.1111/j.1398-9995.2004.00645.x.

50   Benjamin Apelberg et al., "Systematic Review: Exposure to Pets and Risk of Asthma and Asthma-like Symptoms," *Journal of Allergy and Clinical Immunology*, 2001, doi:10.1067/mai.2001.113240.

51   Kyoung Bok Min and Jin Young Min, "Exposure to Household Endotoxin and Total and Allergen-Specific IgE in the US Population," *Environmental Pollution* 199 (2015): 148–54, doi:10.1016/j.envpol.2014.12.012.

52   Bert Brunekreef et al., "Early Life Exposure to Farm Animals and Symptoms of Asthma, Rhinoconjunctivitis and Eczema: An ISAAC Phase Three Study," *International Journal of Epidemiology* 41, no. 3 (2012): 753–61, doi:10.1093/ije/dyr216; Timo T. Hugg et al., "Exposure to Animals and the Risk of Allergic Asthma: A Population-Based Cross-Sectional Study in Finnish and Russian Children," *Environmental Health: A Global Access Science Source* 7 (2008): 28, doi:10.1186/1476-069X-7-28.

53   Audrie Lin et al., "Distinct Distal Gut Microbiome Diversity and Composition in Healthy Children from Bangladesh and the United States," *PLoS ONE* 8, no. 1 (2013), doi:10.1371/journal.pone.0053838.

54   Tanya Yatsunenko et al., "Human Gut Microbiome Viewed across Age and Geography," *Nature*, 2012, doi:10.1038/nature11053.

55   Carlotta De Filippo et al., "Impact of Diet in Shaping Gut Microbiota Revealed by a Comparative Study in Children from Europe and Rural Africa," *Proceedings of the National Academy of Sciences* 107, no. 33 (2010): 14691–96, doi:10.1073/pnas.1005963107.

56   Ulla Uusitalo et al., "Association of Early Exposure of Probiotics and Islet Autoimmunity in the TEDDY Study," *JAMA Pediatrics* 170, no. 1 (2016): 20, doi:10.1001/jamapediatrics.2015.2757.

57   Dan Dang et al., "Meta-Analysis of Probiotics and/or Prebiotics for the Prevention of Eczema," *Journal of International Medical Research* 41, no. 5 (2013): 1426–36, doi:10.1177/0300060513493692.

58   Joohee Lee et al., "Meta-Analysis of Clinical Trials of Probiotics for Prevention and Treatment of Pediatric Atopic Dermatitis," *Journal of Allergy and Clinical Immunology* 121, no. 1 (2008): 116–121.e11, doi:10.1016/j.jaci.2007.10.043; G. Zuccotti et al., "Probiotics for Prevention of Atopic Diseases in Infants: Systematic Review and Meta-Analysis," *Allergy* 70 (2015): n/a–n/a, doi:10.1111/all.12700.

59   Kristin Wickens et al., "A Differential Effect of 2 Probiotics in the Prevention of Eczema and Atopy: A Double-Blind, Randomized, Placebo-Controlled Trial," *Journal of Allergy and Clinical Immunology* 122, no. 4 (2008): 788–94, doi:10.1016/j.jaci.2008.07.011; Katja Doege et al., "Impact of Maternal Supplementation with Probiotics during Pregnancy on Atopic Eczema in Childhood—A Meta-Analysis," *British Journal of Nutrition* 107, no. 1 (2012): 1–6, doi:10.1017/S0007114511003400.

60   H. Vliagoftis et al., "Probiotics for the Treatment of Allergic Rhinitis and Asthma: Systematic Review of Randomized Controlled Trials," *Annals of Allergy, Asthma & Immunology* 101, no. 6 (2008): 570–79, doi:S1081-1206(10)60219-0 [pii]\r10.1016/S1081-1206(10)60219-0.

61   T. Y. Lin et al., "Effect of Probiotics on Allergic Rhinitis in Df., Dp., or Dust-Sensitive Children: A Randomized Double Blind Controlled Trial," *Indian Pediatrics* 50, no. 2 (2013): 209–13, www.ncbi.nlm.nih.gov/pubmed/22728633.

62   Y. S. Chen et al., "Randomized Placebo-Controlled Trial of Lactobacillus on Asthmatic Children with Allergic Rhinitis," *Pediatric Pulmonology* 45, no. 11 (2010): 1111–20, doi:10.1002/ppul.21296; K. H. Lue et al., "A Trial of Adding Lactobacillus Johnsonii EM1 to Levocetirizine for Treatment of Perennial Allergic Rhinitis in Children Aged 7–12 Years," *International Journal of Pediatric Otorhinolaryngology* 76, no. 7 (2012): 994–1001, doi:10.1016/j.ijporl.2012.03.018; Arthur C. Ouwehand et al., "Specific Probiotics Alleviate Allergic Rhinitis during the Birch Pollen Season," *World Journal of Gastroenterology* 15, no. 26 (2009): 3261–68, doi:10.3748/wjg.15.3261.

63   M. B. Azad et al., "Probiotic Supplementation during Pregnancy or Infancy for the Prevention of Asthma and Wheeze: Systematic Review and Meta-Analysis," *BMJ* 347 (December 4, 2013): f6471–f6471, doi:10.1136/bmj.f6471; H. Vliagoftis et al., "Probiotics for the Treatment of Allergic Rhinitis and Asthma: Systematic Review of Randomized Controlled Trials," *Annals of Allergy Asthma & Immunology* 101, no. 6 (2008): 570–79, doi:S1081-1206(10)60219-0 [pii]\r10.1016/S1081-1206(10)60219-0; N. Elazab et al., "Probiotic Administration in Early Life, Atopy, and Asthma: A Meta-Analysis of Clinical Trials," *Pediatrics* 132, no. 3 (2013): e666–76, doi:10.1542/peds.2013-0246.

64    M. B. Azad et al., "Probiotic Supplementation during Pregnancy or Infancy for the Prevention of Asthma and Wheeze: Systematic Review and Meta-Analysis," *BMJ* 347 (December 4, 2013): f6471–f6471, doi:10.1136/bmj.f6471.

65    L. B. Van Der Aa et al., "Synbiotics Prevent Asthma-like Symptoms in Infants with Atopic Dermatitis," *Allergy: European Journal of Allergy and Clinical Immunology* 66, no. 2 (2011): 170–77, doi:10.1111/j.1398-9995.2010.02416.x.

66    Sertac Arslanoglu et al., "Early Dietary Intervention with a Mixture of Prebiotic Oligosaccharides Reduces the Incidence of Allergic Manifestations and Infections during the First Two Years of Life," *Journal of Nutrition* 138, no. 6 (June 1, 2008): 1091–95, www.ncbi .nlm.nih.gov/pubmed/18492839.

67    Ibid.

68    Sertac Arslanoglu et al., "Early Neutral Prebiotic Oligosaccharide Supplementation Reduces the Incidence of Some Allergic Manifestations in the First 5 Years of Life," *Journal of Biological Regulators and Homeostatic Agents* 26, no. 3 Suppl. (2012): 49–59, www.researchgate.net/profile/Paola_Tonetto/publication/258972795_JBRHA26-3S/links/00b49529879926cd7a000000. pdf#page=51.

69    David A. Osborn and John K. H. Sinn, "Prebiotics in Infants for Prevention of Allergy," in *Cochrane Database of Systematic Reviews*, 2013, doi:10.1002/14651858.CD006474.pub3.

70    L. Orivuori et al., "High Level of Fecal Calprotectin at Age 2 Months as a Marker of Intestinal Inflammation Predicts Atopic Dermatitis and Asthma by Age 6," *Clinical and Experimental Allergy* 45, no. 5 (2015): 928–39, doi:10.1111/cea.12522.

71    Roberto Berni Canani et al., "Formula Selection for Management of Children with Cow's Milk Allergy Influences the Rate of Acquisition of Tolerance: A Prospective Multicenter Study," *Journal of Pediatrics* 163, no. 3 (2013), doi:10.1016/j.jpeds.2013.03.008.

72    E. S. Ivakhnenko and S. L. Nian'kovskiĭ, "Effect of Probiotics on the Dynamics of Gastrointestinal Symptoms of Food Allergy to Cow's Milk Protein in Infants," in *Georgian Medical News*, no. 219 (June 2013): 46–52. www.ncbi.nlm.nih.gov /pubmed/23863210.

73    Jeroen Hol et al., "The Acquisition of Tolerance toward Cow's Milk through Probiotic Supplementation: A Randomized, Controlled Trial," *Journal of Allergy and Clinical Immunology* 121, no. 6 (2008): 1448–54, doi:10.1016/j.jaci.2008.03.018.

74    Raakel Luoto et al., "The Impact of Perinatal Probiotic Intervention on the Development of Overweight and Obesity: Follow-up Study from Birth to 10 Years," *International Journal of Obesity* 34, no. 10 (2010): 1531–37, doi:10.1038/ijo.2010.50.

75    Jean Pierre Chouraqui et al., "Assessment of the Safety, Tolerance, and Protective Effect against Diarrhea of Infant Formulas Containing Mixtures of Probiotics or Probiotics and Prebiotics in a Randomized Controlled Trial," *American Journal of Clinical Nutrition* 87, no. 5 (2008): 1365–73, doi:87/5/1365 [pii].

76    Raakel Luoto et al., "Impact of Maternal Probiotic-Supplemented Dietary Counselling on Pregnancy Outcome and Prenatal and Postnatal Growth: A Double-Blind, Placebo-Controlled Study," *British Journal of Nutrition* 103, no. 12 (2010): 1792–99, doi:10.1017 /S0007114509993898.

77    Didier Raoult, "Probiotics and Obesity: A Link?," *Nature Reviews Microbiology* 7, no. 9 (2009): 616–616, doi:10.1038/nrmicro2209.

78    Nathalie Delzenne and Gregor Reid, "No Causal Link between Obesity and Probiotics," *Nature Reviews Microbiology* 7, no. 12 (2009): 901–901, doi:10.1038/nrmicro2209-c2; S. Dusko Ehrlich, "Probiotics—Little Evidence for a Link to Obesity," *Nature Reviews Microbiology* 7, no. 12 (December 1, 2009): 901–901, doi:10.1038/nrmicro2209-c1.

79    Minna Rinne et al., "Probiotic Intervention in the First Months of Life: Short-Term Effects on Gastrointestinal Symptoms and Long-Term Effects on Gut Microbiota," *Journal of Pediatric Gastroenterology and Nutrition* 43, no. 2 (2006): 200–205, doi:10.1097 /01.mpg.0000228106.91240.5b.

80    Carole Rougé et al., "Oral Supplementation with Probiotics in Very Low Birth Weight Preterm Infants: A Randomized, Double-Blind, Placebo-Controlled Trial," *American Journal of Clinical Nutrition* 89, no. 6 (2009): 1828–35, doi:10.3945/ajcn.2008.26919; Rie Olsen et al., "Prophylactic Probiotics for Preterm Infants: A Systematic Review and Meta-Analysis of Observational Studies," *Neonatology*, 2016. doi:10.1159/000441274.

81    P. Manzoni et al., "Oral Supplementation with Lactobacillus Casei Subspecies Rhamnosus Prevents Enteric Colonization by Candida Species in Preterm Neonates: A Randomized Study," *Clinical Infectious Diseases : An Official Publication of the Infectious Diseases Society of America* 42, no. 12 (2006): 1735–42, doi:10.1086/504324.

82    Samuli Rautava et al., "Specific Probiotics in Reducing the Risk of Acute Infections in Infancy—A Randomised, Double-Blind, Placebo-Controlled Study," *British Journal of Nutrition* 101, no. 11 (2009): 1722–26, doi:10.1017/S0007114508116282; K. Kukkonen et al., "Long-Term Safety and Impact on Infection Rates of Postnatal Probiotic and Prebiotic (Synbiotic) Treatment: Randomized,

Double-Blind, Placebo-Controlled Trial," *Pediatrics* 122, no. 1 (2008): 8–12, doi:10.1542/peds.2007–1192; M. B. Azad et al., "Probiotic Supplementation during Pregnancy or Infancy for the Prevention of Asthma and Wheeze: Systematic Review and Meta-Analysis," *BMJ* 347 (December 4, 2013): f6471–f6471, doi:10.1136/bmj.f6471.

83   Travis C. B. Honeycutt et al., "Probiotic Administration and the Incidence of Nosocomial Infection in Pediatric Intensive Care: A Randomized Placebo-Controlled Trial," *Pediatric Critical Care Medicine : A Journal of the Society of Critical Care Medicine and the World Federation of Pediatric Intensive and Critical Care Societies* 8, no. 5 (2007): 452–8, quiz 464, doi:10.1097/01.PCC.0000282176.41134.E6.

# PART 2

---

## DIET FOR OPTIMUM GUT HEALTH

# CHAPTER 6

# INFLAMMATORY FOODS AND FOODS THAT FEED GUT BACTERIA

## CREATING A HEALTHY ENVIRONMENT FOR HEALTHY BACTERIA

The environment you create for the bacteria in your body will dictate what type of bacteria thrive. If you create a healthy environment, you'll harbor healthy bacteria and reap all the benefits. If you create an unhealthy environment, you'll harbor unhealthy bacteria and your health will suffer.

You can almost think of this like a self-perpetuating cycle. If you create a healthy environment, you will harbor healthy bacteria, and then these bacteria will further contribute to a healthier environment. This cycle is very similar to a community of people. If a city has an environment that's favorable for crime, a very high crime rate will result. This will eventually create an environment that's not safe, which will push out local businesses and residents, which will, in turn, make the environment even more favorable for crime.

This cycle will continue until you're left with a very unhealthy community. Local law enforcement could step into this city and repair the environment by enforcing laws, which would make it an appropriate place for families and businesses again. Similarly, we can repair your internal environment, which will allow healthy bacteria to thrive.

Here in part 2, we'll detail diet strategies that can be used to repair your internal environment. We'll talk more about carb intake, food allergies, processed foods, and artificial sweeteners. An entire book could be written about diet and the microbiota. We could travel all over Africa and South America, looking at exotic diets of the native people and how they have different bacteria because of it. We could also get lost in bacteria ratios and names. And we could even speculate about how and why other cultures are healthy because of these different bacteria or bacterial ratios. But haven't we already learned that generalizing from one culture's data isn't the best idea? We know that what we see in another culture might not be good for you. It might even be bad for you. Right? We've learned that before you consider a diet or treatment, it should be put through a clinical trial in humans to ensure its safety and effectiveness.

Just like there has been no miracle antioxidant cure from an exotic rain-forest fruit, there will be no magic bacteria from a rain-forest tribe. But we will examine some core principles regarding gut health and survey the research to find strategies for healing *your* gut and achieving the health benefits that will follow. This information will be cutting-edge, but it will also be practical and grounded.

## SUMMARY OF KEY DIETARY PRINCIPLES

Below are key principles to keep in mind when it comes to diet:

- You must first eat to control inflammation. Eating to control inflammation will create a healthy environment for gut bacteria and thus improve your microbiota.
- You must also eat to control and balance blood sugar. Eating to balance blood sugar will create a healthy environment for gut bacteria, which will improve your microbiota.
- A spectrum exists for carbohydrate and prebiotics intake; some will do better on less, and some will do better on more. We each must determine where we fit on this spectrum.
- A similar spectrum exists for food allergens and food intolerances. We each must determine what our problem foods are.
- Certain food additives can damage your gut and might have a negative impact on your microbiota. These changes correlate with certain diseases and conditions of the gut.

- *For your gut bacteria, environment is more important than food—so you want to eat in a way that produces a healthy environment.*

## FOOD ALLERGENS AND INTOLERANCES

Our discussion on diets returns us to an important concept we touched on earlier:

> *eating to reduce inflammation is more important than eating to feed your gut bugs*

or, said another way,

> *eating to control inflammation will create a healthy environment for gut bacteria and thus improve your microbiota.*

A great way to reduce inflammation is by minimizing exposure to food allergens and foods you're intolerant to. As a response to ingesting an allergen (or intolerant food), your immune system reacts with inflammation. Accordingly, when you eat inflammatory foods, the environment in your gut becomes more favorable for bad bacteria. In this unhealthy/inflammatory environment, we can start to lose good bacteria as they are pushed out by the growing number of bad bacteria. This imbalance is known as **dysbiosis**.[1]

Celiac disease is a condition in which people have a severe allergy to gluten. The allergic reaction to gluten causes inflammation and autoimmunity, which then damages the intestinal tract. It has been shown that celiac patients experience an improvement in their microbiota when following a gluten-free diet.[2] What's interesting here is that a gluten-free diet will often reduce the amount of carbs and prebiotics a patient eats. So, even though people on a gluten-free diet might be eating less of the foods that feed their gut bacteria, their gut bugs still get healthier. Why? Because *eating to reduce inflammation is more important than eating to feed your gut bugs*.

Several studies have shown that those with celiac disease have dysbiosis—no surprise there. However, many of these studies have also shown *increased* microbiota diversity in those with celiac disease. This increased diversity has been shown in the large intestine and in the small intestine.[3] The good news is that the solution here is a practical one. Most of these studies have shown that a gluten-free diet can restore the microbiota to be more like that of healthy controls. Again, this is because eating to control inflammation is more important than eating to feed your gut bugs.

Does this mean grains and gluten are a problem for all people? No. Are gluten and grains the only inflammatory foods you should consider avoiding? No. There are other foods that can be allergenic, such as dairy, corn, soy, and eggs. Let's elaborate on specific foods that can be problematic and investigate whether food-allergy testing can help you determine what foods you should avoid.

## THE QUESTIONABLE USEFULNESS OF FOOD-ALLERGY TESTING

The most important dietary change you can make is to avoid foods that you are allergic to or intolerant of. These two terms are often used interchangeably, but there is a difference. To put it simply, food allergies typically cause reactions that are quite severe and sudden—think of a deadly peanut allergy or severe skin reactions. These are often mediated by an immune system reaction called IgE. Food intolerances are often subtler. A food intolerance might include bloating, fatigue, brain fog, or irritability but can manifest in a wide array of symptoms, even subtle skin reactions,

like pimples, often appearing the next day. Food intolerances are often mediated by other immune reactions, which include IgA, IgM, and IgG. Some food intolerances have nothing to do with your immune system but can still cause you to feel lousy. Since the term "food allergy" is often used to describe both "allergy" and "intolerance," going forward, I will mostly use the term "allergy" to broadly refer to both. The reason avoiding food allergens is so important is because food allergens cause lots of inflammation, and we have already established reducing inflammation is a crucial factor for optimizing your internal environment.

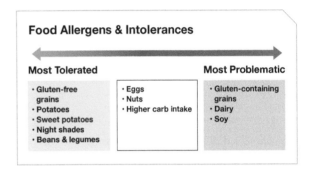

**Food Allergens & Intolerances**

**Most Tolerated** ⟷ **Most Problematic**

| Most Tolerated | | Most Problematic |
|---|---|---|
| · Gluten-free grains<br>· Potatoes<br>· Sweet potatoes<br>· Night shades<br>· Beans & legumes | · Eggs<br>· Nuts<br>· Higher carb intake | · Gluten-containing grains<br>· Dairy<br>· Soy |

Food-allergy testing is a commonly performed but mostly unnecessary test, in my opinion. Several years ago, when we knew less about food allergies, I think this testing had more utility. However, since we have established what the most common food allergies are, we no longer need testing to determine this.

I know there are some who feel quite strongly about food-allergy testing and would not agree with my thinking on this. Here is something to consider: we can always find a reason to do a test, but we should be asking why *not* to do a test, too. This is an important philosophical point. If we try hard enough, we can come up with a few references or mechanisms to support almost any test. But is this really what's best for you? Or might this create "runaway" testing, testing that progressively becomes more and more elaborate and expensive (which, by the way, is the current state of most functional medicine). A better approach may be to search for the vital few tests that are truly essential. For the past three years, I have stopped food-allergy testing in my clinic, and I feel the results I get now are much better because I focus on other more important testing. This is not to say addressing food allergies isn't important; it's number one on my list. However, testing is not needed to sort out food allergies.

If not testing, then what? First, eliminate foods that are known to be problematic, then reintroduce these foods later. A 2015 review paper concluded

> *The most helpful diagnostic test for food intolerance is food exclusion to achieve symptom improvement followed by gradual food reintroduction.*[4]

To translate, the best way to determine what your food intolerances are is to eliminate common food allergens, then gradually reintroduce them. This consensus has been supported by other review papers also.[5] Some studies do show benefit from food-allergy testing, but what you typically see in these studies is a person being diagnosed with a food allergy that could easily be determined without testing by elimination followed by reintroduction. The food allergies most commonly diagnosed through testing are the ones we already know to be common food allergens. When we look at this combined with how expensive food-allergy testing is, it's hard to support testing.

## THERE ARE MANY REASONS WHY FOOD-ALLERGY TESTING IS NOT VERY HELPFUL

Here are some of the reasons:

- There is more to food reactions than just the immune system; we must consider how much certain foods feed bacteria and fungus. Some people react negatively to foods that feed bacteria or fungus—these people do better on the low-FODMAP diet or the Specific Carbohydrate Diet (SCD). Food-allergy testing won't tell you if you're one of those people.

- The effect of a food on your blood sugar is not tested by food-allergy testing.

- Gut inflammation, infections, or excessive stress will cause gut damage (leaky gut). Once you have leaky gut, you will react to many foods. These are false allergies, and they will go away once your gut heals. When I had a parasite, I had twenty-three food allergies! Once I fixed my leaky gut, they all went away. All the food-allergy testing did was stress me out and distract me from finding the underlying cause of my food reactions.

- Food-allergy test results can differ, depending on whether the test is using raw or cooked foods.[6] A certain lab is excited about this because they now offer both cooked and raw allergy testing—for over $1,000! I appreciate that the lab is trying to offer more comprehensive testing, but this is a lot of money for a test that has questionable clinical utility.

- Testing is not always accurate. I would estimate that roughly 50% of the time, the food my patients know they react negatively to come back as OK on their food-allergy tests. And 50% of the time, foods they really seemed to feel good on came back as allergens. This is pretty disappointing after spending $400 to $1,000.

- There are other nonallergenic compounds in foods that can cause reactions. One in particular is histamine. Those who are histamine intolerant can experience brain fog, irritability, flushing, and/or runny nose from overconsumption of histamine-rich foods. These include fermented foods, cured meats, aged cheeses, and citrus fruits.

- Finally, those who have gut inflammation may feel worse if they consume high amounts of fiber or raw foods, as the roughage can cause irritation.

This, of course, is not tested by food-allergy testing.

## WHEN CAN FOOD-ALLERGY TESTING BE BENEFICIAL?

If you need a test to motivate or convince you to avoid a food, then food-allergy testing can be useful. However, I think this will only be a short-term solution. We will work together through a process that will motivate you to avoid foods you react to. We will first be a bit strict with your diet while focusing on healing your gut. Then you will reintroduce foods. You'll find that most foods are fine. But with some foods, you'll notice a negative reaction (fatigue, bloating, mood swings). Any negative reaction you notice soon after introducing a new food makes that food suspect. You'll try that food a few times to make sure it's not a coincidence. By doing this you *experientially* determine what you can and can't eat. This will cause long-term change, because you won't want to eat foods that make you feel bad.

Let's come back to relying on test results. What if you really want to have some dairy, but your test results say no dairy? At first, you will avoid dairy, but it's only a matter of time until some dairy slips in or you cave and just have some dairy. Now, if you eat the dairy and don't notice anything, what are the chances you'll do it again? And then again? And then eventually be back to eating dairy? In my opinion, this is because food-allergy testing as a motivator is based on fear, and fear is not a good long-term motivator—especially when there is no negative experience to reinforce the fear.

Is it hard to remove common allergies? Thankfully, no. The Paleo diet does a great job of removing common food allergens from your diet. The Paleo diet essentially focuses on foods that you could only hunt, fish, or gather. There are a number of Paleo diet books available that walk you

through exactly how to follow the diet. See www.DrRuscio.com/GutBook for a simple handout on how to follow the Whole30 version of the Paleo diet. (Note, the handout states you should try it for thirty days, but for our purposes give it two to three weeks.) Here is a simple overview:

In the Paleo diet, you focus on
- fresh vegetables and fruits;
- fresh meats, fish, and eggs;
- healthy fats/oils;
- nuts and seeds.

And you avoid
- grains,
- beans and legumes,
- processed foods, and
- dairy.

Following this diet is a simple way to cut out the most common allergens. You should follow this diet for two to three weeks and then reevaluate how you feel. If you don't feel much better, try some of the additional dietary modifications listed below. When we cover your action plan in part 5, we will discuss specific guidelines for how diet fits into the larger picture.

## ADDITIONAL ALLERGENS AND FOODS THAT FEED GUT BACTERIA

If you try the Paleo diet and don't see the level of improvement you would like, there are a couple of modifications you can make. Think of it this way: the Paleo-type diet is our starting point. We can modify some rules and restrictions, but only if you need to. The main modifications are the autoimmune Paleo diet and the low-FODMAP diet.

The autoimmune Paleo diet removes some less common food allergens. For some people who don't respond ideally to the standard Paleo diet, this is the missing piece. Remember, fewer allergens equals less inflammation.

The low-FODMAP diet helps to reduce bacterial overgrowth by restricting foods that feed bacteria. Let's elaborate on these.

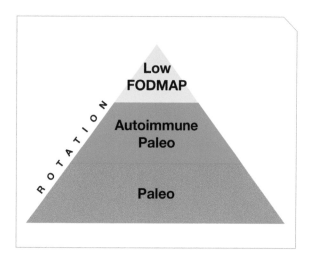

If you haven't tried the Paleo diet for two to three weeks, start there. After you have done the Paleo diet for two to three weeks (or longer), it will be part of your routine, and then adding in the additional restrictions will be very manageable. Take this one step at a time.

Go to www.DrRuscio.com/GutBook for food lists for the Paleo diet, the autoimmune Paleo diet, and the low-FODMAP diet. If you would like more support, like shopping lists, recipes, and sample meal plans, there are many good books available for each of these diets. I recommend first starting with using a basic food list and keeping your meals simple. Then, once you have found the diet you feel best on, find a good cookbook for delicious recipes within that diet.

## THE AUTOIMMUNE PALEO DIET (AIP)

What's the autoimmune Paleo diet (AIP)? It's essentially a slightly more restrictive version of the Paleo diet. The AIP diet restricts the following in addition to the standard Paleo diet restrictions:

- Eggs
- Nuts
- Seeds (including coffee)
- Nightshades (potatoes, tomatoes, eggplants, sweet and hot peppers, and spices derived from peppers)
- Alcohol

What's the purpose of these additional dietary restrictions? The AIP diet restricts even more food allergens, so we can really check the low-allergen box after you've tried it. But dietary theory and actually adhering to a diet are two different things. This diet can be hard, and many people wonder, how strict do you have to be? In my opinion, you don't need to do this 100% to reap the benefits. If you *can* eat strictly according to the diet for two to three weeks, great. Do it. If it feels crushingly difficult, try eliminating a *couple* of foods from the above list for one to two weeks, and see how you feel. Then move on to a couple of more foods, until you work through the list. If you uncover a major allergen, you'll notice that you feel better. If you don't feel very different, you don't need to worry about avoiding the foods you removed. These diets are merely tools to help you discover what foods work and don't work for you.

Another difficult thing about this diet is that you need to avoid pepper spices. You may read on the Internet that you have to strictly avoid all pepper spices for at least a month or you will "fail." I don't agree. I find this drastic warning scares more people out of even trying the diet than it helps with getting started. Here is what I would recommend: avoid pepper spices for *one week*. If you feel a noticeable difference, you'll want to only use them occasionally. If you don't notice anything, then don't worry about this food restriction. If you think you might be feeling better but aren't sure, give it another week and see. Practical, right?

I have observed that those with autoimmune conditions are sometimes scared into thinking this is the diet they *must* follow, because it's called *autoimmune* Paleo. It's certainly worth a shot, but if after a brief trial you don't notice improvement, move on. This diet is an aggregation of avoiding different allergens that have been shown to work for different autoimmune conditions, but it doesn't mean you have to follow *every* rule for *your* autoimmune condition. For example, avoiding nightshades (including peppers) has been shown to be helpful for the autoimmune condition rheumatoid arthritis, but it *hasn't* been shown to help with autoimmune thyroid conditions. It's important that you understand this. Now, might avoiding nightshades help you if you have an autoimmune thyroid condition? Maybe. Give it a try, but don't be scared into thinking because you have an autoimmune thyroid condition, you must follow this diet blindly forever.

Regarding autoimmune conditions, it's also important to mention that diet is only one of several factors that are at play. Some of these other factors, like your early life immune system and microbiota development, are out of your control to modify. So, don't obsess over diet; there is more to autoimmunity than diet.

## THE LOW-FODMAP DIET

We discussed earlier how common bacterial overgrowths are and how, because of this, certain people can do well on diets that starve these bacterial overgrowths. The low-FODMAP diet achieves this. FODMAP stands for fermentable oligosaccharides, disaccharides, monosaccharides, and polyols.

> *The low-FODMAP diet essentially restricts foods (mainly carbohydrates) that can feed bacteria*

or can be hard to digest. With this diet, we are addressing two very important issues: bacterial overgrowth and carbohydrate malabsorption.

Remember, many people with IBS, hypothyroidism, and celiac disease, and those who are overweight, may have bacterial overgrowth in the intestine, so eating to control bacteria can be very helpful. The low-FODMAP diet limits foods that encourage bacterial overgrowth, so it ends up starving the overgrowth.

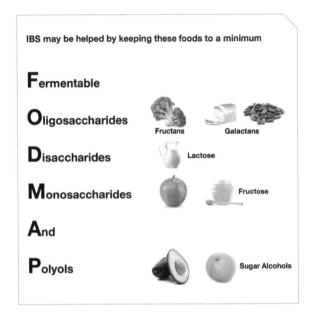

IBS may be helped by keeping these foods to a minimum

**F**ermentable

**O**ligosaccharides — Fructans, Galactans

**D**isaccharides — Lactose

**M**onosaccharides — Fructose

**A**nd

**P**olyols — Sugar Alcohols

Tied in with bacterial overgrowth is the concept of carbohydrate malabsorption. In the intestines, carbs that we can't or don't digest are broken down by our gut bacteria. These carbs feed our gut bugs. When everything is working properly, this doesn't pose a problem. But, as we have discussed, some people have too much bacteria. Eating too many of the carbs that feed gut bugs can exacerbate an existing bacterial overgrowth and cause symptoms like gas, bloating, and diarrhea. Here is the twist: the bacterial overgrowth can damage the area of the intestines that helps digest these carbs. This causes carbohydrate malabsorption, which means you can't digest certain carbs and when you eat them, you have a negative reaction.

So, bacterial overgrowth can cause carbohydrate malabsorption by damaging your intestines. Eating foods that feed bacteria can worsen carbohydrate malabsorption. But this problem works in reverse, too. Some people have intestines that can't digest carbs because they don't release the enzymes needed. Think of someone who is lactose intolerant. They don't digest the carbohydrate found in dairy called lactose because their intestines can't produce the lactase enzyme. When your intestines fail to break down and absorb these carbs, guess who feeds on them? Your gut bacteria. When these people eat carbs they can't break down, they are at increased risk for bacterial overgrowth because these carbs end up overfeeding their gut bacteria. The low-FODMAP diet restricts common carbs that either feed gut bacteria or are more prone to malabsorption—or both. Bacterial overgrowth and carbohydrate malabsorption are two of the main reasons many people do best on a dietary approach that reduces or rebalances intestinal bacteria—instead of blindly feeding them. If this seems a little technical, don't worry; all you need to do is continue to work through our steps.

What can seem counterintuitive about these diets is they call for restricting seemingly healthy foods. For example, on the low-FODMAP diet you avoid apples and cauliflower. But aren't these healthy? Well, yes, these foods are nutritious, but there is more to deciding if a food is good for you than its nutritional value. For some people, these foods can overly encourage bacterial growth and cause problems like gas, bloating, abdominal pain, diarrhea, intestinal damage, and nutrient malabsorption. The goal is to heal your gut so you can eat all of these foods with no negative reaction. But in the short term, while we're healing your gut, you may have to avoid some of these seemingly healthy foods. Remember, a food is only nutritious and healthy for *you* if you can digest it properly. A food might be loaded with nutrition, but if it's damaging to *your* intestines, it will make you sick.

## CONFLICTING INFORMATION ABOUT WHAT A LOW-FODMAP DIET IS

Sometimes patients who have researched the low-FODMAP diet before coming into our office are confused by the lack of agreement among the different food lists they find on the Internet. Some of this stems from the fact that there are two versions of the low-FODMAP diet readily available upon an Internet search: the standard low-FODMAP diet and the Paleo low-FODMAP diet. The Paleo low-FODMAP diet is more restrictive because it adheres to both sets of rules—Paleo and low FODMAP. The standard low-FODMAP diet is easier to follow due to fewer restrictions. The main difference between the two is the standard low-FODMAP diet allows the following foods, while the Paleo low-FODMAP diet does not:

- Potatoes
- Rice
- Low-FODMAP grains
- Oats, quinoa, rice, corn, gluten-free breads
- Low-FODMAP dairy
- Hard cheeses, such as cheddar, Swiss, parmesan, mozzarella, feta
- Kefir, butter, cream, Greek yogurt
- Any lactose-free dairy foods
- Low-FODMAP processed foods
- Soy
- Coffee, chocolate, and alcohol (in small quantities)

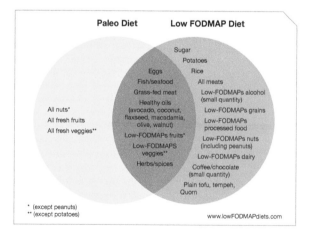

Go to www.DrRuscio.com/GutBook for both the standard low-FODMAP food list and the Paleo low-FODMAP food list.

I have noticed many people do well with gluten-free grains, rice, and potatoes, so being able to eat them, as outlined by the standard low-FODMAP diet, can be helpful.

## HOW TO DETERMINE WHICH VERSION OF THE LOW-FODMAP DIET IS RIGHT FOR YOU

The Paleo low-FODMAP diet is best for you if . . .

- you felt better on the Paleo diet (for example, you notice you feel better when avoiding grains or dairy)

The standard low-FODMAP diet is best for you if . . .

- you didn't notice any improvements when following the Paleo diet
- you are underweight (you may need the potatoes, rice, and grains allowed on the standard low-FODMAP diet)

Remember, if a diet is working for you, you should notice a difference within the first couple of weeks.

## FOOD ROTATION

Food rotation isn't a diet but rather a concept that can be applied to any diet. This simply means you try to vary your diet by not eating the same thing every day. For those who try one of the diets we've discussed and still don't feel 100% better, food rotation can be helpful. It's also a good general dietary principle that pushes you toward more variety in your diet. For example, avoid eating a chicken and spinach salad Monday through Friday for lunch. Instead, try to have one or two days where you do not eat the foods you ate the day before. What might this look like? On Monday, you might focus on eating mostly chicken, duck, spinach, squash, and olive oil, and then you might try to avoid these foods until Thursday. On Tuesday, perhaps you focus on eating salmon, tuna, kale, chard, and rice and cook with coconut oil, and then you try to avoid these foods until Friday. It's most important to rotate your proteins and your carbs (for example, your meats and your vegetables). Spices and oils are less important.

Why is rotation important? If your gut is not healthy, you may develop allergies to whatever you eat repeatedly. Rotating your foods will prevent this because you won't be eating the same things every day. Also, different foods contain different nutrients, and by eating a variety of foods (instead of the same ones over and over), you will ensure you get the many vitamins and nutrients you need.

Sometimes, people can become overwhelmed when they try to rotate their foods. Don't over-complicate it. Just do your best to divide your foods into groups and rotate the groups. It doesn't have to be perfect or exact. Also, the healthier your gut becomes, the less necessary this is. However, it's good to maintain a degree of this indefinitely because it will push you to eat a wide array of foods and thus get a wide array of nutrients.

### DON'T DRIVE YOURSELF CRAZY

Trying to adhere to an increasing number of dietary rules and restrictions can make some people feel like there is nothing they can eat, which can create diet neurosis. This is not necessary and is something you should avoid. While the diets we have discussed have much overlap, there are some subtle differences as well. Sometimes people feel they must comply perfectly with a diet, which can be maddening and nearly impossible.

Please know there is no magic diet, so don't drive yourself crazy trying to perfectly adhere to one diet's rules if it violates another diet's rules. The point of these diets is to help you uncover foods that are causing problems. They are tools to guide awareness, not a list of rigid mandates that cannot be broken. Many patients end up combining rules from the different diets as they have observed a need. For example, they might avoid a few FODMAPs they notice don't agree with them but eat others. They generally eat Paleo but also

notice they feel OK with rice. The way to determine this is to work through these diets gradually, over several weeks, rather than trying to do this all at once. By doing it gradually, you will develop a sense for what rules from a given diet you should follow and what rules you don't need to follow. Take what you need, and leave the rest.

## CONCEPT SUMMARY

- The environment you create for the bacteria in your gut will dictate what type of bacteria thrive.

- For your gut bacteria, environment is more important than food—so you want to eat in such a way that emphasizes a healthy environment.

- You must first eat to control inflammation. Eating to control inflammation will create a healthy environment for gut bacteria and thus improve your microbiota.

- The most helpful diagnostic test for food intolerance is food exclusion to achieve symptom improvement followed by gradual food reintroduction.

- Eating a diet low in allergens is a pillar of a healthy diet.

- You can eat a diet low in allergens by following the Paleo diet or the AIP diet.

- The low-FODMAP diet removes foods that can feed bacterial overgrowth and be hard to digest.

- Remember, if a diet is working for you, you should notice a difference within the first couple of weeks.

1    Claudia Lupp et al., "Host-Mediated Inflammation Disrupts the Intestinal Microbiota and Promotes the Overgrowth of Enterobacteriaceae," *Cell Host and Microbe* 2, no. 2 (2007): 119–29, doi:10.1016/j.chom.2007.06.010; Bärbel Stecher et al., "Salmonella Enterica Serovar Typhimurium Exploits Inflammation to Compete with the Intestinal Microbiota," *PLoS Biol*, 2007, doi:10.1371/journal.pbio.0050244; Laura G. Patwa et al., "Chronic Intestinal Inflammation Induces Stress-Response Genes in Commensal Escherichia Coli," *Gastroenterology* 141, no. 5 (2011): 1842–51, doi:10.1053/j.gastro.2011.06.064; Frederic A. Carvalho et al., "Transient Inability to Manage Proteobacteria Promotes Chronic Gut Inflammation in TLR5-Deficient Mice," *Cell Host and Microbe* 12, no. 2 (2012): 139–52, doi:10.1016/j.chom.2012.07.004.

2    Esther Nistal et al., "Differences of Small Intestinal Bacteria Populations in Adults and Children with/without Celiac Disease: Effect of Age, Gluten Diet, and Disease," *Inflammatory Bowel Diseases* 18, no. 4 (2012): 649–56, doi:10.1002/ibd.21830; Serena Schippa et al., "A Distinctive 'Microbial Signature' in Celiac Pediatric Patients," *BMC Microbiology* 10, no. 1 (2010): 175, doi:10.1186/1471-2180-10-175.

3    Esther Nistal et al., "Differences of Small Intestinal Bacteria Populations in Adults and Children with/without Celiac Disease: Effect of Age, Gluten Diet, and Disease," *Inflammatory Bowel Diseases* 18, no. 4 (2012): 649–56, doi:10.1002/ibd.21830; Yolanda Sanz et al., "Differences in Faecal Bacterial Communities in Coeliac and Healthy Children as Detected by PCR and Denaturing Gradient Gel Electrophoresis," *FEMS Immunology and Medical Microbiology* 51, no. 3 (2007): 562–68, doi:10.1111/j.1574-695X.2007.00337.x; Maria Carmen Collado et al., "Specific Duodenal and Faecal Bacterial Groups Associated with Paediatric Coeliac Disease," *Journal of Clinical Pathology* 62, no. 3 (2009): 264–69, doi:10.1136/jcp.2008.061366; Serena Schippa et al., "A Distinctive 'Microbial Signature' in Celiac Pediatric Patients," *BMC Microbiology* 10, no. 1 (2010): 175, doi:10.1186/1471-2180-10-175; Raffaella Di Cagno et al., "Duodenal and Faecal Microbiota of Celiac Children: Molecular, Phenotype and Metabolome Characterization," *BMC Microbiology* 11, no. 1 (2011): 219, doi:10.1186/1471-2180-11-219.

4    M. C. E. Lomer, "Review Article: The Aetiology, Diagnosis, Mechanisms and Clinical Evidence for Food Intolerance," *Alimentary Pharmacology and Therapeutics*, 2015, doi:10.1111/apt.13041.

5    Barbara K. Ballmer-Weber, "Value of Allergy Tests for the Diagnosis of Food Allergy," *Digestive Diseases* 32, no. 1–2 (2014): 84–88, doi:10.1159/000357077.

6    Aristo Vojdani, "Detection of IgE, IgG, IgA and IgM Antibodies against Raw and Processed Food Antigens," *Nutrition and Metabolism* 6 (2009): 22, doi:10.1186/1743-7075-6-22.

# CHAPTER 7

# GLUTEN, CELIAC DISEASE, AND NONCELIAC GLUTEN SENSITIVITY

## UNDERSTANDING GLUTEN

By adhering to the diets we have covered, you will be able to determine your relationship with gluten. However, because gluten has received so much attention (some of it highly inaccurate), it may be helpful to clarify a few things and provide you with a healthy perspective.

Gluten is a mixture of proteins found in many grains, such as wheat, rye, and barley. As with many controversial subjects, there seems to be two opposing and extreme positions on gluten. On one end, some feel gluten can be the cause of any and every health problem. On the other end, some feel gluten-free diets are a fad and that only those with true celiac disease need to avoid gluten. Where does the confusion come from? In part, it comes from not following the three ways to avoid confusion in the dietary-health controversy we covered in an earlier chapter. When we examine the available research using our three-ways method, we arrive at a very reasonable conclusion.

### A SUMMARY OF THE ISSUE

- Dietary gluten can be problematic for many people, and the problems can manifest with differing levels of severity and a wide array of symptoms.
- Determining your relationship to gluten and other food allergens can be one of the most important steps you can take toward improving your health.
- Nonceliac gluten sensitivity (reacting negatively to gluten even though you are not diagnosed with celiac disease) has been scientifically validated.
- A new clinical condition has emerged called "celiac lite."
- There are other important issues that should be addressed to help you determine your relationship to gluten. These include other food allergies and other food reactions, such as dairy allergy or FODMAP intolerance. This includes other conditions, such as SIBO.

- If you change your diet and still do not improve, there is likely a nondietary problem in your gut that needs to be identified and treated. Often, the problem is SIBO.
- Gluten is *not* a problem for everyone, and there are some documented health benefits to eating grains.

## WHY IS IT IMPORTANT TO DETERMINE IF YOU HAVE A PROBLEM WITH GLUTEN?

If you have a problem with gluten and are consuming it frequently, this could be negatively affecting your health. More importantly, by simply removing a food (in this case gluten-containing foods) from your diet, many problems may disappear. Like the improvements related to gut health we listed earlier, common symptoms and conditions that may be improved by removing gluten (and thus improving your gut health) are[1]

- autoimmune conditions (Hashimoto's thyroiditis, Grave's disease, multiple sclerosis, arthritis);
- skin conditions (psoriasis, eczema, canker sores);
- IBS;
- abdominal bloating and pain;
- constipation;
- brain fog;
- depression;
- weight gain.

## SOUNDS TOO GOOD TO BE TRUE— IS THIS GLUTEN-FREE HYPE?

Let's use high-level science to help sort this out. There is no debate that those with a full-blown clinical allergy to gluten (that is, those with celiac disease) must avoid gluten. But what about those who do not have celiac disease but still feel like they have a problem with gluten? To date, there have been five RCTs (remember, RCTs are randomized clinical trials—high-level research)

regarding nonceliac gluten sensitivity (NCGS). NCGS is a condition reported by those without celiac disease who feel they still have a problem with gluten.

Four of these five studies have found that

> ## *gluten can in fact be problematic for those who do not have celiac disease.*[2]

The fifth study found reactions may stem from FODMAPs and not the gluten itself.[3] FODMAPs are high in prebiotics and can feed bacteria in the gut. Bacteria feeding can make you feel worse if you have a preexisting bacterial overgrowth like SIBO. This one study suggested it was not the gluten in grains that caused the reaction but rather the bacteria-feeding FODMAPs.

The fact that FODMAPs can be problematic shouldn't be surprising, based upon what we have already discussed. However, this fifth study created quite a media frenzy and led many to proclaim, "See, gluten-free is a fad! It's not the gluten; it's the FODMAPs!" But what have we learned to help us avoid confusion like this? We learned we should avoid drawing conclusions based on one study and examine the entire body of evidence. Right? When we look at the entire body of evidence, we see that four out of five studies showed that gluten can be problematic for those without celiac disease. One of these five studies suggested FODMAPs actually caused the reactions and it's not the gluten. However, included in these five studies were two studies that clearly showed that

> ## *FODMAPs did not cause the reactions—gluten did.*

These two studies isolated for the effects of gluten by having the subjects eat gluten that was FODMAP-free, thus removing any impact from FODMAPs. When eating FODMAP-free gluten, these people still reacted, suggesting it was actually the gluten causing the reaction.[4] So, although, yes, one study found FODMAPs were to blame for the reaction, there is more data (specifically two studies) suggesting that gluten itself can be a problem.

What does all this mean? It means we should craft a dietary plan that accounts for both gluten and FODMAPs. It means there is more to a healthy diet than avoiding food allergens like gluten and that eating to balance bacteria (as you do on a low-FODMAP diet) is also important. This is exactly what we will do in our action steps in part 5.

What is important to mention about all five of these studies is that they took into account the placebo effect, so the negative reactions people reported were not imagined or "all in their heads." While the design of each study varied slightly, the general setup was as follows:

1. Study subjects go gluten-free and notice they feel better.
2. Subjects are then given either a gluten-free placebo or gluten, unaware of which they are receiving.
3. The rate of negative reactions was significantly higher in those who received gluten compared to those who received the placebo.

## INTRODUCING CELIAC LITE

There are differing levels of gluten sensitivity. The most severe sensitivity is called celiac or celiac disease and is an autoimmune disease. For those with celiac disease, there is no debate about whether they must adhere to a gluten-free diet. However, there are some people who are not diagnosed with celiac disease but who feel they have a gluten sensitivity. These people are often classified as nonceliac gluten sensitive.

As researchers have attempted to better understand gluten allergy, a new diagnosis has been suggested for those who are in between celiac disease

and nonceliac gluten sensitive. This diagnosis is called "celiac lite." Those who are celiac lite are people who are not positive for celiac disease upon routine screening but who, when tested further, have other celiac markers come back positive.

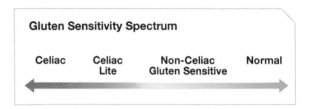

We are finding there is a spectrum of gluten sensitivity. Please don't forget this spectrum includes some who have no problem with gluten—just because gluten is a problem for some doesn't mean it's a problem for all.

## WHAT ABOUT TESTING TO FIGURE THIS OUT?

Testing is where things get messy. As alluring as black-and-white test results can be, there is a major challenge with testing to determine if you are gluten sensitive. It's not black and white. There are other factors that could be damaging your gut, causing your symptoms, and perhaps making you look like a celiac lite patient during testing. These factors are[5]

- other food allergies;
- SIBO;
- poor secretion of digestive acids and enzymes;
- H. pylori bacterial infections;
- use of pain-relief medications (such as Advil, Motrin, and Tylenol).

To complicate things even further, there are several other compounds that can make wheat and grains a problem, compounds that will not show up on testing, like FODMAPs.[6] Furthermore, one well-performed clinical trial found no negative changes in *any* laboratory marker in a group of patients who started eating gluten and felt noticeably worse.[7]

So, finding laboratory support is not guaranteed.

Maybe you have tried going gluten-free and didn't feel any better, or maybe you're just trying to determine whether you need to avoid gluten as a general health practice. We will sort out what your relationship with gluten should be when we work through our action plan in part 5. We do not need a test to sort this out. If, however, you still want to test for celiac disease, NCGS, and celiac lite, there is quite a robust testing algorithm that has been proposed—but you will have to subject yourself to quite a bit of poking and prodding to figure this out. First, you'll need to be tested for HLA haplotypes and celiac disease auto-antibodies. Then, depending on the results of that test, you'll undergo a duodenal biopsy. That will be followed up with additional cultures, gluten challenges, and clinical work.[8]

The best strategy is to simply follow the action plan we will cover in part 5.

## WHO SHOULD BE MOST CAUTIOUS WITH GLUTEN?

Avoiding gluten according to your level of intolerance is the most reasonable recommendation regarding gluten. In other words, the more of a reaction you notice to gluten, the more you should avoid it. Gauging your reaction to gluten can be difficult if you have other issues present. For example, the signs of a gluten reaction and the signs of SIBO are fairly similar. How can you tell where your reaction might be coming from? As we work through our action plan in part 5, we'll first have you remove gluten from your diet. Next, you'll address any bacterial imbalances. Finally, you'll reintroduce gluten to evaluate your tolerance.

There is one group of people who might want to be more cautious with gluten: those with autoimmune conditions. Some autoimmune conditions, like thyroid autoimmunity, respond well to a gluten-free diet *if the person also has celiac disease*. If you don't have celiac disease, your autoimmunity might still benefit from being gluten-free, but the data here are inconclusive. However, many people with autoimmune conditions *do* report feeling better when gluten-free. Of course, if you have a family history of celiac disease, you should be extra cautious regarding gluten consumption.

Is a gluten-free diet a cure-all for autoimmune conditions? No. Some autoimmune conditions do *not* respond to a gluten-free diet. We'll cover that later. If you have an autoimmune condition, I wouldn't put all your eggs in this one gluten-free basket. As we work to improve your gut health, you will be taking substantial steps toward improving autoimmunity. Gluten is part of the picture, but there is much more to it.

## FOR YOUR SANITY

All too often I see patients who have been scared into avoiding gluten without ever determining what their individual tolerability for gluten is. These people have been convinced that *everyone* must practice a celiac disease–like level of avoidance. Just because *some* people have a disease fueled by even small amounts of gluten doesn't mean *everyone* must avoid it completely. This is like saying because some people have alcoholism, we all need to avoid alcohol completely *(there goes the occasional glass of wine with friends).*

On the surface, avoiding gluten completely may not seem like a big deal; however, I've seen this create significant stress. For example, you might shy away from social engagements because you're afraid of dietary challenges. The anxiety, which can impair your relationships and sense of well-being, has even been documented in the published literature.[9] A suboptimal social life can quite dramatically impede healing, especially for women, as we will discuss later.

Theoretically, if gluten isn't a problem for everyone, we should have evidence suggesting grains are safe. Right? (Note, many grains, including wheat and rye and barley, contain gluten.) If you are firmly of the "we should all avoid grains 100% of the time" camp, remember it's healthy to question our beliefs. One review of observational studies found "higher intakes of cereal fiber, particularly from whole-grain sources, are associated with lower total percent body fat and percent trunk fat mass in older adults."[10] These findings were supported by another study examining results from a national nutritional survey called the NHANES.[11]

Two systematic reviews with meta-analyses have shown people who consume grains can be healthier. Whole grains specifically demonstrated a protective effect against heart disease.[12] And whole grains improved bowel function, lowered cholesterol, reduced weight, and may have increased well-being.[13] It's important to mention that these studies are mostly observational, so it might not be the grains that are causing the health effects. People who are trying to be healthier might increase grain consumption as part of adopting other healthy lifestyle practices, like eating less processed food and exercising. Even so, if grains were a universal poison, we wouldn't see these effects.

I have all my patients on a gluten-free diet for their first thirty days. However, after that I listen to each patient's response to determine if the patient can or can't have gluten. Some need to avoid it strictly; others have more freedom. And there are some that clearly feel *better* on grains. I used to be a bit dogmatic on the issue of grains. However, as I've been listening to and monitoring my patients, I've clearly seen some do better *with* grains, which has opened my mind. I want my patients to have the fewest dietary restrictions possible and to have a healthy, non-fear-based relationship with food. This is the point I am

trying to make, and this is where you'll be after we develop your action plan.

If you notice you can tolerate some gluten with no negative reaction, don't stress yourself out trying to practice 100% avoidance. Simply do your best. If you do notice a bad reaction, you'll want to avoid gluten more strictly. Please remember that although eating gluten-free can certainly be helpful for many, others won't have a problem with gluten: a problem for some doesn't mean a problem for all. Each ecosystem has different requirements.

## SOME LAST WORDS ABOUT GLUTEN

Dietary gluten can be problematic for many people, and this problem can manifest with differing levels of severity and a wide array of symptoms. Determining your relationship to gluten can be one of the most important steps you can take toward improving your health, but it's not the only one. Other factors, like other food allergies and bacterial overgrowth, can hinder your body's response to a gluten-free diet.

## CONCEPT SUMMARY

- Problems with dietary gluten can manifest with differing levels of severity and a wide array of symptoms.

- Determining your relationship to gluten and other food allergens can be one of the most important steps you can take toward improving your health.

- Nonceliac gluten sensitivity (reacting negatively to gluten even though you are not diagnosed with celiac disease) has been scientifically validated.

- A new clinical entity has emerged called "celiac lite."

- There are other important food allergies, reactions, and conditions that should be sorted out along with gluten for optimum results. These include FODMAP intolerance and SIBO.

- If you change your diet and still do not improve, there is likely a nondietary problem in your gut (often SIBO) that needs to be identified and treated.

- Gluten is *not* a problem for everyone, and there are some documented health benefits to grains.

1    Antonio Di Sabatino et al., "Small Amounts of Gluten in Subjects with Suspected Nonceliac Gluten Sensitivity: A Randomized, Double-Blind, Placebo-Controlled, Crossover Trial," *Clinical Gastroenterology and Hepatology* 13, no. 9 (2015): 1604–12, doi:10.1016/j.cgh.2015.01.029.

2    Jessica R. Biesiekierski et al., "Gluten Causes Gastrointestinal Symptoms in Subjects without Celiac Disease: A Double-Blind Randomized Placebo-Controlled Trial," *American Journal of Gastroenterology* 106, no. 3 (2011): 508–14, doi:10.1038/ajg.2010.487; Antonio Carroccio et al., "Nonceliac Wheat Sensitivity Diagnosed by Double-Blind Placebo-Controlled Challenge: Exploring a New Clinical Entity," *American Journal of Gastroenterology* 107, no. 12 (2012): 1898–1906, doi:10.1038/ajg.2012.236; Antonio Di Sabatino et al., "Small Amounts of Gluten in Subjects with Suspected Nonceliac Gluten Sensitivity: A Randomized, Double-Blind, Placebo-Controlled, Crossover Trial," *Clinical Gastroenterology and Hepatology* 13, no. 9 (2015): 1604–12, doi:10.1016/j.cgh.2015.01.029; Bijan Shahbazkhani et al., "Nonceliac Gluten Sensitivity Has Narrowed the Spectrum of Irritable Bowel Syndrome: A Double-Blind Randomized Placebo-Controlled Trial," *Nutrients* 7, no. 6 (2015): 4542–54, doi:10.3390/nu7064542.

3    Jessica R. Biesiekierski et al., "No Effects of Gluten in Patients with Self-Reported Nonceliac Gluten Sensitivity after Dietary Reduction of Fermentable, Poorly Absorbed, Short-Chain Carbohydrates," *Gastroenterology* 145, no. 2 (2013), doi:10.1053/j.gastro.2013.04.051.

4    Antonio Di Sabatino et al., "Small Amounts of Gluten in Subjects with Suspected Nonceliac Gluten Sensitivity: A Randomized, Double-Blind, Placebo-Controlled, Crossover Trial," *Clinical Gastroenterology and Hepatology* 13, no. 9 (2015): 1604–12, doi:10.1016/j.cgh.2015.01.029; Bijan Shahbazkhani et al., "Nonceliac Gluten Sensitivity Has Narrowed the Spectrum of Irritable Bowel Syndrome: A Double-Blind Randomized Placebo-Controlled Trial," *Nutrients* 7, no. 6 (2015): 4542–54, doi:10.3390/nu7064542.

5    J. Molina-Infante et al., "Systematic Review: Noncoeliac Gluten Sensitivity," *Alimentary Pharmacology and Therapeutics,* 2015, doi:10.1111/apt.13155; Ujjal Poddar, "Pediatric and Adult Celiac Disease: Similarities and Differences," *Indian Journal of Gastroenterology,* 2013, doi:10.1007/s12664-013-0339-9.

6    J. Molina-Infante et al., "Systematic Review: Noncoeliac Gluten Sensitivity," *Alimentary Pharmacology and Therapeutics,* 2015, doi:10.1111/apt.13155.

7    Jessica R. Biesiekierski et al., "Gluten Causes Gastrointestinal Symptoms in Subjects without Celiac Disease: A Double-Blind Randomized Placebo-Controlled Trial," *American Journal of Gastroenterology* 106, no. 3 (2011): 508–14, doi:10.1038/ajg.2010.487.

8    J. Molina-Infante et al., "Systematic Review: Noncoeliac Gluten Sensitivity," *Alimentary Pharmacology and Therapeutics,* 2015, doi:10.1111/apt.13155.

9    Susy Rocha et al., "The Psychosocial Impacts Caused by Diagnosis and Treatment of Coeliac Disease," *Revista Da Escola de Enfermagem* 50, no. 1 (2016): 65–70, doi:10.1590/S0080-623420160000100009.

10   N. M. McKeown et al., "Whole-Grain Intake and Cereal Fiber Are Associated with Lower Abdominal Adiposity in Older Adults," *Journal of Nutrition* 139, no. 10 (2009): 1950–55, doi:10.3945/jn.108.103762.

11   Carol E. O'Neil et al., "Whole Grain and Fiber Consumption Are Associated with Lower Body Weight Measures in US Adults: National Health and Nutrition Examination Survey, 1999–2004," *Nutrition Research* (New York, NY) 30, no. 12 (2010): 815–22, doi:10.1016/j.nutres.2010.10.013.

12   Gang Tang et al., "Meta-Analysis of the Association between Whole-Grain Intake and Coronary Heart Disease Risk," *American Journal of Cardiology* 115, no. 5 (2015): 625–29, doi:10.1016/j.amjcard.2014.12.015.

13   P. G. Williams, "The Benefits of Breakfast Cereal Consumption: A Systematic Review of the Evidence Base," *Advances in Nutrition: An International Review Journal* 5, no. 5 (2014): 636S–673S, doi:10.3945/an.114.006247.

# CHAPTER 8

# CARBS AND YOUR GUT

## HOW CARBS AFFECT YOUR GUT

We've covered dietary strategies regarding food allergens and foods that feed your gut bacteria. Let's now discuss how eating to control blood sugar makes the environment healthy and therefore allows healthy gut bugs to thrive.

We have already discussed that there is a spectrum of carb intake: some do better on a lower-carb diet, and some do better on a higher-carb diet. But don't our gut bacteria need carbs for food? Doesn't this make a lower-carb diet bad for your gut bacteria? This is an understandable assumption, but, as we covered earlier, different guts need different levels of carb intake.

For example, it has been shown that eating a lower-carb diet that controls blood sugar can help improve your microbiota. Let's look at a study where a group of overweight individuals were placed on a high-protein, reduced-calorie diet for six weeks. What's interesting about this study is that microbiota testing was performed on all subjects. Based on their test results, individuals were labeled either low- or high-microbiota diversity.

Those who entered the study with high diversity tended to be healthier and responded best to the diet. Those who entered with lower diversity were not as healthy and did not respond as favorably to the diet. Triglycerides, inflammation, and blood sugar were the main markers tracked. Here is where it gets interesting. The low-diversity group saw their microbiota become more like the high-diversity group after going on a higher-protein, lower-calorie diet. The diet essentially increased protein, fruit, and vegetable consumption, while decreasing carbs, breads, starches, and fat.[1] Was this a special diet? No. It simply hits a few important dietary principles and is in alignment with our create-a-healthy-environment-in-order-to-have-healthy-bacteria paradigm.

How much of an effect did being high- or low-microbiota diversity have? Was it meaningful? Well, not really. The effect of diet was far more powerful than the effect of microbiota. Yes, the microbiota predicted if a participant would respond better or worse to the diet, but the overall effect of the diet was far more powerful. This means if your goal is weight loss, finding the right diet for you is more important than what type of microbiota you have. This is in alignment with what we learned from the high-level science examining the microbiota in obesity, right? Obesity researchers have commented there is no consistent relationship between the microbiota and obesity. So, it shouldn't be surprising that in this study the differences seen in the microbiota didn't make much of a difference.

Let's look at some specifics of the diet that was used in the study:

The diet decreased
- calories, by about 650 per day;
- carbs, cutting them in half to about 94 grams per day;
- breads, starches, and sugars;
- fat, cutting it in half.

It increased
- protein;
- total fiber, increasing from 15 to 23 grams per day;
- fruits and vegetables.

This diet looked very much like a Paleo-type diet: protein was increased, as were fiber, fruits, and vegetables; grains and processed foods were decreased. The nice thing about this type of diet is you can eat to control your blood sugar (by decreasing carb intake, especially breads, starches, and sugars) and feed your gut bacteria (by eating more fruits and vegetables).

It doesn't have to be either/or. If you cut certain carbs while increasing vegetables and fruits, you will decrease your carb intake while increasing your fiber intake. Are you wondering which box this is in? The high-carb-diet box or low-carb-diet box? This diet would be considered a moderate-to-lower-carb diet, but the labels aren't that important.

The diet in this study improved the microbiota by decreasing carbs and increasing fiber. Can improving blood sugar levels *without* increasing your fiber still cause an improvement in your microbiota? If so, this would truly show that environment alone (in this case blood sugar levels) can improve your microbiota and that improving the microbiota is not dependent upon feeding your gut bacteria (with fiber).

It has been shown that type 2 diabetic mice treated with the drug metformin experience improvements in blood sugar levels and in their microbiota.[2] But this was an animal study that used a drug, so this might not translate to humans and diet. Remember our rule from before? Demand human-outcome studies.

In another study, the microbiotas of children with type 1 diabetes were compared to healthy controls. It was found that the diabetic children had high Bacteroides bacteria, while the healthy children had high Prevotella. The diabetics then began treatment with insulin and were monitored for two years. Treatment here is natural, because children with type 1 diabetes are merely given insulin. Insulin is a hormone we all produce, but, sadly, type 1 diabetic children can't. After two years, the two groups were again compared, and the diabetic children's microbiota now looked like the healthy children's![3] Similar results have been seen after treating rheumatoid arthritis patients with anti-inflammatory drugs[4] and in inflammatory bowel disease patients who were treated with similar anti-inflammatory drugs.[5]

In both these cases the microbiota normalized after treatment. This supports other evidence that optimizing your environment can improve the health of your gut bacteria, even without doing any work to feed your gut bacteria.

In the studies using anti-inflammatory drugs on patients with rheumatoid arthritis, the subjects had overzealous immune systems, a condition that creates a hostile environment for gut bacteria. By using a treatment that calms the immune system, patients become healthier and their microbiotas improve. We have already discussed ways to reduce inflammation with diet, and later we will cover more powerful *natural* anti-inflammatory strategies that can reduce inflammation and calm your immune system.

## CARBS, WEIGHT LOSS, AND YOUR GUT BACTERIA

Feeding your gut bacteria to lose weight is a theory that is excitedly being discussed by many microbiota enthusiasts. But what happens when we test this theory? And how do we test this theory? Think for a minute. How can we assess whether feeding gut bacteria is a viable method for weight loss or if this is just media-sound-bite theory? If you said, "In clinical trials in humans," you nailed it!

What do we see when we look at the clinical trials objectively? We see that while all healthy diets can lead to weight loss, diets that focus on feeding your gut bacteria are not the most effective method for weight loss. A systematic review with meta-analysis has shown that low-carb diets are better for weight loss than higher-carb (lower fat) diets. Again, higher-carb diets feed your gut bacteria, and lower-carb diets may starve your gut bugs.[7]

Lower-carb diets, then, may actually *decrease* gut bacteria.

## Maybe starving rather than feeding your gut bugs is a good thing for weight loss and diabetes.

Maybe by starving gut bugs, we can starve certain bacterial overgrowths/imbalances and then allow the other bacteria a chance to thrive. In fact, this has been demonstrated! A study of type 2 diabetic patients showed that a low-carb diet *caused* a healthier microbiota! Remember, first eat to control blood sugar. For many, a lower-carb diet is best because it regulates their blood sugar.

In another study, one comparing diets with three different levels of carb intake (high, medium, and very low), researchers found that the lower the carb intake, the better the weight loss. The very low-carb group lost the most weight but also saw a decrease in some of their gut bacteria and SCFA (short-chain fatty acids, which are produced by gut bacteria).[8]

**SUMMARY OF STUDY RESULTS OF HOW CARB-INTAKE LEVEL AFFECTS WEIGHT LOSS**

| Carbs/day | Weight loss | Change in gut bacteria |
|---|---|---|
| high: 360g | 0 lbs | none |
| moderate: 181g | 8.7 lbs | none |
| very low: 22g | 14 lbs | decrease in bacteria and SCFA |

The fact that the group that went very low carb experienced the best clinical results (weight loss) but did see some bacterial loss reinforces our principle: eating to control your blood sugar is more important than eating to feed your gut bugs. This concept is strongly reinforced when we consider that the best trials using therapies that feed gut bacteria (prebiotics, fiber) don't produce anywhere near the amount of weight loss when compared to a dietary strategy—such as a lower-carb diet—that starves gut bacteria.

Here's something interesting about this study we just discussed. If participants ate the moderate-carb diet, they lost weight, but there wasn't a significant impact on their gut bacteria. Other studies have reinforced that around 170–180 grams of carbs per day won't greatly affect your gut bacteria.[9] Might this be why people lost more weight on the very low-carb diet—because the very low-carb diet reduced bacterial overgrowth? Again, maybe these people had too many bacteria, so eating in a way that starved bacteria helped rebalance the gut and led to weight loss.

Inflammation might be another key reason why antibacterial approaches, like low-carb diets or treating bacterial overgrowth, seem to work well for weight loss. Perhaps people who gain weight do so because they have gut inflammation, and this inflammation is caused by bacterial overgrowths. Inflammation can then cause weight gain via a variety of mechanisms: water retention, decreased fat metabolism, decreased thyroid hormone function, insulin resistance, stress hormone imbalances, disrupted sleep, and increased cravings, to name a few. Perhaps this is why many patients who treat gut imbalances like SIBO and SIFO lose weight without making any additional dietary or exercise changes.

We have good support for our concept of eating to control blood sugar before feeding gut bacteria. Before you jump on the low-carb bandwagon, remember that some people can lose weight on any healthy diet. Remember the A to Z Weight Loss Study where Dr. Gardner compared high-carb and low-carb diets? Gardner showed people can lose weight on any diet, but those with a poor ability to process carbs might do better on a lower-carb diet. If you work through the process of decreasing carbs and then later slowly increase

your carb intake, a process we'll discuss a little later, you will settle in at your ideal carb intake.

> **GUT GEEKS**
> *There is some evidence that certain bacteria we think are healthy (specifically F. prausnitzii, which is believed to have anti-inflammatory properties) increase on a low-carb diet.*[10]

What about using special fiber or prebiotic supplements to feed gut bacteria to lose weight? Unfortunately, the results here have been disappointing. The best weight-loss results, which were obtained in obese subjects who had a lot of weight to lose, have shown about 2.3 pounds of weight loss with prebiotic supplementation.[11] These results can be considered almost negligible. We will go into this in more detail in part 4, when we cover specific gut treatments like probiotics, supplemental fiber, and prebiotics.

# CUTTING THROUGH THE CARB CONFUSION— FINDING YOUR IDEAL CARB INTAKE

Let's now cover specifically what you can do to determine if you should eat a lower-carb, moderate-carb or higher-carb diet.

Here is a summary of how you'll find your ideal carb intake. We'll go into more detail in part 5.

- You will first spend a few weeks determining the diet you feel best on: Paleo, AIP, or low FODMAP. When you follow one of those three diets, you will naturally tend to reduce your carb intake.
- During this time, we will check to make sure you're eating a lower-carb diet. Most people feel best when eating roughly 100–150 grams of carbs per day or less. Don't get overly concerned about exact

numbers, but do check to see roughly how many grams of carbs you are eating per day, and adjust accordingly if you are significantly over 100–150.

- Later, when we get to step 5 (of our eight-step action plan, which you'll learn about in part 5), you will increase your carb intake, and we will determine what level of carb intake you feel best at. We follow this sequence because many do better with lower-carb diets initially but then later, once their guts heal, need more carbs. Why? Because as the gut heals, people can better digest carbs and have fewer bacterial imbalances, which makes them better able to tolerate carbs.
- Throughout this process, you should eat regular meals—every three to five hours—unless you notice you feel notably better when skipping meals.

What do we mean by "carbs"? The term is often used loosely, which creates confusion for some people. Generally speaking, carbs include bread, pasta, cereal, fruits, and vegetables (including potatoes and winter squashes). The other food categories are proteins (chicken and fish, for example) and fats (such as olive oil and coconut oil).

Within the carb family, some foods contain more carbohydrates than others. For example, one medium potato contains about 37 grams of carbs, whereas an equivalent serving of broccoli contains about 13 grams. When we restrict carbs, as in a lower-carb diet, we usually restrict the types of foods that are the most carb dense. For example, we might limit potatoes and focus on broccoli.

The following foods are carb dense and should be limited on a lower-carb diet:

- Grains (breads, cereals, rice, oatmeal, quinoa)
- Starches (potatoes, sweet potatoes, winter squashes)
- Fruits (limit all fruits except berries, which have the lowest sugar content)

To put it simply, vegetables and berries tend to be the lowest in carbs, so focus on them if you are trying to follow a lower-carb eating plan.

## THE TWO MAIN REASONS CARB AND BLOOD SUGAR REGULATION ARE IMPORTANT

There are two main reasons why carb and blood sugar regulation are important:

- Stable blood sugar promotes healthy weight, metabolism, energy, and stress hormones
- *Appropriate* carb intake will help optimize your microbiota

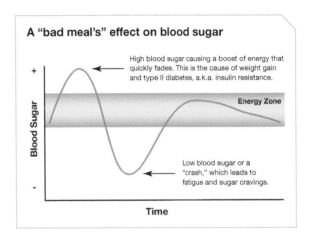

A "bad meal's" effect on blood sugar

High blood sugar causing a boost of energy that quickly fades. This is the cause of weight gain and type II diabetes, a.k.a. insulin resistance.

Energy Zone

Blood Sugar

Low blood sugar or a "crash," which leads to fatigue and sugar cravings.

Time

So far, we've focused our discussion on controlling carb intake to optimize your microbiota, but let's briefly discuss the concept of carb intake as it relates to blood sugar regulation. When you eat a meal that doesn't contain the right balance of carbs (for you), it can cause you to have ups and downs in your blood sugar. As you see in the diagram, this can first lead to a blood sugar high, which can cause weight gain and insulin resistance. Then, after the high, comes the low. Blood sugar lows are a major reason for cravings, and if you can avoid these lows, you will have better energy, fewer cravings, and often weight loss. Avoiding these lows can even prevent anxiety, irritability, and brain fog.

Blood sugar lows can also occur if you go too long without eating. Regardless of how you get there, recurring blood sugar lows can be very hard on your body hormonally. When blood sugar lows occur, your body releases more of the stress hormone cortisol. Over time, this can cause a condition known as "adrenal fatigue"—a term I don't love but will use to keep things simple. What is adrenal fatigue? To put it simply, adrenal fatigue occurs when your body has been under prolonged stress, which then causes imbalances in your stress hormones. The imbalanced stress hormones can cause weight gain, fatigue, insomnia, irritability, brain fog, light-headedness, and low libido, just to name a few effects. Eating to stabilize your blood sugar is a huge step toward balancing your stress hormones and improving how you feel.

## CARB CONFUSION

There is much debate about whether we should eat a lower-carb or higher-carb diet. I think the debate exists because no single answer is correct for all people. You may go online and research healthy diets and see wildly conflicting opinions regarding carbs. Some swear by low-carb diets; others swear that you must have more carbs in your diet to be healthy. If you go to a low-carb website and read the message boards, you'll likely see people sharing their own stories of improving their health with a low-carb diet. Head over to a website advocating high-carb eating, and you will likely see people reporting how their health improved after going high carb. Confused?

What ends up happening is the people who do better on a low-carb diet aggregate in one camp and the people who do better on a higher-carb diet aggregate in another camp. Then they argue over who is "right." I think a much healthier approach is to recognize there is a spectrum of carb intake, from high to low, and we all need to determine where we fit on this spectrum. This puts the *person* first rather than putting *dietary ideology* first. If

you listen to your body, you will find the ideal dietary approach regarding carbs.

## DEFINING HIGH CARB VERSUS LOW CARB

How do we define low carb versus high carb? To be truthful, I am not overly concerned with these definitions because they just reinforce the line of thinking that you are either pro low carb or pro high carb. But there are a few guidelines that are helpful:

- High carb—more than 175 grams per day
- Moderate carb—100–175 grams per day
- Low carb—less than 100 grams per day
- Very low carb—less than 50 grams per day

These differing carb intakes connect to latitudinal regions of the world. Before the advent of supermarkets, different foods were available at different latitudes. This regional food availability influenced the genes of our ancestors. If your heritage is that of an equatorial region, you may do better with a higher-carb diet; whereas if your heritage is of a more northern region, you may do better with a lower-carb diet.

Here is a world map that highlights the Mediterranean region, which is between the zones for high carb and low carb.

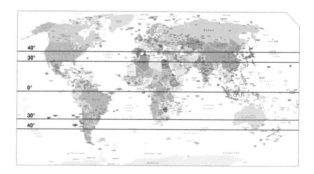

- High carb—equatorial (0°–30°)
- Moderate carb—Mediterranean or semiequatorial (30°–40°)
- Low carb—northern (>40°)

There are a number of free carb-counting tools available on the Internet. The Atkins Center offers a few here: www.atkins.com/how-it-works/free-tools. MyFitnessPal is another helpful tool. You can also simply search for something like "amount of carbs in an apple" to get an idea how many grams of carbs are contained in a certain food.

As you start one of our diets (Paleo, AIP, or low FODMAP) make sure you're aware of how many carbs you are eating. This will ensure you're not eating too many. Again, most people end up naturally reducing their carb intake when starting one of these diets, but it's good to check. Then, in step 5, we will perform a carb reintroduction. People who have an imbalance in the gut like SIBO or SIFO, or who have IBD (ulcerative colitis or Crohn's disease) might have problems with a higher carb intake. However, once their guts heal they might need more carbs. For example, what if you are an athlete with a lot of muscle mass but you have SIBO as well? At first you will need to lower your carb intake to heal your gut. But once your gut is healed, you might feel best on a moderate or higher carb intake. The carb-reintroduction step will allow you to determine the best amount of carbs for your body.

## COMPARISON OF SAMPLE DAILY MENUS FOR LOW-, MODERATE-, AND HIGH-CARB DIETS

*Breakfast*
- **Low carb**—three-egg omelet with mushrooms, tomato, and half an avocado
- **Moderate carb**—three-egg omelet with mushrooms, tomato, and hash browns
- **High carb**—two-egg omelet with mushrooms, tomato, hash browns, gluten-free toast, fruit

*Lunch*
- **Low carb**—chicken breast with skin, spinach salad with mushrooms, red onion, hard-boiled egg, bacon, red wine Dijon mustard dressing
- **Moderate carb**—chicken breast without skin, spinach salad with mushrooms, red onion, hard-boiled egg, bacon, ¼ cup slivered almonds, sliced strawberries, red wine vinegar Dijon mustard dressing
- **High carb**—smaller chicken breast without skin, spinach salad with mushrooms, red onion, hard-boiled egg, ¼ cup slivered almonds, sliced strawberries, red wine vinegar Dijon mustard dressing, rice or quinoa

*Dinner*
- **Low carb**—steak, cauliflower mash, steamed broccoli, green salad with sliced celery, green onion, cucumber, cherry tomatoes, olive oil vinaigrette dressing
- **Moderate carb**—steak, cauliflower mash, steamed broccoli and carrots, green salad with sliced celery, green onion, cucumber, cherry tomatoes, apples, olive oil vinaigrette dressing
- **High carb**—steak, baked potato, corn on the cob, green salad with sliced celery, green onion, cucumber, cherry tomatoes, apples, olive oil vinaigrette dressing

The main difference is that if you're on a low-carb-intake diet, you generally avoid the dense carbs, so no potatoes, rice, breads, or winter squashes and limited fruits. A moderate-carb intake allows a small amount of these at each meal. The high-carb intake has a full serving of these at each meal. That is really it. We don't have to make the diet any more complicated than that. If you follow that general principle, you'll be fine. It can be easy to feel overwhelmed, so stick to the simple concepts, and don't get overly analytical with the details.

However, there is one other principle that is important to understand. As carb intake goes up, it's best to bring down the fat slightly—fat is the main nutrient that changes. What this looks like is this: as your carbs increase, have a *slightly* smaller serving of protein and choose meats that have less fat. For example, chicken with skin on or chicken thighs would be higher fat; skinless chicken breast would be lower fat. You should also use less fat in food prep (cooking oils) and as a dressing, as your carb intake increases. It's really that simple. You often hear about diets that are either low carb or low fat, and this is why: fats and carbs should generally be consumed in opposing amounts, more fat equals fewer carbs and vice versa. You almost never hear someone recommending a high-carb, high-fat diet. Again, don't get overwhelmed by details here. Just understand that if you end up with a lower-carb intake, you can have a fair amount of fat in your diet. If you end up eating a higher-carb diet, then you should compensate by eating fewer high-fat foods. It's that simple. Specific numbers and ratios are not needed.

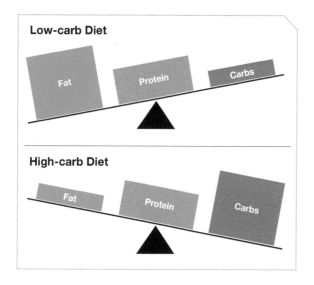

Just as you may notice your ability to tolerate potential food allergens increases after you heal your gut, the same can happen with carbs. You may notice that potato causes you to bloat one month into this process, but a few months later you may notice that you actually feel better when you eat some potato. Remember, our goal is to be able to eat the broadest diet, and this process will help you get there.

The removal and later reintroduction of allergens and of carbs has a lot of overlap. That is, when you cut out common allergens, you inadvertently end up reducing your carbs at the same time. Correspondingly, when you reintroduce potential allergens, you usually end up increasing your carb intake. If you cut out bacterial-feeding foods like high FODMAPs, you tend to reduce carbs even more.

> *As you start on one of our diets, whether it's Paleo, autoimmune Paleo, or low FODMAP, you'll end up reducing your carb intake.*

## HOW TO KNOW WHERE YOU FALL ON THE CARB SPECTRUM

**THE FOLLOWING SUGGEST YOU MAY DO BETTER WITH FEWER CARBS, AROUND 100 GRAMS/DAY OR FEWER:**

1. You have tried a lower-carb diet and felt good.
2. You have a family history of diabetes.
3. You have diabetes or prediabetes (type 2).
4. You are overweight.
5. You crave carbs or can't stop eating carbs/sugars once you start eating them.
6. You are of a more northern descent than equatorial descent (for example, Irish versus Venezuelan).

**THE FOLLOWING SUGGEST YOU MAY DO BETTER WITH MORE CARBS, AROUND 150 GRAMS/DAY OR MORE:**

1. You have tried a higher-carb diet and felt good.
2. You are an athlete or highly active.

3. You need to gain weight.

4. You are of a more equatorial descent than northern descent (for example, Venezuelan versus Irish).

## SAFE CARB SOURCES

If you notice you feel better with a moderate to higher carb intake, use this list of higher-carb foods that tend to work well for most:

- White rice
- White potato
- Sweet potato
- Gluten-free bread products
- Oats
- Plantains
- Cassava, taro, yucca
- Rutabaga
- Corn (non-GMO)

To review, we have already covered a few reasons why some do better on high-carb diets and others do better on low-carb diets. These reasons include

- differences in insulin sensitivity;
- gene origin (the latitude);
- underlying imbalances in the gut (SIBO and SIFO).

The general approach we will take is to first limit carb intake and then later reintroduce carbs in step 5.

## DOES LOW-CARB INTAKE NEGATIVELY AFFECT MY THYROID?

In short, no. This point often gets confused on the Internet. When you eat a lower-carb diet, some of your thyroid hormones can shift as part of a natural adjustment to changing your diet. This adjustment is usually accompanied by weight loss and better energy, so don't assume that a shift is necessarily negative. Also, one study even showed an improvement of thyroid autoimmunity after following a diet that restricted carbs.[12] It's true that long-term low-calorie diets may cause a negative shift in thyroid hormones, but that's not what we're doing here, so no need to worry.

We've discussed what to eat, but how about meal frequency?

# MEAL FREQUENCY AND FASTING

## HOW FREQUENTLY SHOULD YOU EAT?

### Small frequent meals

To regulate your blood sugar, it's typically best to eat somewhat frequently, every three to five hours. Some people will clearly do better with this approach. These are the same people who notice if they go more than three to five hours without food, they might get irritable, binge eat, become fatigued, or have brain fog. Going too long without eating is a major reason why people make poor food choices. This is because when your blood sugar gets low, you tend to crave sweets and carbs.

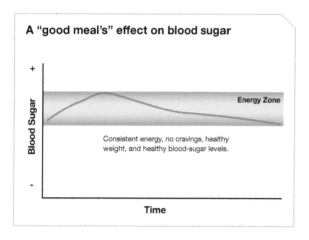

**A "good meal's" effect on blood sugar**

Energy Zone

Blood Sugar

Consistent energy, no cravings, healthy weight, and healthy blood-sugar levels.

Time

Here is an example: You intended to have the healthy chicken salad you brought from home for lunch at noon. You had been feeling great all morning and at ten said to yourself, "I feel great, and I can do this healthy-eating thing." But you got distracted and didn't eat at noon but instead ate at two thirty. At two thirty there was a much different internal dialogue occurring. You felt much less motivated and a little tired, and your thinking was fuzzy. The healthy salad you brought from home didn't have the same appeal as it did at ten, and the cafeteria pizza seemed irresistible. You caved and ate the cafeteria pizza and immediately regretted it. Can you guess why all of the above happened? Because you were experiencing a blood sugar low. By eating somewhat frequently, you can regulate and balance your blood sugar and prevent all the negative symptoms associated with blood sugar lows.

### Large, infrequent meals and fasting

There is another important piece to consider here, especially when looking at this from the angle of healing the gut. Sometimes, periodic fasting (essentially skipping a meal or meals) can give the gut a chance to rest and heal. The analogy I use with my patients is healing a sprained ankle. If you run three miles per day with a sprained ankle, how effectively would it heal? If your gut is "injured" and you're eating three meals a day, how well will your gut heal? Some people feel much better when they don't eat frequent meals but rather only eat two meals per day. In fact, for some people, this one change can make a world of difference. Some clinical studies have shown fasting to benefit both IBS[13] and IBD.[14]

"But isn't it true that skipping meals will slow my metabolism? And what about breakfast being the most important meal of the day?" These are fair questions. Again, what do we do when we have differing opinions on an issue? We look to both sides of the science to obtain an unbiased answer. So then, what *does* the science say?

A meta-analysis examining the effect of fasting (skipping meals) on body composition found a small benefit but did comment that the data were limited.[15] Reminder, a meta-analysis is the highest level of science. Meta-analyses summarize available clinical trials and provide an aggregate score of the finding, like the restaurant-scoring system on Yelp.

One systematic review essentially concluded that there does appear to be health benefits to fasting or skipping meals.[16] Another systematic review found that fasting may or may not be helpful for weight loss.[17]

What we see is a trend in the data that fasting either has no negative impact or even has a slight benefit when it comes to body composition. Does skipping meals slow your metabolism? The answer appears to be probably not. But remember, not everyone feels better when skipping meals. We'll work through our personalized action steps later to help you determine the best fit for you. If you feel better skipping breakfast, skip it. If you feel worse skipping breakfast, eat.

Sometimes, people express concern that they will develop a nutrition deficiency from a short fast. This is very misguided. Fasting has been shown to have many health benefits and is well documented to have the ability to allow various gut and inflammatory conditions to improve. How does this tie into nutrient deficiency? If your gut is not working properly, you will not be absorbing nutrients well to begin with—nutritional deficiencies are known to occur in many digestive conditions, even if a person is eating healthy foods. A short fast can actually help you become *better* nourished in the long run as it can increase your absorption of nutrients.

## FINDING THE RIGHT MEAL FREQUENCY FOR YOU

Should you eat smaller frequent meals or skip some meals and eat fewer larger ones? When we begin getting into our Great-in-8 Action Plan, the first step will be experimenting with fasting to help you determine what works best for you. But here are the basic points that will help you determine if you should eat small frequent meals (every three to five hours) or larger infrequent meals (skipping one or more meals per day).

You will do better skipping meals (fasting) if
- you have noticed you feel better when skipping meals;
- you find you are not hungry at certain mealtimes;
- you felt good on the modified fast (we will discuss this next).

You will do better with frequent meals if
- you have noticed you feel worse when skipping meals (fatigued, irritable, hungry, foggy-headed);
- you are hungry at or before mealtimes;
- you felt poorly on the modified fast.

## A MODIFIED FAST

The first step in our Great-in-8 Action Plan (which we will detail in part 5) consists of performing a modified fast. A modified fast is a liquid-only fast that can be incredibly reparative for your gut. Short-term liquid fasting can give your gut a break and aid in healing the same way avoiding activity can help heal an ankle sprain.

There are two options available for the modified fast—choose whichever one appeals most to you. One is a cleansing lemonade, and the other is a homemade broth. See the ***Modified Fast*** handout on www.DrRuscio.com/GutBook for specific instruction on exactly how to make the fasting solution. To perform the modified fast, your only source of calories for two to four days will be the fasting solution you've chosen.

The first day is a transition day. Not everyone feels better on day one. It's usually by the second day that improvements are noticeable. Often, patients report improved energy, mental clarity, digestive symptoms, weight, sleep, and mood. For most people, modified fasting seems to work well and can be used again in the future if they experience a flare-up of their symptoms. However, occasionally someone feels tired or hungry or has some other negative reaction that lasts the entire fast. For these people, it's generally best to avoid fasting. If you're one of these people, simply move along to the next part of step 1, the diet. How long you perform the modified fast depends on how you are responding. If you are responding well, go for the full four days. If you are having a reaction that doesn't abate after the second day, stop at day two.

Before I tried a liquid fast, I was sure I wouldn't be able to do it. I was very wrong. My energy, sleep, and mental clarity were incredible. This can be a powerful healing tool for you to keep in your toolbox. It's not a guarantee, but giving the fast a trial is well worth it. Remember, we are not performing the fast now; I just wanted to introduce you to this concept.

## HOW MANY CALORIES SHOULD YOU EAT?

In my opinion, the best way to determine how many calories you should eat is by listening to your body. This is good news, because it means you do not need to count calories. I am not a supporter of calorie counting for two reasons: it's tedious, and it doesn't reinforce listening to your body. Learning to listen to your body is a principle that will help you determine the healthiest diet for you.

> *The most powerful thing you can do to improve your health is to learn to listen to your own body and stop listening to everyone else.*

It may interest you to know that when starting on a healthier diet, one that helps balance blood sugar, people tend to decrease their calorie intake without even knowing it. This is likely because when you regulate your blood sugar, you avoid blood sugar lows. Blood sugar lows cause cravings, poor food choices, and overeating. So, if we focus on a healthy diet, your calories will take care of themselves. Also, it has been shown that people tend to self-regulate how much they eat at each meal depending on how many meals they eat. For example, if someone eats four meals a day, the meals tend to be smaller; if someone only eats two meals a day, those meals tend to be larger. Eat until you feel satisfied. Don't leave the table feeling hungry, but don't leave the table feeling gorged.

We have covered inflammatory foods, food allergens, carb intake, and meal frequency. These are the major concepts regarding diet. Let's next discuss food additives and processed foods.

## CONCEPT SUMMARY

- You must eat to control and balance blood sugar. Eating to balance blood sugar will create a healthy environment for gut bacteria and thus improve your microbiota.

- A spectrum exists for carbohydrate and prebiotic intake: some will do better on less, and some will do better on more. We each have to determine where we fit on this spectrum.

- A similar spectrum exists for food allergens and food intolerances. We each have to determine what our problem foods are.

- Eating a diet that regulates blood sugar is another pillar of a healthy diet.

- The two main reasons carb and blood sugar regulation are important are stable blood sugar promotes healthy weight, metabolism, energy, and stress hormones and appropriate carb intake will help optimize your microbiota.

- Differences in insulin sensitivity, the latitude your genes originate from, and underlying imbalances in the gut are all reasons why some do better on a high-carb diet and some do better on a low-carb diet.

- A low-carb diet avoids dense carbs like potatoes, rice, breads, and squashes and limits fruit to berries.

- A moderate-carb diet allows a small amount of these carbs at each meal.

- A high-carb diet has a full serving of high-carb foods at each meal.

- As carb intake goes up, you should bring down the protein and fat intake slightly. Fat is the main nutrient that changes.

- Start with a more restrictive diet of low-allergen foods and lower carbs, and as the gut heals slowly work to bring both of these back into the diet.

- Eating to control your blood sugar is more important than eating to feed your gut bugs.

- In order to regulate your blood sugar, it's typically best to eat somewhat frequently, every three to five hours. However, some people do better when they skip meals (practice fasting).

- A modified fast is a liquid-only diet that can aid in gut healing and repair.

- The best way to determine how many calories you should eat is by listening to your body, not by calorie counting.

1   Aurélie Cotillard et al., "Dietary Intervention Impact on Gut Microbial Gene Richness," *Nature* 500, no. 7464 (2013): 585–88, doi:10.1038/nature12480.

2   H. Lee and G. Ko, "Effect of Metformin on Metabolic Improvement and Gut Microbiota," *Applied and Environmental Microbiology* 80, no. 19 (2014): 5935–43, doi:10.1128/AEM.01357-14.

3   María Esther Mejía-León et al., "Fecal Microbiota Imbalance in Mexican Children with Type 1 Diabetes," *Scientific Reports* 4, no. 3814 January (2014), doi:10.1038/srep03814.

4   Xuan Zhang et al., "The Oral and Gut Microbiomes Are Perturbed in Rheumatoid Arthritis and Partly Normalized after Treatment," *Nature Medicine* 21, no. 8 (2015): 895–905, doi:10.1038/nm.3914.

5   David Busquets et al., "Anti-Tumour Necrosis Factor Treatment with Adalimumab Induces Changes in the Microbiota of Crohn's Disease," *Journal of Crohn's & Colitis* 9, no. 10 (2015): 899–906, doi:10.1093/ecco-jcc/jjv119.

6   Marta Caretto et al., "Preventing Urinary Tract Infections after Menopause without Antibiotics," *Maturitas*, 2017, doi:10.1016/j.maturitas.2017.02.004.

7   Deirdre K. Tobias et al., "Effect of Low-Fat Diet Interventions versus Other Diet Interventions on Long-Term Weight Change in Adults: A Systematic Review and Meta-Analysis," *Lancet Diabetes and Endocrinology* 3, no. 12 (2015): 968–79, doi:10.1016/S2213-8587(15)00367-8.

8   Wendy R. Russell et al., "High-Protein, Reduced-Carbohydrate Weight-Loss Diets Promote Metabolite Profiles Likely to Be Detrimental to Colonic Health," *American Journal of Clinical Nutrition* 93, no. 5 (2011): 1062–72, doi:10.3945/ajcn.110.002188.

9   Grant D. Brinkworth et al., "Comparative Effects of Very Low-Carbohydrate, High-Fat and High-Carbohydrate, Low-Fat Weight-Loss Diets on Bowel Habit and Faecal Short-Chain Fatty Acids and Bacterial Populations," *British Journal of Nutrition* 101, no. 10 (2009): 1493–1502, doi:10.1017/S0007114508094658.

10  Alan W. Walker et al., "Dominant and Diet-Responsive Groups of Bacteria within the Human Colonic Microbiota," *ISME Journal* 5, no. 2 (2011): 220–30, doi:10.1038/ismej.2010.118.

11  Jill A. Parnell and Raylene A. Reimer, "Weight Loss during Oligofructose Supplementation Is Associated with Decreased Ghrelin and Increased Peptide YY in Overweight and Obese Adults," *American Journal of Clinical Nutrition* 89, no. 6 (2009): 1751–59, doi:10.3945/ajcn.2009.27465.

12  T. N. Hustoft et al., "Effects of Varying Dietary Content of Fermentable Short-Chain Carbohydrates on Symptoms, Fecal Microenvironment, and Cytokine Profiles in Patients with Irritable Bowel Syndrome," *Neurogastroenterology and Motility* 29, no. 4 (2017), doi:10.1111/nmo.12969.

13  Motoyori Kanazawa and Shin Fukudo, "Effects of Fasting Therapy on Irritable Bowel Syndrome," *International Journal of Behavioral Medicine* 13, no. 3 (2006): 214–20, doi:10.1207/s15327558ijbm1303_4.

14  Hamid Tavakkoli et al., "Ramadan Fasting and Inflammatory Bowel Disease," *Indian Journal of Gastroenterology: Official Journal of the Indian Society of Gastroenterology* 27, no. 6 (2008): 239–41, www.indianjgastro.com/IJG_pdf/nov2008/nov08_SR2_pg239_acknowledge241.pdf.

15    Brad Jon Schoenfeld et al., "Effects of Meal Frequency on Weight Loss and Body Composition: A Meta-Analysis," *Nutrition Reviews* 73, no. 2 (2015): 69–82, doi:10.1093/nutrit/nuu017.

16    Benjamin D. Horne et al., "Health Effects of Intermittent Fasting: Hormesis or Harm? A Systematic Review," *American Journal of Clinical Nutrition*, 2015, doi:10.3945/ajcn.115.109553.

17    Hollie A. Raynor et al., "Eating Frequency, Food Intake, and Weight: A Systematic Review of Human and Animal Experimental Studies," *Frontiers in Nutrition* 2 (2015), doi:10.3389/fnut.2015.00038.

# CHAPTER 9

## PROCESSED FOOD, FOOD ADDITIVES, AND FOOD QUALITY

## A DIET THAT FOCUSES ON FRESH, WHOLE, AND UNPROCESSED FOODS

It probably goes without saying that if you are trying to improve your health, you should focus on whole, fresh foods and avoid processed foods. However, there are a few points here that are important for us to cover, especially as this relates to your gut health.

We have already discussed the important concepts of eating a diet that is low in allergens and foods to which you have intolerances and that regulates blood sugar. Eating fresh, whole, unprocessed, and organic foods is important but not as important as avoiding allergens and regulating blood sugar. The reason I rank these is to help you prioritize if you can't make all these changes at once. In fact, I think for most people, it's best to gradually work into these changes so they feel manageable. The goal here is not to overwhelm

yourself but rather to gradually bring these practices into your everyday life. Again, if you can only do one, focus on the right type of food (low allergens, controls blood sugar) before you concern yourself with food quality (organic, grass fed, and so on). Here are a few tips and reminders:

- Whole foods take precedence over organic
  - » Fresh conventional beans over canned organic beans
  - » A nonorganic chicken salad over a prepackaged organic dinner
- Focus on unprocessed meats, fresh vegetables, healthy fats, and some fruits. Worry about the quality once this feels routine

Let's use potatoes as an example: A whole potato is unprocessed (think baked potatoes or homemade mashed potatoes). Organic, sea-salt-flavored potato chips are minimally processed. Standard potato chips that are sour cream and onion flavored are the most processed and contain emulsifiers or other ingredients that negatively affect your gut. If you stick to buying foods that are not processed, you will end up avoiding many unhealthy foods. Think of it like this:

## if you couldn't hunt it, fish it, or gather it, you shouldn't buy it.

Another example that may help here is to imagine shopping at a farmers' market. What would you see? TV dinners? Soy burgers? Likely not. You would mostly see fresh fruits and vegetables, whole chickens, various cuts of meat, eggs, and nuts. Yes, there would be some processed stuff, like salami or jams, but for the most part, foods will be minimally processed, and (bonus) they will be local.

When you *do* buy packaged foods, look for ones that have a shorter ingredient list and ingredients that you can pronounce. Usually, the shorter and simpler the list, the "cleaner" the food. Here are two examples of potato chips from earlier. As is typical, the shorter list contains simpler ingredients, and the longer list contains some words you have likely never heard before. Once you start reading labels, you will see it's fairly easy to distinguish a minimally processed food from a highly processed food. Of course, nonprocessed

whole foods contain only one ingredient. For example, the only ingredient in a carrot is carrot. A chicken only contains chicken.

## EATING OUT

Don't use eating out as an excuse to eat poorly. You can eat out, have a delicious meal, and still eat healthy foods. However, don't avoid eating out due to fear of deviating from your diet. Eating out is an important social practice, and it should be a fun time with friends and family! Just avoid the major no-nos: gluten, desserts, processed foods, dairy. Sometimes you have to strike a balance, but this shouldn't be too hard to figure out. Let's say you and a friend are out for dinner. Here are a few tips and thoughts:

- Have the waiter hold the bread, or just don't eat the bread.
- Avoid breaded foods.
- Ask if there is a gluten-free option.
- Ask for a side of veggies or a side salad instead of pasta.
- Avoid dishes that contain heavy amounts of dairy (but if you get a salad with a few flakes of cheese, don't freak out).
- Opt for dishes that focus on meat and vegetables.
- Remember, you can always ask the waiter to mix and match.
  - » "Can I have the seared tuna? Please hold the rice. And could I do a side salad of the baby spinach salad?"
  - » "Can I have the bacon burger on a lettuce wrap?" If the waiter says, "I'm sorry we don't offer lettuce wraps," you can reply, "OK, how about on a bed of lettuce?" If the answer is "We don't have beds of lettuce," you can ask, "OK, can I order a side salad, and can you serve my burger on top of that without the bun?" (Sometimes you have to help a lackluster waiter with his or her serving skills.)

**Ingredients:** Potatoes, Safflower and/or Sunflower and/or Canola Oil, Sea Salt.

**Ingredients:** Corn, Vegetable Oil (Sunflower, Canola, and/or Corn Oil), Maltodextrin (Made From Corn). Salt, Cheddar Cheese (Milk, Cheese Cultures, Salt, Enzymes), Whey, Monosodium Glutamate, Buttermilk, Romano Cheese (Part-Skim Cow's Milk, Cheese Cultures, Salt, Enzymes), Whey Protein Concentrate, Onion Powder, Corn Flour, Natural and Artificial Flavor, Dextrose, Tomato Powder, Lactose, Spices, Artificial Color (Including Yellow 6, Yellow 5, and Red 40), Lactic Acid, Citric Acid, Sugar, Garlic Powder, Skim Milk, Red and Green Bell Pepper Powder, Disodium Inosinate, and Disodium Guanylate.
**CONTAINS MILK INGREDIENTS.**

» "Can I have the lemon chicken, but instead of pasta can I do vegetables?"

- Don't obsess over trace amounts of anything, unless you know you are extremely sensitive.

If you are eating Paleo or low FODMAP, eating out can be more challenging but still totally doable. Just do your best. Remember, one meal that isn't perfect will not make or break your health. Also, remember that social time is important for healing. If you have a fun night out with a good friend but eat non-AIP and non-low FODMAP, you will most likely still come out on top because the therapeutic effect of social time will outweigh the effect of one off-plan meal. Yes, maybe you will be a little gassy, but you will have fed your soul. If you do have a negative reaction to a certain food, this is a good learning opportunity to determine what you can and cannot eat.

This all seems fairly reasonable, right? As long as you understand the principles of your healthy diet, you can create your own meals at home or when eating out. Don't be afraid to ask waiters or chefs to deviate from their norm—after all, you are paying them! Just be kind in your requests.

# PROCESSED FOOD AND YOUR GUT

It's widely agreed that processed foods aren't good for you, but do they affect your microbiota? More importantly, could poor-quality food have a negative effect on your microbiota and cause subsequent ill health?

How do processed foods specifically affect your microbiota? We lack the robust clinical trials needed to more definitively answer the question. So, we will use the best data we have. We don't need an extensive body of evidence to support the recommendation to avoid processed foods. Fortunately, we do have some very interesting studies regarding the effects of processed foods on your general gut health.

## EMULSIFIERS AND ADDITIVES

There are several types of food additives used in processed foods. One type of additive that is worth mentioning is emulsifiers, sometimes known as surfactants. Emulsifiers are used to add texture and increase shelf life, but they might have some undesirable effects on your gut.

Your gut is lined with a mucous membrane—it is the most thin and sensitive in your small intestine. This membrane is very important in preventing leaky gut, infection, and inflammation. One of the reasons emulsifier additives are bad for your gut is because they can break down this mucous membrane. Some studies have shown that even trace amounts of these emulsifiers can cause bacteria to leak through your gut and into your bloodstream, a process known as bacterial translocation.[1]

How much of an effect does this have on your gut and overall health? We don't really know. Again, we don't have the robust clinical trials to be able to say with accuracy. But let's look at the best information we do have and use this to generate a recommendation.

In 2015, a review paper was published in the journal *Autoimmunity Reviews*. The paper examined the available evidence and suggested food additives irritate the gut, which causes leaky gut, which then causes autoimmune disease. This paper discussed how specific food additives (glucose, salt, emulsifiers, solvents, gluten, transglutaminase, and nanoparticles) may all cause leaky gut and subsequent autoimmunity.

This same paper cites a systematic review with meta-analysis in which the researchers showed that exposure to compounds often found in processed foods is a risk factor for developing autoimmune disease. The authors continued by stating that those with a family history of autoimmunity should avoid processed foods.[2]

Japan offers some interesting observational data to help us assess the impact increased processed-food consumption has on gut health. In Japan, as annual sales of emulsifier-containing processed foods increased, so did the incidence of Crohn's disease.[3] As we've discussed, Crohn's disease is an inflammatory and autoimmune condition that affects both the small and large intestine. These are merely observations, so we can't say for sure the processed food *caused* the increase in Crohn's disease. However, it would seem wise to exercise caution, nonetheless.

Have we learned anything from our furry friends on this? Yes. Feeding mice "relatively low concentrations of two commonly used emulsifiers, namely carboxymethylcellulose and polysorbate-80, induced low-grade inflammation and obesity/metabolic syndrome . . . and promoted robust colitis."[4] So, mice fed small amounts of emulsifiers became inflamed, overweight, and had autoimmunity in their intestines.

Was there a microbiotal impact? Yes. An altering of the microbiota was observed in this mouse study. Also, when the gut bacteria of these emulsifier-fed mice were then transplanted into other mice, the other mice started to develop the same diseases.

We have discussed SIBO and how it can plague people with the symptoms of IBS (gas, bloating, constipation, diarrhea, abdominal pain). This leads us to another animal study in which the emulsifier carboxymethylcellulose (CMC) caused SIBO in mice! Not only did the emulsifier additive cause SIBO, it also caused inflammation and allowed bacteria to sneak their way into deep pockets in the lining of the intestines, called crypts.[5] Some of these changes were similar to those we see in Crohn's disease. This led the authors to conclude "Because of its ubiquity in products and its unrestricted use in food of the industrial world, CMC

is an ideal suspect to account for the rise of IBD [Crohn's and ulcerative colitis] in the twentieth century."

A nice visual of what this looks like comes from the 2015 review paper discussed earlier.[6] This diagram shows how the food industry takes common foods like baked goods, meat, fish, confection, oils, beverages, and convenience foods and adds sugar, salt, gluten, emulsifiers, and other additives to them. These foods can then cause leaky gut (due to the autoimmunogenic additives), which can then fuel autoimmune disease.

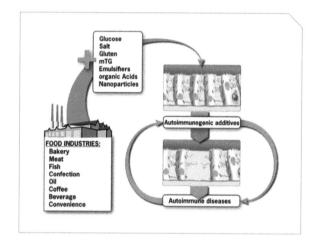

Based on what we *do* know, what is the most practical advice we can give? A 2013 review published in *Alimentary Pharmacology and Therapeutics* made a conclusion based upon the best available evidence. They recommend *reasonable* avoidance of processed foods, which often contain emulsifiers, especially high-fat processed foods, because they may contain higher levels of emulsifiers.[7] This recommendation was for those with IBD; however, because we know these emulsifiers can have a negative impact on your gut, and your gut strongly affects your overall health, I feel it's prudent to recommend reasonable avoidance for everyone.

The authors of the 2015 review paper published in *Autoimmunity Reviews* also concluded that those with autoimmune disease or a family history of autoimmune disease should consider decreasing processed foods to mitigate risk.[8] Does this mean you have to freak out and never eat anything processed, ever, in your entire life? No. Please do not take these things to the extreme. But do avoid processed foods as much as you can.

Is there a list of food additives to avoid? There are so many additives—a single additive can have several names, and new additives are being added to processed foods every day—that making a list isn't practical. The best strategy is to focus on eating whole, fresh, unprocessed foods.

# THE IMPACT OF ARTIFICIAL SWEETENERS ON YOUR MICROBIOTA, HEALTH, AND WEIGHT

Artificial sweeteners are another example of why sticking to whole and unprocessed foods is a good idea. So, how might artificial sweeteners affect your microbiota? By now I hope you are starting to think of this question in two parts. First, how might artificial sweeteners affect your microbiota? Second, and perhaps more importantly, do these changes have any meaningful health impact?

Artificial sweeteners are calorie-free sweeteners that provide a sweet taste without the accompanying calories. They are often used in diet sodas and other diet drinks but are making their way into processed foods. Artificial sweeteners include

- saccharin (Sweet 'N Low);
- aspartame (NutraSweet, Equal);
- acesulfame-K;
- sucralose (Splenda);
- neotame.

Artificial sweeteners are another controversial issue. As with most controversies, it exists because you can find studies supporting the pro views *and* the con views. The way to get to the truth is to examine the entire body of evidence and see what the data shows. Then apply a little common sense. Let's look at a brief overview of the issues.

## THE EFFECT OF ARTIFICIAL SWEETENERS ON YOUR MICROBIOTA

It's important to mention that artificial sweeteners will have significant contact with your gut microbiota. This is because they are mostly unabsorbed, meaning they make their way through your entire digestive tract, then out the other end, bumping into your microbiota all the way.

To date, there is only one study that looks at the effect of artificial sweeteners on your microbiota, published in 2014 in the journal *Nature*.[9] The researchers examined the effect of artificial sweeteners in animals and, more importantly, in humans.

### ANIMAL FINDINGS

Two groups of mice were fed artificial sweeteners (AS). In addition, the mice were fed either normal mouse food or unhealthy mouse food (high-fat chow). The group on the AS and unhealthy diet soon developed higher blood sugar levels; the group being fed AS and normal mouse food did not. What is interesting here is after being given antibiotics, blood sugar levels of the AS-and-unhealthy-diet group normalized, even though they were still on the unhealthy diet. Antibiotics can kill the overgrowth of unwanted bacteria in the gut. Since antibiotics normalized the glucose, this implies the AS combined with poor diet caused changes in gut bacteria that then caused blood sugar problems. This could then be remedied by killing these bad bacteria with antibiotics. Perhaps this is why we see blood sugar levels improve in humans after using antibiotics for SIBO.

Next, gut bacteria (microbiota) samples were taken from the AS-plus-unhealthy-diet mice and then transplanted into the intestines of normal mice. The normal mice then developed blood sugar imbalances, suggesting it was alterations in gut bacteria that caused the problems. Testing confirmed significant differences in the gut bacteria between these two groups of mice.

This is all very interesting, but this study has some holes. There wasn't a good control group here. Meaning, the effect could have been from just the unhealthy diet. Since there was no group *only* eating an unhealthy diet, we don't know what caused the negative effect in the mouse group eating AS and an unhealthy diet. Let's zoom out and look at the simpler human part of this study.

## HUMAN FINDINGS

Through dietary observation of 381 subjects, researchers found that increased AS use was associated with metabolic syndrome, larger waistlines, and elevated fasting blood glucose and hemoglobin A1C (hemoglobin A1C is a two-to-three-month average of blood sugar levels). Microbiota testing was performed, and it showed significant differences between the microbiotas of AS users and nonusers. Note that these differences were not biased by weight, meaning it wasn't the heavier subjects that had different microbiota, but rather it was those who consumed *more AS* that had different microbiotas.

> **GUT GEEKS**
>
> *These changes included increased Enterobacteriaceae, deltaproteobacteria, and actinobacteria. AS may also have caused increased bacteroides and decreased clostridiales. Some of these changes may cause you to absorb more calories from your diet.*

Here is the most interesting and relevant part of this study: To test if AS consumption *caused*

glucose imbalances (elevated blood sugar), seven subjects who did not normally consume AS were given AS for seven days. These subjects then had their blood glucose monitored. Four of the seven subjects experienced worsening of their glucose levels (determined by a glucose-tolerance test), whereas the other three saw no change. This led the researchers to suggest there are "AS responders" and "AS nonresponders." AS responders are those who experience negative metabolic response to AS, such as elevations of blood sugar. Perhaps this is why we see some conflicting findings in AS studies, because not everyone is affected by AS in the same way.

Finally, it was shown that before the experiment started, AS responders had different microbiotas than AS nonresponders. It was shown that after consuming AS, AS responders experienced a shift in their microbiotas, while AS nonresponders did not. This implies that the AS causes a negative change in the microbiotas in responders, which then causes unfavorable changes in metabolism. When the microbiotas of the AS responders were then transplanted into mice, the mice experienced a worsening of their glucose levels. When the microbiotas of AS nonresponders were transplanted into another group of mice, these mice were fine. Again, this implies that the AS was causing the changes in the microbiota, which were then causing glucose problems.

In the closing comments of this study, the authors noted that AS sweeteners might be fueling the same problems they are trying to prevent: weight gain, high blood sugar, and so on.

We have examined some preliminary data showing AS may damage your microbiota and metabolism. But you should never draw a conclusion from one study (remember—that's one of our rules), so let's now take a look at the larger body of evidence that has examined what effect AS has on your weight. Let's see if we can determine what the overall trend is here. Does AS tend to cause weight gain, or does it help with weight loss? Or does it do nothing?

## THE EFFECT OF ARTIFICIAL SWEETENERS ON YOUR HEALTH AND YOUR WEIGHT

Most observational studies show increased consumption of artificial sweeteners correlates with increased risk of being overweight, metabolic syndrome, and type 2 diabetes. In fact, in many cases your risk of these health problems is the same whether you drink regular soda or artificially sweetened soda.[10]

But just because we can observe the effect of something doesn't mean it causes the problem. When there is a crime, we could observe there are usually cop cars present, but this doesn't mean the cop cars caused the problem. Those who are already unhealthy might gravitate toward artificial sweeteners in attempts to lose weight. This could give us a false observation. With this in mind, it's very important to mention that even after researchers control for these false observations, it still appears increased consumption of artificial sweeteners correlated with increased weight gain.[11]

This suggests artificial sweeteners *cause* weight gain.

But even more meaningful than these well-executed observational studies would be the results of clinical studies. So, what do the clinical studies say? Controlled clinical trials generally show no effect from artificial sweeteners, good or bad. There is some evidence that children may gain less weight if using artificial sweeteners, but this does not appear to be the case for adults.

The reason for this is an interesting one. It appears that when children consume artificial sweeteners, their brains think they have eaten a meal, so the children actually eat fewer calories when they consume their next meal. However, this doesn't seem to be the case in adults, maybe because by the time we reach adulthood, we have forgotten how to listen to our hunger signals.

Conversely, there is some observational evidence that shows artificial sweeteners may lead to overeating in adults. Some researchers are concerned about this, especially because artificial sweeteners combined with added sugar (a common practice in packaged foods) may lead to uncontrolled overeating. These are observations but noteworthy nonetheless.

Clinical trial findings on the effect of artificial sweeteners are highlighted by the San Antonio Longitudinal Study of Aging. The study tracked 749 people over a nine-year period in an attempt to see what effect artificially sweetened soda use had on people's waistlines. This study controlled for potentially misleading variables, like overweight people using more artificial sweeteners because they are trying to lose weight. What did they find? They found that the more artificially sweetened soda people consumed, the larger their waistlines became. Over the nine-year period, those who did not use artificially sweetened soda gained 0.8 inches, while heavy AS-soda users gained 3.1 inches. There was no correlation between regular soda use and waistline size.

Here is where it gets even more interesting and ties back in with a point from earlier. Those who were overweight and using AS soda experienced *double* the waist-size increase compared to those who were overweight and not using AS soda! This suggests that AS may in fact interfere with satiation (feeling full) and that use of AS by those who are overweight may be making an underlying problem of overeating worse. The researchers commented that if you need to sweeten your food or drink, lightly sweetening with natural sweeteners (fruit juices) may be the best approach.[12]

My conclusion, and that of some of the researchers, is

> *because little benefit has been shown and potential detriment has been documented, caution with artificial sweetener use is warranted.*

My philosophy is that when science shows no consensus, I default to favoring the ancestral option. Artificial sweeteners are a modern invention, so I lean toward considering them guilty until proven innocent. On the other hand, my view of foods and lifestyle practices that have been present for the majority of our evolution is that they are innocent until proven guilty. Of course, modern medicine has proven many new inventions to be miraculously beneficial, so it's important we remain open to change and progress. But when we don't have enough evidence to prove safety, I revert to my basic philosophy.

Will an occasional dose of artificial sweeteners kill you or make you gain three inches on your waist? Probably not. Should you use artificial sweeteners daily? Probably not. Limit them to occasional use, use sweeteners in general minimally, and when you need to use a sweetener, opt for natural ones (sugar, juice, honey). I would consider natural, calorie-free sweeteners, like stevia, guilty until proven innocent because they were not regularly consumed throughout the majority of our evolution.

Before leaving this section on food quality and food additives, there is one final item we'll discuss: over-the-counter pain relievers like Advil and Motrin (these are known as NSAIDs). It has been shown that NSAID drugs (such as Advil and aspirin) "are responsible for a marked reduction of lactobacilli, which act in the maintenance of . . . mucosal permeability . . . mucus production, and immune system modulation."[13] To put it simply, NSAIDs like Advil and Motrin decrease good bacteria in your gut and cause leaky gut, lead to less

protective mucus production, and may negatively affect your immune system. The negative effect on the immune system is likely because that mucous membrane is an important immune system barrier. When the mucus gets broken down, your immune system can go haywire. Aspirin has also been shown to cause leaky gut and injury to your intestinal mucosa.[14]

If you are in chronic pain, what should you do? This is a difficult question to answer because there can be many causes for and many types of pain: headaches, joint pain, muscle pain, nerve pain, and so on. Seek out the counsel of a health-care provider who can identify and treat the underlying cause of the problem. There are some natural anti-inflammatories that work very well, like curcumin, Boswellia, and fish oil. As we work to improve the health of your gut, many pain and inflammatory issues will improve, so you will likely be able to stop or at least decrease your use of pain medication.

We just covered some key dietary principles that all support an overarching principle: eating to optimize your internal environment is the key to a healthy gut and gut bacteria. Remember, healthy environment equals healthy bacteria. We have also established some things to avoid, like food additives. Let's continue with our theme of optimizing your environment to optimize your health.

## CONCEPT SUMMARY

- Eating fresh, whole, unprocessed, and organic foods is important but not as important as avoiding allergens and regulating your blood sugar.

- Focus on the right type of food (low allergens, controls blood sugar) before you concern yourself with food quality (organic and grass fed, for example).

- Whole foods take precedence over organic.

- Focus on unprocessed meats, fresh vegetables, healthy fats, and some fruits (berries); worry about the quality once this has become routine.

- If you couldn't hunt it, fish it, grow it, or gather it, you shouldn't buy it.

- Healthy food will have a larger impact on your health (weight, body composition, energy) than exercise will. They are both important, but focus on food first.

- Don't be too hard on yourself; start the process of working to rebalance your life gradually.

- Certain food additives can damage your gut and might have a negative impact on your microbiota.

These changes correlate with certain diseases and conditions of the gut.

- Because little benefit has been shown and potential detriment has been documented, caution with artificial sweetener use is warranted.

- It has been shown that NSAIDs (such as Advil and aspirin) are responsible for a reduction in certain good gut bacteria that act in the maintenance of gut-lining health (preventing leaky gut), mucus production, and immune system modulation.

- Seek the council of a health-care provider who can help detect the underlying cause of your chronic pain. There are natural anti-inflammatories that work very well, like curcumin, Boswellia and fish oil.

1    Yvette Merga et al., "Mucosal Barrier, Bacteria and Inflammatory Bowel Disease: Possibilities for Therapy," *Digestive Diseases* 32, no. 4 (2014): 475–83, doi:10.1159/000358156.

2    Carolina Barragán-Martínez et al., "Organic Solvents as Risk Factor for Autoimmune Diseases: A Systematic Review and Meta-Analysis," *PLoS ONE* 7, no. 12 (2012), doi:10.1371/journal.pone.0051506; A. Lerner and T. Matthias, "Changes in Intestinal Tight Junction Permeability Associated with Industrial Food Additives Explain the Rising Incidence of Autoimmune Disease," *Autoimmunity Reviews* 14 (June 2015): 479–89, doi: 10.1016/j.autrev.2015.01.009.

3    Carol L. Roberts et al., "Hypothesis: Increased Consumption of Emulsifiers as an Explanation for the Rising Incidence of Crohn's Disease," *Journal of Crohn's and Colitis* 7, no. 4 (2013): 338–41, doi:10.1016/j.crohns.2013.01.004.

4    Benoit Chassaing et al., "Dietary Emulsifiers Impact the Mouse Gut Microbiota Promoting Colitis and Metabolic Syndrome," *Nature* 519, no. 7541 (2015): 92–96, doi:10.1038/nature14232.

5    Alexander Swidsinski et al,. "Bacterial Overgrowth and Inflammation of Small Intestine after Carboxymethylcellulose Ingestion in Genetically Susceptible Mice," *Inflammatory Bowel Diseases* 15, no. 3 (2009): 359–64, doi:10.1002/ibd.20763.

6    A. Lerner and T. Matthias, "Changes in Intestinal Tight Junction Permeability Associated with Industrial Food Additives Explain the Rising Incidence of Autoimmune Disease," *Autoimmunity Reviews* 14 (June 2015): 479–89, doi: 10.1016/j.autrev.2015.01.009.

7    E. Richman and J. M. Rhodes, "Review Article: Evidence-Based Dietary Advice for Patients with Inflammatory Bowel Disease," *Alimentary Pharmacology and Therapeutics*, 2013, doi:10.1111/apt.12500.

8    A. Lerner and T. Matthias, "Changes in Intestinal Tight Junction Permeability Associated with Industrial Food Additives Explain the Rising Incidence of Autoimmune Disease," *Autoimmunity Reviews* 14 (June 2015): 479–89, doi: 10.1016/j.autrev.2015.01.009.

9    Jotham Suez et al., "Artificial Sweeteners Induce Glucose Intolerance by Altering the Gut Microbiota," *Nature*, 2014, doi:10.1038/nature13793.

10   Susan E. Swithers, "Artificial Sweeteners Produce the Counterintuitive Effect of Inducing Metabolic Derangements," *Trends in Endocrinology and Metabolism*, 2013, doi:10.1016/j.tem.2013.05.005.

11   Ibid.

12    Sharon P. G. Fowler et al., "Diet Soda Intake Is Associated with Long-Term Increases in Waist Circumference in a Biethnic Cohort of Older Adults: The San Antonio Longitudinal Study of Aging," *Journal of the American Geriatrics Society* 63, no. 4 (2015): 708–15, doi:10.1111/jgs.13376.

13    L. Montenegro et al., "Nonsteroidal Anti-Inflammatory Drug Induced Damage on Lower Gastro-Intestinal Tract: Is There an Involvement of Microbiota?," *Curr Drug Saf* 9, no. 3 (2014): 196–204, doi:10.2174/1574886309666140424143852.

14    Wojciech Marlicz et al., "Nonsteroidal Anti-Inflammatory Drugs, Proton Pump Inhibitors, and Gastrointestinal Injury: Contrasting Interactions in the Stomach and Small Intestine," *Mayo Clinic Proceedings*, 2014, doi:10.1016/j.mayocp.2014.07.015; Polychronis Pavlidis and Ingvar Bjarnason, "Aspirin Induced Adverse Effects on the Small and Large Intestine," *Current Pharmaceutical Design* 21, no. 35 (2015): 5089–93, www.ingentaconnect.com/content/ben/cpd/2015/00000021/00000035/art00007.

# CHAPTER 10

## HOW IMPORTANT IS DIETARY FIBER? YOU MIGHT BE SURPRISED . . .

## PROS AND CONS OF INCREASING DIETARY FIBER

You have likely heard that fiber is "healthy," but there is more to fiber than simply saying it's healthy or not healthy. One important question to ask is, are the purported health benefits seen with higher-fiber diets exclusively due to the fiber content? Probably not. When people start to eat a healthier diet, many factors change, including the amount of fiber they eat. If someone cuts out processed foods and sugar-sweetened beverages and replaces them with fruits, vegetables, and healthy meats and fats, many things happen, such as

- decreased sugar intake;
- decreased calorie intake;
- decreased carbohydrate intake;
- decreased additive intake;
- decreased processed fats (trans fats);

- increased fiber (fruits, vegetables, grains);
- increased protein;
- increased nutrients and vitamins;
- increased healthy fats.

It's important to understand that some of the health benefits of a higher-fiber diet appear to be due to other factors that accompany the diet and not necessarily the fiber itself. Also, remember that fiber can feed bacteria in the gut and therefore increase their numbers, which can be a problem for some.[1]

### FIBER TIP

In step 5 of our Great-in-8 Action Plan, you will work to broaden your diet, and as you do this, your fiber intake will increase. This is achieved as you start to eat more vegetables, fruits, and grains, if you tolerate them upon reintroduction. However, if you have IBS, SIBO, IBD, or just general digestive tract inflammation, too much fiber might aggravate your gut. So, if you start eating lots of vegetables and dietary fiber and notice your gut is bothered by this, you may want to eat a little less until your gut heals and then slowly work to see how much fiber you can tolerate. If your gut is sensitive, focusing on softer fibers can be helpful. Avoid lots of raw veggies, and opt for veggies that are softened via steaming or sautéing. Also, avoid the skins and seeds of fruits and vegetables, which are rougher and can be irritating. Again, focus on things that are soft.

Depending on how step 5 of our Great-in-8 Action Plan goes, you may have some concerns. If you end up settling into a diet that is lower in carbs and/or fiber, you might feel uneasy about not eating lots of the "healthy fiber" that everyone proclaims is so good for you. Maybe you feel better on a little less fiber but can't help second-guessing yourself because it seems everywhere you turn, you hear someone talking about how fiber feeds your gut bacteria and we need lots of healthy gut bacteria to be healthy. We have covered numerous reasons why this is simply not true for some. To help give you even more confidence, we'll take a dive into the pool of research on fiber, the research that actually matters to you, the research that asks questions like the following:

- What happens when someone like you eats more or less fiber?
- If *you* eat more or less fiber, can you affect your chances of developing certain diseases, like colon cancer or heart disease?

We will not get sidetracked by what happens when an obscure group of hunter-gatherers in Africa, who live nothing like you do and have digestive systems nothing like yours, eat a diet you could never eat. When we resurface, you will have a practical, non-fad-driven perspective on dietary

fiber. Let's get you the info you need to get healthy and then move on. We will cover dietary fiber's impact on

- digestive-tract cancer;
- IBD (inflammatory bowel disease);
- IBS (irritable bowel syndrome);
- diabetes;
- heart disease;
- obesity.

# DIETARY FIBER'S IMPACT ON SPECIFIC CONDITIONS

In the rest of this chapter, we'll work through each condition that might be affected by a lower-fiber diet. For each condition, I will

- summarize the data that shows fiber is helpful for that condition;
- summarize the data showing fiber is *not* helpful for that condition;
- provide a summary of fiber's impact on that condition.

There are a few conditions for which there is so little data that only a conclusion is needed. If you want a less detailed look at each condition, simply read the conclusion paragraph at the end of each topic. If you'd like to skip to the overall summary of fiber's impact on these conditions, go to "Fiber Conclusion—Do You Really Need to Feed Your Gut Bugs with Fiber?" at the end of the chapter.

## DIGESTIVE-TRACT CANCERS

Digestive cancers might be the most important issue involving fiber. Why? Because it's the only area where eating a lower-fiber diet might be problematic. We know that lower-fiber and/or lower-carb approaches can work well for weight loss, diabetes, metabolic syndrome, IBS, and IBD.

But what if you are successfully managing one of these conditions with a lower-fiber or lower-carb approach but you're afraid that if you don't consume enough roughage, you will have an increased risk of colorectal or other digestive tract cancers? This is an important question and one that requires significant, detailed attention.

### Digestive-tract cancers—dietary fiber helpful

Several systematic reviews and meta-analyses have shown that increased fiber consumption protects against colorectal cancer.[2] Increased fiber consumption has also been shown to be protective against stomach and esophageal cancer.[3] A meta-analysis showed an increased dietary fiber consumption was protective against cancer, heart disease, and death from any cause.[4] Other meta-analyses have shown similar results.

Is there a more beneficial fiber type—fruit, vegetable, or grain? Review papers show increased consumption of fruits and vegetables are associated with decreased gastrointestinal cancer risk.[5] A meta-analysis looking at twenty studies and nearly eleven thousand subjects found that dietary fruit fiber, vegetable fiber, and cereal grain fiber *all* protected against colorectal cancer.[6]

However, some research suggests grain fibers are slightly more protective. A meta-analysis of twenty-five studies found dietary-fiber intake was protective, with the greater fiber intake leading to greatest protection. Specifically, total fiber, cereal fiber, and whole-grain fiber were found to be protective, whereas fruit and vegetable fiber consumption did not show protection.[7]

A meta-analysis of prospective cohort studies found that cereal fiber and, to a lesser extent, vegetable fiber were protective against death from any cause. Fruit fiber consumption provided no protection, however. The researchers controlled for other healthy lifestyle variables that sometimes accompany increased fiber consumption, and this relationship was still present.[8]

So, essentially what we see is all fiber types seem to offer protection; however, grain fibers might be slightly more protective. It's also possible that the reason why we see more protection from grains is because, worldwide, healthy diets centered around whole grains are more common than healthy diets centered around fruits and vegetables; therefore, we simply have more data on grains. If we had more data on fruit- and vegetable-centered diets, we might find them equally protective or maybe even more protective than grains. In a moment, we will compare grain-centered diets to fruit- and vegetable-centered diets and see reinforcement of the idea that fruit- and vegetable-centered diets appear healthier.

Grains have received a lot of bad press lately, especially those containing gluten. Rightfully so—if you have a problem with gluten, you should avoid it, as we have already discussed. However, I fear some have become overzealous in their anti-grain and antigluten sentiments. There are studies showing increased grain consumption correlates with better health. A meta-analysis of eleven studies and over 1.7 million people found that whole-grain consumption was protective against colorectal cancer.[9] Another meta-analysis found that whole-grain consumption was protective against cardiovascular disease, cancer, and ***overall chance of death***.[10]

A meta-analysis of fourteen clinical trials found dietary fiber consumption caused a slight but significant decrease in the inflammatory marker C-reactive protein. Many of the fibers were derived from grain; eight of the fourteen studies used fibers containing gluten.[11]

If grains were a universal poison, we wouldn't see all these benefits. This doesn't mean you have to consume gluten-containing grains, or any grains, but it does mean you shouldn't be fearful of all grains in any quantity.

### Digestive-tract cancers—dietary fiber no effect

But what if you don't do well on grains? Or what if you are eating a lower-fiber or low-carb diet because too much fiber or too many carbs cause symptoms like bloating, weight gain, or high blood sugar? While there is much data showing fiber to be protective, there is also much data showing fiber offers no benefit.

A systematic review of forty-three studies examined the association between cereal-fiber intake, whole-grain intake, or both to cancer risk. The vast majority of the studies found that neither cereal fiber nor whole-grain consumption protected against cancer.[12]

In another study over eighty-eight thousand women were followed for sixteen years to assess dietary-fiber intake's impact on colorectal cancer. No association between fiber intake and colorectal cancer was found.[13]

Another study examined the diet of 816 people with colorectal cancer compared to healthy controls. Increased fiber consumption did not protect against colorectal cancer. However, both rice and fruit consumption appeared protective against colorectal cancer. Vegetable intake had no association; however, a high intake of nonrice cereals *increased* risk of colorectal cancer.[14]

The diets of forty-eight thousand men were analyzed for a relationship between dietary factors and colon cancer. No association between fiber or vegetable intake and colon cancer was found.[15] A systematic review with meta-analysis found no significant association between overall fiber intake and small-intestinal cancer.[16] The *British Journal of Nutrition* performed a systematic review and did not find oat consumption to be protective against colon cancer.[17]

Are you starting to see there is quite a bit of data showing that fiber isn't the colorectal-cancer-preventing miracle it is sometimes portrayed to be? I hope so. I'll list just a few more points regarding fiber and colorectal cancer.

According to a systematic review from the prestigious Cochrane Database, dietary fiber did not protect against colorectal cancer or colorectal cancer recurrence. This study examined five randomized clinical trials.[18] In another review of clinical trials, it was found there was inconsistent evidence regarding dietary fiber's role in prevention of colorectal cancer.[19]

We discussed earlier how those who increase their fiber intake may simultaneously be changing their behaviors in other health-improving ways. For example, someone might increase his or her fiber intake, stop smoking, and start exercising all at the same time. The *Journal of the American Medical Association* examined thirteen prospective cohort studies, involving 725,628 people, and the relationship between fiber intake and colorectal cancer risk. The researchers adjusted for these other variables, like exercising. They found no protective effect of fiber intake (of any kind) on colorectal cancer.[20]

### Digestive-tract cancers and dietary fiber conclusion

OK . . . what to do? Simply continue to follow the steps in our Great-in-8. Our goal will be to get you on the broadest diet possible, one that includes a broad array of foods that provide fiber and carbohydrates. However, if you end up on a diet that is lower in carbs or fiber, you shouldn't live in fear. Although some evidence shows dietary fiber protects against digestive tract cancers, there is an equivalent amount of data showing fiber does *not* protect against digestive tract cancers—probably because there are different types of gut ecosystems requiring differing amounts of fiber. It is likely that any healthy diet that avoids processed foods and focuses on whole, fresh foods will reduce chances of colon cancer. This is likely why a recent trial found both the Paleo diet and the Mediterranean diet decreased colon-cancer risk, even though these diets differ in their carb and fiber content.[21] So, if you don't feel well when you eat certain high-fiber or higher-carb foods, don't force yourself to eat them—ignore the dogma. Do your best to work toward the broadest diet you can, minimize processed-food consumption, and you'll be fine. Whatever diet you end up on, you'll be armed with the information you need to follow it with confidence.

## IBD

### *IBD—dietary fiber helpful*
A meta-analysis of observational studies of dietary-fiber intake has shown a reduced risk of IBD with an increased intake of dietary fiber.[22] There also appears to be a dose response, meaning the more dietary fiber you eat, the greater the protection. The rough approximations regarding specific intakes from this study are high fiber equals 24 g per day, low fiber equals 4 g per day.

Nineteen studies examining twenty-six hundred IBD patients found fiber intake to be protective against developing IBD.[23] However, once you *have* IBD, it appears that there is no benefit of increased fiber consumption in decreasing disease activity.[24]

Dietary surveys from over sixteen hundred patients found that avoiding fiber or eating lower fiber increased the risk of having a flare-up if you have Crohn's disease. There was no association with ulcerative colitis, however.[25] Other studies have found adding some fiber to the diet may help with Crohn's disease.[26]

### *IBD—dietary fiber no effect*
A systematic review of twelve clinical trials found exclusion diets (meaning food allergens have been removed) and the low-FODMAP diet to be effective treatments for IBD.[27] Note, the low-FODMAP diet restricts certain types of fiber.

One review article found a low intake of insoluble fiber might be helpful for IBD.[28] The British Dietetic Association's dietary guidelines for managing Crohn's disease recommends elemental or semielemental diets as a preliminary treatment consideration.[29] A major reason the elemental/semielemental diets are effective is their low-fiber content.

### *IBD dietary fiber conclusion*
Increasing dietary fiber may be helpful for IBD and Crohn's disease in particular. However, eating a lower-fiber diet has been shown to be helpful, too. The best strategy if you have IBD is to start with a lower-fiber (10 g per day) approach, especially if you are in a flare. Then, slowly work your way up. What might this look like? Initially, it might involve the hybrid use of elemental/semi-elemental-liquid shakes interspersed with whole foods that are lower in fiber and/or lower in FODMAPs. Then, as you become stable, gradually increase your fiber intake—just as we will during our reintroduction step. If you notice you start to react once your fiber intake hits a certain level (for example, at 20 g or 30 g), scale back. For those with IBD, the most typical reactions will be more frequent stools, looser stools or even diarrhea, and bowel urgency. Regarding counting your grams of fiber, I would only recommend doing this until you get a sense of how much fiber you can and can't tolerate. Then, simply follow the intuition you have developed. This process is outlined in our Great-in-8, so if you're confused now, don't worry. Simply continue with our plan.

One side note before we leave the topic of fiber and IBD—a concept that helps us think in a less fiber-centric way—we discussed earlier how some are afraid to eat a lower-fiber diet because they think it will increase their risk of colon cancer. We discussed how this doesn't appear to be true, because there is about as much evidence showing fiber intake *doesn't* influence cancer risk as data showing fiber intake is protective. It's important to keep in mind that having inflammatory bowel disease increases risk of colon cancer. Also, the level of the disease's activity increases risk: the more active, the more risk;[30] the less active the disease, the less risk. So, if you have to eat a lower-fiber diet to manage your IBD, you should mitigate your colon-cancer risk. It's more important to eat a diet that manages the inflammation of IBD than it is to eat a diet that feeds your gut bugs. We always want you to reach for the broadest diet possible; however, if you end up on a limited diet, it's OK. This comes back to our principle of first eating to reduce inflammation rather than eating to feed your gut bugs.

## IBS

### IBS—dietary fiber helpful

A systematic review of sixty-five dietary studies examined the effect of dietary-cereal-fiber intake and bowel function. They found that increased intake of cereal fiber increased stool bulk and reduced constipation.[31] Similarly, increased dietary fiber improved constipation, according to a review of fifty-one studies.[32]

An analysis to determine if dietary fiber is a cost-effective treatment for constipation found that even a small increase in dietary-fiber intake could reduce health-care costs related to constipation.[33]

A meta-analysis of grain-fiber consumption found increased grain-fiber consumption caused more frequent bowel movements, more fecal weight, and aided in remission of functional bowel disorders. There were no negative bowel side effects.[34]

### IBS—dietary fiber no effect

The British Dietetic Association performed a systematic review of eighty-six studies to generate dietary recommendations for IBS.[35] They concluded that the first step should be nutritional coaching on healthy eating (reduce sugar, processed foods, alcohol, and caffeine, and eat more

fruits and vegetables). If this first step doesn't work, the second step is a low-FODMAP diet (by the way, this is exactly what we are doing in our Great-in-8). They also summarized eleven studies examining dietary-fiber intake's effect on IBS (abdominal pain, bloating, constipation, and diarrhea). Increasing dietary-fiber intake was helpful in three studies, while it caused either no change or detriment in eight studies.

A small clinical trial tracked twelve subjects who had IBS and went on a low-fiber diet.[36] These subjects saw a reduction in the hydrogen gas that can be produced by small-intestinal bacterial overgrowth (SIBO) and a significant reduction in symptoms.[37]

We have covered how fiber can help with constipation, but what about diarrhea? Two review papers that provide clinical guidelines for doctors concluded that increasing fiber should not be done in those with diarrheal-type IBS (diarrhea, gas, pain, bloating).[38]

Two studies have shown that a low-carb diet (remember, low-carb diets tend to be lower in fiber) helps to reduce gastroesophageal reflux disease (GERD), reflux, and heartburn.[39] What's interesting here is a systematic review has found there is a strong overlap between IBS and GERD.[40] With this in mind, it's not surprising that the low-FODMAP diet, which has been shown to be helpful for IBS, has been shown helpful for GERD as well.

### IBS and dietary fiber conclusion

Increasing dietary fiber can help or harm those with IBS. Those with constipation have the greatest chance of benefit. Those with diarrhea should be careful, because they have the highest chance of harm. Reducing dietary-fiber intake can also help with IBS. If you are someone who is highly symptomatic, the best strategy is to start with a lower-fiber diet and then slowly increase fiber intake to find what level works best for you. If you are someone who only has minor symptoms, there is a smaller chance of a negative reaction to fiber, and you probably won't need to worry about your fiber intake. Working through the Great-in-8 will help guide you toward your ideal intake.

## DIABETES, HEART DISEASE, AND OBESITY

### Diabetes, heart disease, and obesity—dietary fiber helpful

A 2016 meta-analysis concluded that a higher intake of fruits and vegetables was associated with lower risk of type 2 diabetes.[42] Not surprisingly, it has been concluded that the greater the quantity and variety of fruit and vegetable intake, the lower the risk of type 2 diabetes.[43]

Another meta-analysis has shown that fiber intake protects against type 2 diabetes.[44] Fruit and vegetable fiber appears to be more protective than cereal fiber. This is likely because cereal fibers often contain more grams of carbs than fruits and vegetables.

When we say "increased fruit, vegetable, and whole-grain consumption" is protective, this usually means it's protective compared to a standard American diet or other type of unhealthy diet. Said another way, we are looking at how helpful the standard nutritional advice of "increase consumption of fruits, vegetables, and whole grains" is compared to a terrible diet of processed food, added sugar, and trans fats. But what if we start comparing different types of healthy diets? This could help us understand which healthy diet is the healthiest, right? When comparing healthy diets, three diets are typically compared:

- Traditional lower-fat, higher-carb diets
- Paleo diets
- Lower-carb diets

How does this relate to fiber, though? Any healthy diet plan tends to have more fiber than a standard American diet or a generally unhealthy diet filled with processed foods. However, the traditional lower-fat/higher-carb diets have the highest amounts of fiber.[45]

The lower-carb diets have the lowest amounts of fiber, and the Paleo diet falls somewhere in between. So, if the relatively lower-fiber diets are shown to be healthier, it supports the thinking that fiber is not the be-all and end-all of a healthy diet. Recent research in diabetes, heart disease, and obesity has performed these comparisons and provides some interesting insights. Also, remember that the traditional higher-carb/lower-fat diets are the most similar to what the Africans eat—yes, they eat grains! (For a refresher, revisit chapters 2 and 3.)

### Diabetes, heart disease, and obesity—dietary fiber not helpful

We discussed earlier how you should first eat to control blood sugar and not worry about feeding your gut bacteria with prebiotics/fiber. Well, the *American Journal of Clinical Nutrition* examined twenty-two studies and found a diet that controls blood sugar is better at reducing inflammation than a diet that increases fiber.[46]

A clinical trial comparing a low-carb diet to a more traditional low-fat diet found the low-carb diet worked better for treating type 2 diabetes.[47] Another clinical trial comparing low-fat versus low-carb diets for type 2 diabetes found they both worked, but low-carb worked better.[48] A Paleo diet has been shown to work better than a conventional lower-fat/higher-grain diet for type 2 diabetes.[49]

Again, there are many studies showing traditional low-fat/high-carb diets that increase fiber, fruit, vegetable, and whole-grain intake all help with heart disease and obesity,[50] but let's continue to look at what happens when we compare different healthy diets to see if we can find the healthiest diet.

A recent trial found that a Paleo diet improves cholesterol levels to a greater extent than traditional heart-healthy (low-fat) dietary recommendations.[51] Another study found consuming a Paleo-type diet for only two weeks improved several cardiovascular risk factors compared to a healthy reference diet (traditional low-fat diet) in subjects with metabolic syndrome.[52]

A Paleo diet caused better improvements to blood sugar control and several cardiovascular risk factors compared to a diabetes diet (traditional lower-fat/higher-carb diet) in patients with type 2 diabetes.[53] A systematic review with meta-analysis shows the Paleo diet is more effective for metabolic syndrome than standard nutritional-recommendation diets, which are typically lower-fat and higher-carb/fiber.[54]

What about the best diet for weight loss? While all healthy diets are helpful, it appears lower-carb diets have a slight edge for weight loss. A systematic review with meta-analysis of fifty-three studies found that low-carb diets are better for weight loss than low-fat diets.[55]

Throughout this book, we have been discussing the importance of looking at clinical research to guide our health-care decisions rather than speculating from theory or mechanism. Low-fat diets are a good illustration of this. The *mechanistic theory* says that because fat contains more calories than a carbohydrate or protein (fat has nine calories per gram, protein has four calories per gram, and carbohydrate has four calories per gram), you should eat less fat, which will then make you consume fewer calories, and you will then lose weight. However, what do we see when we look at the *clinical research*? Clinical research points to higher-fat/lower-carb diets working better for weight loss. So, the theory said one thing, but the real world showed something else.

### Diabetes, heart disease, and obesity conclusion

When we look at the traditional healthy diet of increased fruits, vegetables, and whole grains (which are higher in carbs and fiber) compared to more contemporary healthy diets, like Paleo or lower carb (which are lower in carbs and fiber), what do we see? We see all healthy diets can improve your health, but when we compare different healthy diets, it appears a Paleo diet or a lower-carb diet is more effective. Paleo and lower-carb diets tend to be lower in carbs and relatively lower in fiber. This perfectly reinforces our principle that it's more important to eat to control your blood sugar (by eating a lower-carb or Paleo diet) than it is to eat to feed your gut bugs (by eating a diet that is high in fiber and carbs). If you're doing better on a lower- or moderate-carb approach, don't feel pressured by the fiber enthusiasts to change. Listen to your body. Keep in mind that some will do better on a higher-carb diet. How do you determine what your ideal carb and fiber intake is? Start eating a lower-carb/fiber diet, and then gradually work your way upward to find your ideal intake. This is exactly what we will work through in our Great-in-8, with the initial dietary changes in step 1, and then in step 5, the reintroduction.

# FIBER CONCLUSION— DO YOU REALLY NEED TO FEED YOUR GUT BUGS WITH FIBER?

When we take a look at both sides of the evidence, it's clear to see fiber can be a double-edged sword. It may help some, and it may harm others. For high-risk diseases like digestive tract cancers, fiber has not been consistently shown to help. For metabolic conditions like diabetes, obesity, and heart disease, it appears eating to control blood sugar (which often happens via a lower-fiber diet) is more important than eating to increase fiber. For those with constipation, there is a good chance upping your fiber will help you become more regular. For those with IBS or IBD, fiber may or may not be helpful, so it's worth cautiously trying to increase your intake.

Sorry to deprive you of the easy "this is good/ that is bad" dichotomy, but fiber is not a black-and-white issue. What this all really boils down to is you should simply work through our Great-in-8 steps to find your personalized ideal diet—that is, to find the ideal amount of "rain" for your gut eco-system. Then, be confident with where you end up. Remember to periodically expand your dietary boundaries so you're on the broadest diet possible. Do this, and you will thrive.

Information is very powerful. Imagine if my opinion was that dietary fiber was bad. I could

then write this book citing *only* the information that supports my assertion that dietary fiber is bad. You would then finish this book thinking, "Man, I should really start avoiding dietary fiber." But remember some of the benefits of dietary fiber we just covered, especially for those with constipation, for example? If I had chosen to include only the information that supports my opinion, you would have none of the "fiber is helpful" data. You would be misinformed! I can't emphasize enough the importance of searching for and learning from those who appear to have a reasonable view, those who are willing to look at both sides of an issue to give you a well-informed opinion. If you carry this principle forward with you, you can save yourself much confusion and frustration.

In part 1, we obtained a solid understanding of how important your gut is, how your gut works, how your gut can affect many systems of your body, and how problems in your gut may underlie your health ailments. We gained an appreciation for how all guts are different and have unique needs, just like different ecosystems require differing amounts of rainfall. We discussed early life factors that are important in shaping your gut microbiota and your immune system.

Here in part 2, we detailed dietary strategies for optimum gut health, including inflammatory foods, food allergens, carbs, fiber, and prebiotic intake. We discussed fasting, meal frequency, and processed foods. We then ended part 2 with a detailed and unbiased overview of dietary fiber's impact on your health.

Let's move on to part 3, where we'll discuss the environmental and lifestyle factors required for optimum gut and overall health.

# CONCEPT SUMMARY

- Supplemental and dietary fiber can be helpful for some, but the health benefits of fiber have been exaggerated.

- Generally speaking, carbs, fiber, and prebiotics occur in foods together. When you eat to increase or decrease one of them, you tend to increase or decrease all of them.

- When comparing different healthy diets, those that are lower in carbs often outperform healthy diets that are higher in carbs. However, all healthy diets are helpful.

- We will sequentially experiment with adding in fiber, prebiotics, and resistant starch. This will help some but cause reactions in others, so be cautious here, and listen to your body.

1   S. Macfarlane et al., "Review Article: Prebiotics in the Gastrointestinal Tract," *Alimentary Pharmacology and Therapeutics*, 2006, doi:10.1111/j.1365-2036.2006.03042.x; S. Hooda et al., "454 Pyrosequencing Reveals a Shift in Fecal Microbiota of Healthy Adult Men Consuming Polydextrose or Soluble Corn Fiber," *Journal of Nutrition* 142, no. 7 (2012): 1259–65, doi:10.3945/jn.112.158766; Evelyne M. Dewulf et al., "Insight into the Prebiotic Concept: Lessons from an Exploratory, Double-Blind Intervention Study with Inulin-Type Fructans in Obese Women," *Gut* 62, no. 8 (2013): 1112–21, doi:10.1136/gutjnl-2012-303304.

2   Salman Azeem et al., "Diet and Colorectal Cancer Risk in Asia—A Systematic Review," *Asian Pacific Journal of Cancer Prevention* 16, no. 13 (2015): 5389–96, doi:10.7314/APJCP.2015.16.13.5389; Federica Turati et al., "Fruit and Vegetables and Cancer Risk: A Review of Southern European Studies," *British Journal of Nutrition* 113 Suppl., no. S2 (2015): S102–10, doi:10.1017/S0007114515000148; Qiwen Ben et al., "Dietary-Fiber Intake Reduces Risk for Colorectal Adenoma: A Meta-Analysis," *Gastroenterology* 146, no. 3 (2014), doi:10.1053/j.gastro.2013.11.003; D. Aune et al., "Dietary Fibre, Whole Grains, and Risk of Colorectal Cancer: Systematic Review and Dose-Response Meta-Analysis of Prospective Studies," *BMJ* 343, no. nov10 1 (2011): d6617–d6617, doi:10.1136/bmj.d6617; Kun Chen et al., "Meta-Analysis of Risk Factors for Colorectal Cancer," *World Journal of Gastroenterology* 9, no. 7 (2003): 1598–1600, ovidsp.ovid.com/ovidweb.cgi?T=JS&PAGE=reference&D=med4&NEWS=N&AN=12854172.

3   Zhizhong Zhang et al., "Dietary-Fiber Intake Reduces Risk for Gastric Cancer: A Meta-Analysis," *Gastroenterology* 145, no. 1 (2013), doi:10.1053/j.gastro.2013.04.001; Lingli Sun et al., "Dietary-Fiber Intake Reduces Risk for Barrett's Esophagus and Esophageal Cancer," *Critical Reviews in Food Science and Nutrition*, 2015, doi:10.1080/10408398.2015.1067596; Helen G. Coleman et al., "Dietary Fiber and the Risk of Precancerous Lesions and Cancer of the Esophagus: A Systematic Review and Meta-Analysis," *Nutrition Reviews* 71, no. 7 (2013): 474–82, doi:10.1111/nure.12032.

4   Lihua Liu et al., "Fiber Consumption and All-Cause, Cardiovascular, and Cancer Mortalities: A Systematic Review and Meta-Analysis of Cohort Studies," *Molecular Nutrition and Food Research*, 2015, doi:10.1002/mnfr.201400449.

5   Federica Turati et al., "Fruit and Vegetables and Cancer Risk: A Review of Southern European Studies," *British Journal of Nutrition* 113 Suppl., no. S2 (2015): S102–10, doi:10.1017/S0007114515000148.

6   Qiwen Ben et al., "Dietary-Fiber Intake Reduces Risk for Colorectal Adenoma: A Meta-Analysis," *Gastroenterology* 146, no. 3 (2014), doi:10.1053/j.gastro.2013.11.003.

7   D. Aune et al., "Dietary Fibre, Whole Grains, and Risk of Colorectal Cancer: Systematic Review and Dose-Response Meta-Analysis of Prospective Studies," *BMJ* 343, no. nov10 1 (2011): d6617–d6617, doi:10.1136/bmj.d6617.

8   Youngyo Kim and Youjin Je, "Dietary-Fiber Intake and Total Mortality: A Meta-Analysis of Prospective Cohort Studies," *American Journal of Epidemiology*, 2014, doi:10.1093/aje/kwu174.

9   P. Haas et al., "Effectiveness of Whole-Grain Consumption in the Prevention of Colorectal Cancer: Meta-Analysis of Cohort Studies," *International Journal of Food Sciences and Nutrition* 60, no. September (2009): 1–13, doi:10.1080/09637480802183380.

10  G. C. Chen et al., "Whole-Grain Intake and Total, Cardiovascular, and Cancer Mortality: A Systematic Review and Meta-Analysis of Prospective Studies," *American Journal of Clinical Nutrition* 104, no. 1 (2016): 164–72, doi:10.3945/ajcn.115.122432.

11    Jun Jiao et al., "Effect of Dietary Fiber on Circulating C-Reactive Protein in Overweight and Obese Adults: A Meta-Analysis of Randomized Controlled Trials," *International Journal of Food Sciences and Nutrition* 66, no. 1 (2015): 114–19, doi:10.3109/09637486.2014.959898.

12    Nour Makarem et al., "Consumption of Whole Grains and Cereal Fiber in Relation to Cancer Risk: A Systematic Review of Longitudinal Studies," *Nutrition Reviews* 74, no. 6 (2016): 353–73, doi:10.1093/nutrit/nuw003.

13    Charles S. Fuchs et al., "Dietary Fiber and the Risk of Colorectal Cancer and Adenoma in Women," *New England Journal of Medicine* 340, no. 3 (1999): 169–76, doi:10.1056/NEJM199901213400301.

14    Kazuhiro Uchida et al., "Dietary Fiber, Source Foods, and Colorectal Cancer Risk: The Fukuoka Colorectal Cancer Study," *Scandinavian Journal of Gastroenterology* 45, no. 10 (2010): 1223–31, doi:10.3109/00365521.2010.492528.

15    Alberto Ascherio et al., "Intake of Fat, Meat, and Fiber in Relation to Risk of Colon Cancer in Men," *Cancer Research* 54, no. 9 (1994): 2390–97, doi:10.1519/JSC.0000000000000496.

16    Caoimhe M. Bennett et al., "Lifestyle Factors and Small Intestine Adenocarcinoma Risk: A Systematic Review and Meta-Analysis," *Cancer Epidemiology* 39, no. 3 (2015): 265–73, doi:10.1016/j.canep.2015.02.001; Arthur Schatzkin et al., "Prospective Study of Dietary Fiber, Whole-Grain Foods, and Small Intestinal Cancer," *Gastroenterology* 135, no. 4 (2008): 1163–67, doi:10.1053/j.gastro.2008.07.015.

17    Frank Thies et al., "Oats and Bowel Disease: A Systematic Literature Review," *British Journal of Nutrition* 112 Suppl. (2014): S19–30, doi:10.1017/S0007114514002281.

18    T. Asano and R. S. McLeod, "Dietary Fibre for the Prevention of Colorectal Adenomas and Carcinomas," *Cochrane Database of Systematic Reviews*, no. 2 (2002): CD003430, doi:10.1002/14651858.CD003430.

19    Ningoi Hou et al., "Prevention of Colorectal Cancer and Dietary Management," *Chinese Clinical Oncology* 2, no. 2 (2013): 13, doi:10.3978/j.issn.2304-3865.2013.04.03.

20    Yikyung Park et al., "Dietary-Fiber Intake and Risk of Colorectal Cancer: A Pooled Analysis of Prospective Cohort Studies," *JAMA: Journal of the American Medical Association* 294, no. 22 (2005): 2849–57, doi:10.1001/jama.294.22.2849.

21    Kristine A. Whalen et al., "Paleolithic and Mediterranean Diet Pattern Scores and Risk of Incident, Sporadic Colorectal Adenomas," *American Journal of Epidemiology* 180, no. 11 (2014): 1088–97, doi:10.1093/aje/kwu235.

22    Xiaoqin Liu et al., "Dietary-Fiber Intake Reduces Risk of Inflammatory Bowel Disease: Result from a Meta-Analysis," *Nutrition Research*, 2015, doi:10.1016/j.nutres.2015.05.021.

23    Jason K. Hou et al., "Dietary Intake and Risk of Developing Inflammatory Bowel Disease: A Systematic Review of the Literature," *American Journal of Gastroenterology* 106, no. 4 (2011): 563–73, doi:10.1038/ajg.2011.44.

24    Linda Wedlake et al., "Fiber in the Treatment and Maintenance of Inflammatory Bowel Disease: A Systematic Review of Randomized Controlled Trials," *Inflammatory Bowel Diseases* 20, no. 3 (2014): 576–86, doi:10.1097/01.MIB.0000437984.92565.31.

25    Carol S. Brotherton et al., "Avoidance of Fiber Is Associated with Greater Risk of Crohn's Disease Flare in a Six-Month Period," *Clinical Gastroenterology and Hepatology* 14, no. 8 (2016): 1130–36, doi:10.1016/j.cgh.2015.12.029.

26    Carol S. Brotherton et al., "A High-Fiber Diet May Improve Bowel Function and Health-Related Quality of Life in Patients with Crohn's Disease," *Gastroenterology Nursing* 37, no. 3 (2014): 206–16, doi:10.1097/SGA.0000000000000047.

27    Ashley Charlebois et al., "The Impact of Dietary Interventions on the Symptoms of Inflammatory Bowel Disease: A Systematic Review," *Critical Reviews in Food Science and Nutrition* 56, no. 8 (2016): 1370–78, doi:10.1080/10408398.2012.760515.

28    E. Richman and J. M. Rhodes, "Review Article: Evidence-Based Dietary Advice for Patients with Inflammatory Bowel Disease," *Alimentary Pharmacology and Therapeutics*, 2013, doi:10.1111/apt.12500.

29    J. Lee et al., "British Dietetic Association Evidence-Based Guidelines for the Dietary Management of Crohn's Disease in Adults," *Journal of Human Nutrition and Dietetics* 27, no. 3 (2014): 207–18, doi:10.1111/jhn.12176.

30    C. Pohl et al., "Chronic Inflammatory Bowel Disease and Cancer," *Hepato-Gastroenterology* 47, no. 31 (2000): 57–70; Janoš Terzić et al., "Inflammation and Colon Cancer," *Gastroenterology* 138, no. 6 (2010), doi:10.1053/j.gastro.2010.01.058; Lidija Klampfer, "Cytokines, Inflammation, and Colon Cancer," *Current Cancer Drug Targets* 11, no. 4 (2011): 451–64, doi:10.2174/156800911795538066.

31    Jan de Vries et al., "Effects of Cereal Fiber on Bowel Function: A Systematic Review of Intervention Trials," *World Journal of Gastroenterology* 21, no. 29 (2015): 8868–77, doi:10.3748/wjg.v21.i29.8952.

32    Stefan A. Mueller-Lissner and Arnold Wald, "Constipation in Adults," *BMJ Clinical Evidence* 2010 (July 5, 2010): www.ncbi.nlm.nih .gov/pubmed/21418672.

33    Mohammad M. H. Abdullah et al., "Dietary Fibre Intakes and Reduction in Functional Constipation Rates among Canadian Adults: A Cost-of-Illness Analysis," *Food and Nutrition Research* 59 (2015), doi:10.3402/fnr.v59.28646.

34    Jing Zhu et al., "Meta-Analysis on the Relationship among Fiber of Grain and Intestinal Motility and Symptoms," [In Chinese.] *Journal of Hygiene Research* 44, no. 1 (January 2015): 1–7, www.ncbi.nlm.nih.gov/pubmed/25958626.

35    Y. A. McKenzie et al., "British Dietetic Association Systematic Review and Evidence-Based Practice Guidelines for the Dietary Management of Irritable Bowel Syndrome in Adults (2016 Update)," *Journal of Human Nutrition and Dietetics* 29, no. 5 (2016): 549–75, doi:10.1111/jhn.12385.

36    Keith L. E. Dear et al., "Do Interventions Which Reduce Colonic Bacterial Fermentation Improve Symptoms of Irritable Bowel Syndrome?," *Digestive Diseases and Sciences* 50, no. 4 (2005): 758–66, doi:10.1007/s10620-005-2570-4.

37    Ibid.

38    Anastasia Rivkin and Sergey Rybalov, "Update on the Management of Diarrhea-Predominant Irritable Bowel Syndrome: Focus on Rifaximin and Eluxadoline," *Pharmacotherapy*, 2016, doi:10.1002/phar.1712; Oliver Grundmann and Saunjoo L. Yoon, "Irritable Bowel Syndrome: Epidemiology, Diagnosis, and Treatment: An Update for Health-Care Practitioners," *Journal of Gastroenterology and Hepatology* 25, no. 4 (2010): 691–99, doi:10.1111/j.1440-1746.2009.06120.x.

39    Gregory L. Austin et al., "A Very Low-Carbohydrate Diet Improves Gastroesophageal Reflux and Its Symptoms," *Digestive Diseases and Sciences* 51, no. 8 (2006): 1307–12, doi:10.1007/s10620-005-9027-7; W. S. Yancy et al., "Improvement of Gastroesophageal Reflux Disease after Initiation of a Low-Carbohydrate Diet: Five Brief Case Reports," *Alternative Therapies in Health and Medicine* 7, no. 6 (2001).

40    Igor Nastaskin et al., "Studying the Overlap between IBS and GERD: A Systematic Review of the Literature," *Digestive Diseases and Sciences*, 2006, doi:10.1007/s10620-006-9306-y.

41    S. S. Rao et al., "Systematic Review: Dietary Fibre and FODMAP-Restricted Diet in the Management of Constipation and Irritable Bowel Syndrome," *Alimentary Pharmacology and Therapeutics* 41, no. 12 (2015): 1256–70, doi:10.1111/apt.13167.

42    P. Y. Wang et al., "Higher Intake of Fruits, Vegetables, or Their Fiber Reduces the Risk of Type 2 Diabetes: A Meta-Analysis," *Journal of Diabetes Investigation*. 7, no. 1 (2016): 56–69, doi:10.1111/jdi.12376.

43    A. J. Cooper et al., "A Prospective Study of the Association between Quantity and Variety of Fruit and Vegetable Intake and Incident Type 2 Diabetes," *Diabetes Care* 35, no. 6 (2012): 1293–1300, doi:10.2337/dc11-2388.

44    InterAct Consortium, "Dietary Fibre and Incidence of Type 2 Diabetes in Eight European Countries: The EPIC-InterAct Study and a Meta-Analysis of Prospective Studies," *Diabetologia* 58, no. 7 (2015): 1394–1408, doi:10.1007/s00125-015-3585-9.

45    Yunsheng Ma et al., "A Dietary Quality Comparison of Popular Weight-Loss Plans," *Journal of the American Dietetic Association* 107, no. 10 (2007): 1786–91, doi:10.1016/j.jada.2007.07.013; Leach, Jeff, "Paleo versus Vegetarian—Who Eats More Fiber?," *Human Food Project*, July 10, 2015, http://humanfoodproject.com/paleo-versus-vegetarian-who-eats-more-fiber/.

46    Anette E. Buyken et al., "Association between Carbohydrate Quality and Inflammatory Markers: Systematic Review of Observational and Interventional Studies," *American Journal of Clinical Nutrition*, 2014, doi:10.3945/ajcn.113.074252.

47    Laura R. Saslow et al., "A Randomized Pilot Trial of a Moderate Carbohydrate Diet Compared to a Very Low Carbohydrate Diet in Overweight or Obese Individuals with Type 2 Diabetes Mellitus or Prediabetes," *PLoS ONE* 9, no. 4 (2014), doi:10.1371/journal .pone.0091027.

48    Jeannie Tay et al., "Comparison of Low- and High-Carbohydrate Diets for Type 2 Diabetes Management: A Randomized Trial," *American Journal of Clinical Nutrition* 102, no. 4 (2015): 780–90, doi:10.3945/ajcn.115.112581.

49    U. Masharani et al., "Metabolic and Physiologic Effects from Consuming a Hunter-Gatherer (Paleolithic)-Type Diet in Type 2 Diabetes," *European Journal of Clinical Nutrition* 69, no. 8 (2015): 944–48, doi:10.1038/ejcn.2015.39.

50    Janice I. Harland and Lynne E Garton, "Whole-Grain Intake as a Marker of Healthy Body Weight and Adiposity," *Public Health Nutrition* 11, no. 6 (2008), doi:10.1017/S1368980007001279; P. Pietinen, "Intake of Dietary Fiber and Risk of Coronary Heart Disease in a Cohort of Finnish Men. The Alpha-Tocopherol, Beta-Carotene Cancer Prevention Study," *Circulation*, 94:2720–27, 1996, http:// onlinelibrary.wiley.com/o/cochrane/clcentral/articles/187/CN-00134187/frame.html; Yihua Wu et al., "Association between Dietary-Fiber Intake and Risk of Coronary Heart Disease: A Meta-Analysis," *Clinical Nutrition* 34, no. 4 (2015): 603–11, doi:10.1016 /j.clnu.2014.05.009; Mark A. Pereira et al., "Dietary Fiber and Risk of Coronary Heart Disease: A Pooled Analysis of Cohort Studies,"

*Archives of Internal Medicine* 164, no. 4 (2004): 370–76, doi:10.1097/01.ieb.0000142783.97667.b5; Yang Yang et al., "Association between Dietary Fiber and Lower Risk of All-Cause Mortality: A Meta-Analysis of Cohort Studies," *American Journal of Epidemiology* 181, no. 2 (2015): 83–91, doi:10.1093/aje/kwu257.

51   Robert L. Pastore et al., "Paleolithic Nutrition Improves Plasma Lipid Concentrations of Hypercholesterolemic Adults to a Greater Extent Than Traditional Heart-Healthy Dietary Recommendations," *Nutrition Research* 35, no. 6 (2015): 474–79, doi:10.1016/j.nutres.2015.05.002.

52   Inge Boers et al., "Favourable Effects of Consuming a Palaeolithic-Type Diet on Characteristics of the Metabolic Syndrome: A Randomized Controlled Pilot-Study," *Lipids in Health and Disease* 13, no. 1 (2014): 160, doi:10.1186/1476-511X-13-160.

53   Tommy Jönsson et al., "Beneficial Effects of a Paleolithic Diet on Cardiovascular Risk Factors in Type 2 Diabetes: A Randomized Crossover Pilot Study," *Cardiovascular Diabetology* 8, no. 1 (2009): 35, doi:10.1186/1475-2840-8-35.

54   E. W. Manheimer et al, "Paleolithic Nutrition for Metabolic Syndrome: Systematic Review and Meta-Analysis," *American Journal of Clinical Nutrition* 102, no. 4 (2015): 922–32, doi:10.3945/ajcn.115.113613.

55   Deirdre K. Tobias et al., "Effect of Low-Fat Diet Interventions versus Other Diet Interventions on Long-Term Weight Change in Adults: A Systematic Review and Meta-Analysis," *Lancet Diabetes and Endocrinology* 3, no. 12 (2015): 968–79, doi:10.1016/S2213-8587(15)00367-8.

# PART 3

---

# LIFESTYLE AND ENVIRONMENT FOR OPTIMUM GUT HEALTH

# CHAPTER 11

# ENVIRONMENTAL TOXINS, SUN, VITAMIN D, AND NATURE

## IMPROVE YOUR ENVIRONMENT (EXTERNAL AND INTERNAL); OPTIMIZE YOUR HEALTH

Here in part 3, we will discuss lifestyle factors and how they affect your gut and microbiota. These factors include sleep, sun exposure, stress, and the importance of community. We will explore external environmental factors that can alter your internal environment. This will include the most important points regarding exposure to toxins, the impact of nature and exercise, and a series of early life factors that can improve the developing immune systems and microbiotas of infants and children.

### THE GREAT-IN-8 ACTION PLAN

1. Reset—reset your diet and lifestyle
2. Support—support your gut with probiotics and digestive enzymes/acid
3. Remove—remove/reduce unwanted gut bacteria with antimicrobial herbs
4. Rebalance—rebalance gut bacteria after treatment with antimicrobial herbs
5. Reintroduce—reintroduce foods you removed in step 3
6. Feed—feed the good bacteria
7. Wean—wean yourself off the supplements in your plan
8. Maintenance and fun—maintain your improvements, and enjoy your newfound health

So far, we have covered the dietary aspect that we will work through in step 1. We've also discussed the reintroduction of foods in step 5. We discussed how this reintroduction will increase carb, fiber, and prebiotic intake, which feeds good bacteria. We will take that concept a step further in step 6. By the end of our discussion here in part 3, we will have all the knowledge we need for steps 1, 5, and 6. In part 4, we'll cover more direct gut treatments, which are the focus of steps 2, 3, and 4. Then, it's on to part 5, where we put the plan into action. Let's continue.

The current interest in the microbiota has fueled much important research and showcased a very important concept—your gut has a massive impact on your overall health. However, as I have said before, along with this good comes the bad. The bad is the overspeculation, which produces the recommendation of unproven testing and supplements and the making of false health claims. Fortunately, there is a very powerful and important method for improving your microbiota health that is essentially free, is practical, and has been scientifically documented to have positive health impacts. This method is the optimization of your environment. Let's discuss some simple and important lifestyle steps you can take to improve your environment and thus optimize your gut, microbiota, and overall health.

Here are the important environmental factors that can optimize your microbiota health:

- ☐ Limiting toxins
- ☐ Sun exposure and vitamin D
- ☐ Time in nature (forest bathing)
- ☐ Exercise

## LIMITING TOXINS

Although we are still early in our understanding, some studies are exploring the link between lifestyle factors and gut microbiota.[1] Let's start with the impact of toxins on your microbiota. Smoking, of course, is a source of toxin exposure and has an influence on gut microbiota. Smoking has been shown to increase the Bacteroides bacteria group in individuals with Crohn's disease, compared to

healthy individuals.[2] Smoking cessation has also been shown to affect your microbiota; however, exactly what these changes mean is still unclear.[3]

It has been shown that particles from air pollution can make their way into your small intestine.[4] Once inside, these particles can alter your microbiota and immune system.[5] This has led some researchers to question whether the environmental pollution seen in industrialized countries might contribute to the increases in inflammatory bowel disease (Crohn's disease and ulcerative colitis) seen in these countries.

It shouldn't take much to convince you that minimizing your exposure to environmental toxins is probably a good idea for your overall health. This might include using an air filter, drinking filtered water, having plants in your home (they filter air), and using natural cleaning agents and skin-care products. Skin-care products can be tricky. This website will help you research the purity of your skin-care products: www.ewg.org/skindeep/.

Don't overthink this. Simple changes can make a big difference. Filtering your water and using natural cleaning and skin-care products are great places to start. Keep this simple.

## SUN EXPOSURE AND VITAMIN D

Currently, we know little about how sun exposure directly affects your microbiota. Fortunately, you are probably more concerned with how sun exposure can improve your health. This is where we have some very useful information.

Sun exposure has been shown to protect against digestive tract disease and inflammation, specifically diverticulitis and inflammatory bowel disease.[6] It has also been shown that children getting sun exposure have decreased occurrence of eczema and runny nose.[7]

Your body produces vitamin D in response to sun exposure, so you might ask, "Can't I just avoid the sun and get my vitamin D from a supplement?" This is an understandable question. In 2013, the *European Journal of Cancer* published a systematic review showing sun exposure confers cancer-protective effects that have nothing to do with vitamin D levels. In fact, this study concluded that you must have *chronic exposure to the sun* in order to obtain the benefit! The table below summarizes the results. While we do see that vitamin D levels directly protect against *some* cancers (colorectal, breast), we also see vitamin D levels had no effect on other cancers and that only sun exposure was protective against prostate cancer and non-Hodgkin's lymphoma.[8]

CancerIndex.org created a diagram based on Kentucky Cancer Registry data that shows the top distribution of cancer sites. Their data agree with other CDC data.[9]

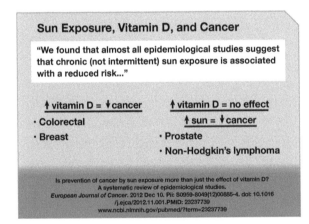

Collectively, we see two cancers protected against by sun exposure (prostate and non-Hodgkin's lymphoma) and two cancers protected against by vitamin D (colorectal and breast). It's reasonable to say that

## sun exposure may help prevent cancers that are more common

## and more dangerous than skin cancer.

(skin cancers are ranked number ten). Does this mean you should go crazy with sun exposure? No. What it does mean is we might want to rethink fearing the sun and follow my guidelines for reasonable and safe sun exposure, which we will discuss below.

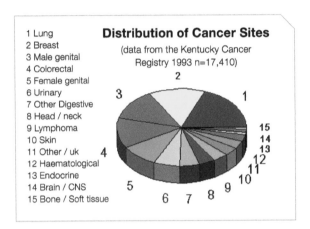

More recently, even stronger data has been published supporting that the sun should not be completely avoided. In 2016, the journal *Dermato-Endocrinology* performed a review of data from North America. They examined the association between sun exposure and cancer and concluded:

> *We found that cancer incidence for all invasive cancers and for eleven of twenty-two leading cancers significantly decreased with increased solar radiation [sun exposure].*[10]

In other words, sun exposure protected against invasive cancer and even protected against eleven of the twenty-two most common cancers! They found no association between sun exposure and melanoma of the skin.

Does sun exposure really make that much of a difference? A large study of Swedish women suggests it does. A group of 29,518 Swedish women were followed for twenty years. Their sun exposure and health status were tracked. The findings here were remarkable. When women who had sun exposure were compared to women who avoided the sun, the women who avoided the sun had twice the risk of death from any cause compared to those who obtained sun exposure. The women who got sun did not have an increased skin-cancer risk.[11]

This was not the only study to show that time in the sun protects against death from any cause, including cardiovascular disease.[12] It is interesting to note skin cancer's relationship to vitamin D. One study found that those who had higher vitamin D levels had less aggressive skin cancer.[13] Other researchers have theorized this is because sun exposure produces vitamin D in your skin.[14] The vitamin D in your skin then protects your skin against cancer on a cellular level. So what *might* happen is this: reasonable sun exposure protects the skin from cancer up to a point, but if you are excessive in your exposure and exceed this point, your skin-cancer risk increases. To put it simply, you should obtain far more sun exposure than modern dermatology dogma suggests. This brings up the important point of appropriate use versus overexposure. It has of course been demonstrated that overexposure to the sun increases our risk of skin cancer. But what does overexposure look like? Excessive use of tanning beds, spending hours every day in the sun, and, of course, sunburns are examples of excessive exposure. So, while, yes, extreme sun exposure is bad, avoiding the sun altogether is bad, too.

Would it be helpful to study humans living in a more natural hunter-gatherer habitat to determine how much vitamin D is produced in a "natural" level of sun exposure? Maybe. A group of researchers traveled to East Africa to study the Maasai and the Hadza, who are hunter-gatherers. They found the average blood levels of vitamin D were about 46 ng/mL, so this might be a good level to shoot for.[15] There seems to be some

agreement here, as other papers have also concluded 48 ng/mL is an ideal level.[16]

OK, let's get back to the issue at hand. How much sun should you get? Well, it's common sense but worth repeating: you should never burn. I will provide you with perhaps the most conservative recommendation on sun exposure, from the Endocrine Society's 2011 clinical guidelines for vitamin D.[17] The Endocrine Society's recommendations are based on levels of vitamin D needed for bone health. These levels may be *less* than the levels needed to obtain other health benefits from vitamin D. I have used the Endocrine Society's position paper to calculate recommendations for sun exposure. Please note, these are not the Endocrine Society's official recommendations. These are my extrapolations of how to meet their vitamin D requirements from sun exposure.

## RECOMMENDATIONS FOR DETERMINING HOW MUCH SUN EXPOSURE YOU SHOULD GET

An adult wearing a bathing suit and exposed to one minimal erythemal dose (MED) of sunlight produces the equivalent of ingesting between 10,000 and 25,000 IUs of vitamin D (we will say 17,500 average). An MED is the amount of exposure needed to produce a slight pinkness of the skin the day after exposure. If just your arms and legs are exposed to an MED, you produce 6,000 IUs.

Keep the following in mind when it comes to supplemental dosing:
- An adult *maintenance* dose for supplementation of vitamin D is 2,000 IUs per day or 14,000 per week (some studies have successfully used higher maintenance doses—3,500 per day).
- An adult *treatment* dose (to correct deficiency) is 6,000 IUs per day or 50,000 IUs per week.

Your skin tone makes a slight difference with these recommendations. If you are dark-skinned, you will need slightly more than what is listed. If you are light-skinned, you will need slightly less. But, again, in the larger context, it's possible that all people will do better with slightly more sun exposure than the amounts listed, because these recommendations get you to the minimum levels, not optimal. Of course, if you have a strong family history of skin cancers, you may want to shoot for the lower end of exposure.

What role does vitamin D from your diet play? A serving of the foods highest in vitamin D (cod-liver oil or salmon, for example) contains 1,000 UIs at best. The effect, then, is somewhat negligible, and it may be very difficult to obtain all your vitamin D from your diet.

A few additional notes from the Endocrine Society

- wearing sunscreen with SPF 30 reduces vitamin D synthesis by more than 95%;
- people with dark skin require three to five times longer in the sun;
- 20 to a 100% of those in the United States, Europe, and Canada are vitamin D deficient;
- The major source of vitamin D is exposure to sunlight; foods are not a robust source.

> *You may be wondering why we would want higher levels than those recommended by the Endocrine Society.*

Vitamin D has shown promise in modulating the immune system and thus having a favorable effect on immune-related disorders such as

- type 1 diabetes,
- rheumatoid arthritis,
- autoimmune thyroid disease,
- multiple sclerosis,
- IBD, and
- certain cancers.

For example, the Endocrine Society cites a study in which infants who were given 2,000 IUs of vitamin D per day for the first year of life reduced their risk of developing type 1 diabetes by 88% when they were monitored for the next thirty-one years of their lives.[18]

If you plan to be in the sun for several hours, I would recommend allowing yourself enough time *sunblock-free* to obtain your MED. Then, use protection—either sunblock or clothing. If you are in doubt, always err on the side of safety. You are better off getting less sun than burning. You can always get more sun another day.

## VITAMIN D SUPPLEMENTATION

We have covered the importance of sun exposure for health. We have covered how supplementing with vitamin D can't replace time in the sun as well. But you may have heard doctors proclaiming vitamin D supplementation as the next miracle treatment. So, which is it? Well, I think medicine got a little overexcited at the potential of vitamin D based on the early studies. It seems every illness we studied was associated with low levels of vitamin D. Could vitamin D be the next wonder supplement?

This brings us back to an important concept we have visited throughout this book: if something is *associated* with a disease, it does not mean it *causes* that disease. Remember our cop-car analogy? Just because police are found at the scene of a crime doesn't mean they caused the crime. As more research on vitamin D flooded the scientific journals, we started to see a picture emerge. Yes, there was clearly an association between low vitamin D levels and ill health. But supplementing ill people with vitamin D did not reverse their ill health like we thought it would. It *is* a good idea to get your vitamin D levels into my recommended range (40–50 ng/mL), but megadosing yourself with supplements with the expectation of a health miracle just hasn't been borne out by the research.

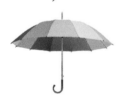 In 2014, the *BMJ* (*British Medical Journal*) released what's called an umbrella review. An umbrella review looks at all available systematic reviews and meta-analyses. It is supremely high-level scientific data. What did they find? Some of the most salient points are listed below:

- Low vitamin D levels are associated with several diseases.
- When supplementing people who have these diseases *and* who have low vitamin D levels, we did not see the improvement we were hoping for.
- We don't have good data about treating autoimmune conditions with vitamin D supplementation.
- "Low vitamin D status is more likely to be a marker of ill health than a cause of disease."[19]

This sentiment has been echoed by other systematic review papers.[20] However, this is not to say there is no benefit to vitamin D supplementation, as some studies have shown there is.[21] There are two exciting vitamin D–related studies that are worth mentioning. One study showed that vitamin D supplementation could successfully treat the symptoms of IBS.[22] Another showed those supplementing with vitamin D experienced a decrease in thyroid autoimmunity.[23] Neither of these studies used alarmingly high doses of vitamin D. We should be a bit more reasonable with our approach to vitamin D supplementation and look at supplementation as a consideration when our lifestyle sources (sun exposure) aren't sufficient.

## WHAT IF YOUR VITAMIN D LEVEL IS ALWAYS LOW?

We see low vitamin D levels in sick people, but supplementing vitamin D does not appear to reverse their illnesses.[24] This suggests that vitamin D deficiency is not *causing* the illness, but rather that low vitamin D levels might be *caused by* illness. Said another way, your health problem, let's say a digestive problem, might be causing your low vitamin D level. The reason for your chronically low amount of vitamin D might be an underlying illness or inflammatory problem that needs to be addressed. This line of thinking is starting to appear in the published medical literature.[25] If you have tried to increase your vitamin D level through sun exposure and supplementation and have noticed it barely budges, it may be a good idea to check in with your doctor or a good functional-medicine doctor for an evaluation.

## VITAMIN D RECOMMENDATIONS

The "normal" range for vitamin D is 30–100 ng/mL at most labs. I like to see patients in between 40 and 50 ng/mL. If they have an autoimmune condition, then shooting for as high as 50–60 ng/mL may be appropriate. Ideally, try to obtain vitamin D from the sun.

Do you need to take vitamin D during the winter? Not necessarily. Our bodies were designed to store enough vitamin D in our liver and fat cells to last us through the winter. If you do a good job obtaining sun exposure through the spring and summer, you should have plenty of reserve for the winter.

If you do need a supplement, it's important to use a balance of vitamin D and vitamin $K_2$. In the clinic, I use a vitamin D supplement that is balanced with adequate vitamin D and vitamin $K_2$. I usually recommend a conservative dose of 2,000 to 4,000 IUs of vitamin D per day. I do this when someone is deficient, in some who have an autoimmune disease, and sometimes during the winter, depending on how much sun a person gets during the summer.

I hope this discussion helps you determine how to address and prevent vitamin D deficiency. It appears the view of sun exposure as an evil and highly cancerous activity needs serious reexamination. Research is indicating that the risk/rewards analysis favors moderate sun exposure (as outlined earlier) rather than overzealous sun avoidance. Be careful not to burn, but also remember it's OK to enjoy the sun responsibly. Use vitamin D supplementation as a fallback, and supplement reasonably, not excessively.

## TIME IN NATURE (FOREST BATHING)

While you're working to optimize your sun exposure, you will, of course, be spending time outside. With this in mind, let's discuss the impressive health benefits of time in nature. In 2014, a group of researchers in Japan studied the effect of time in nature versus time in a city. The researchers divided the study subjects into two groups. One group took a leisurely fifteen-minute walk in a forest and the other group a leisurely fifteen-minute walk in a city. What the researchers found was very interesting: those taking a walk in a forest experienced increased vigor, energy, improved mood and feelings of vitality, while those in the city did not.[26]

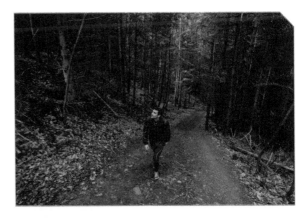

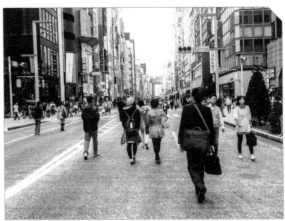

OK, you might *feel* better from a walk in the forest. That's nice. But does this translate into any other health benefits? Yes. A number of studies have shown you live longer and have a lower chance of disease (even heart disease) and death if you live in or spend time in a natural environment. According to an article in *Proceedings of the National Academy of Sciences*, "Numerous studies demonstrate that living close to the natural rural or coastal environment, often denoted 'green space' or 'blue space,' respectively, is beneficial for human health. It reduces overall mortality, cardiovascular disease, and depressive symptoms and increases subjective feelings of well-being. . . . There is suggestive evidence that living close to the natural environment . . . has long-term health benefits."[27]

Other studies have shown that
- having access to nature increased life expectancy of seniors;[28]
- visiting a forest, but not a city, boosts your immune system and increases anticancer cells;[29]
- time in nature decreases negative thoughts.[30]

We observe that certain immune disorders are more common in urban than rural settings, such as
- allergies;[31]
- inflammatory bowel disease (ulcerative colitis, Crohn's disease);[32]
- multiple sclerosis;[33]
- psychiatric disorders.[34]

These findings—that time in nature improves health—have been replicated by an overwhelming number of studies.[35]

Is it possible the reason time in nature is health promoting is because people are more prone to be active (exercise) when in nature? Great question. It has been shown that the health improvements from nature may be *independent* of exercise.[36]

After hearing this, I hope you're motivated to spend time in nature every week. But how does this time in nature affect your microbiota? A 2013 paper provides a few interesting facts that answer this question:

- Living closer to agricultural lands increases bacterial diversity on the skin.
- Pets increase bacterial load in houses.
- People living together start to share microbiota traits.
- Opening windows allows more bacterial exposure than ventilation systems.[37]

This paper also describes "pseudocommensals." These are microbes, like bacteria, from the environment that do not colonize you (meaning they do not take up residence in your gut) but have transient effects. For example, when you take a walk in nature, there are bacteria from the soil that get into the air. You inhale these bacteria, and they pass through your lungs and gut and eventually either leave your body or die. They are just temporary passersby, but while you're exposed to them, they may help tone your immune system. It's my thinking that nearly constant exposure to these bacteria is probably best. This might be why we see a positive effect from living on a farm; however, sometimes we see negative effects if you only periodically visit a farm. Constant exposure may train the immune system, whereas occasional exposure may be perceived as an attack. Environment provides exposure to bacteria. Perhaps this is why time in nature is sometimes referred to as forest bathing. Maybe you are literally bathing yourself in healthy bacteria (in healthy pseudocommensals). And these bacteria are having a positive effect on your overall health. This is likely why the hunter-gatherer-like Africans who have high exposure to environmental bacteria have more diverse bacteria in their microbiotas—because of their constant contact with nature and the bacteria (pseudocommensals) nature provides.

All of this hints at an underlying theme:

> *the more exposure you have to a natural environment, the more bacteria from that environment you are exposed to, which then has a beneficial impact on your microbiota and immune system.*

This is exemplified by another study, one that examined skin health in teenagers.[38] The researchers looked at two groups of teens, those with allergic skin disorders (psoriasis, eczema, dermatitis) compared to those with healthy skin. The teens with skin disorders had a lower diversity of plant life around their homes, which correlated with a lower diversity of bacteria on their skin (the skin microbiota). The authors hypothesize that rich environmental bacteria influences healthy bacteria on your skin, and that this then influences your immune system and may either cause or prevent disease.

Here are a few additional interesting points from this study:

- Healthy teenagers who had more land/plant diversity around their homes had more bacteria on their skin and more anti-inflammatory compounds in their blood; they had fewer allergic/immune skin disorders (eczema/psoriasis/dermatitis).
- Wild plants were significantly more protective than houseplants.
- It was the diversity of bacteria not the total number that made a difference.
- Subjects had grown up in the same dwelling their entire childhood.

As these points suggest, the more diverse the plant life you are exposed to when spending time in nature, the better.[39] This simply means walking through a man-made field of grass is not as good as walking through a naturally occurring forest teeming with various types of plant life.

Are these positive effects all about bacteria? No. The chemicals responsible for the scent of trees, known as phytoncides, lower blood pressure and decrease stress hormones in rats.[40] Also, a high level of negative ions in the air correlates with less depression (according to a systematic review with meta-analysis),[41] and natural environments are known to have higher levels of negative ions.

I hope it's becoming clear that nature has a large influence on your microbiota and overall health. Bear in mind that these studies are *not* all observational. Remember, simply observing something doesn't always tell us about what causes a problem or how to treat it. Some of the studies above (such as the Japanese forest-walking study) have clearly shown taking time in nature *causes* a beneficial health response. This is a big deal. If you're not feeling well, you have a simple, free, proven method of improving your mood, energy, and overall health, maybe in as little as fifteen minutes a few times a week.

## EXERCISE

A common recommendation I make to patients is to get outdoor exercise, preferably with a friend. This could simply be a walk in nature. We know why being outside is important, and we will discuss why time with friends is important (although this shouldn't really be a hard sell). Let's now discuss the impact of exercise on your microbiota and overall health.

The impact exercise has on your microbiota is another area we are just starting to study. However, a handful of studies again show how important the environment is for your microbiota. Here is an important distinction, though: in this case, environment does not mean your surroundings but rather the internal environment you create in your body.

> **Exercise improves your internal environment, and this internal environment allows healthy bacteria (your microbiota) to flourish.**

Undeniably, the best study we have regarding the impact of exercise on your microbiota comes from the journal *Gut* in 2014. This study compared activity level and diet of professional rugby players to that of nonathletes of similar size, sex, and age.

The rugby players were found to have microbiotas that were more diverse and what we think of as healthier. More specifically, this study found increased exercise and protein consumption correlated with increased bacterial diversity![42] What is fascinating about this study is that protein doesn't really feed the microbiota/gut bacteria, so the results might indicate exercise was the main driver of the improved microbiotas. This suggests exercise is an extremely powerful environmental input for your microbiotal health. The rugby players did eat more calories overall, which may have had an effect. However, the researchers concluded that exercise and protein consumption appeared to be the primary associations with the healthier microbiotas seen in the rugby players. In other words, the improvement wasn't due to things like the rugby players eating more carbs, fiber, or prebiotics, for example.

What is happening here? How does exercise improve your microbiotal health? When looking at the big picture, I think we will continue to find that healthy diet and lifestyle practices are the most important factors in influencing your microbiotal health. Why? Because these healthy practices have been shown to have the most powerful impact on your health. It would follow then that they would have the largest impact on your microbiota. But let's look at some specifics of how exercise might have a beneficial impact on your microbiota.

Your gut contains many sensors called "toll-like receptors" or TLRs. These TLRs are responsible for monitoring contents in the gut. They help us distinguish good stuff from bad stuff, such as good bacteria from bad bacteria. Exercise may modulate these sensors (specifically TLR4s) and even prevent them from telling your immune system to attack things it shouldn't.[43] Remember, too much "attack" signaling can occur in autoimmune and inflammatory conditions. These TLRs are sensors for the contents in your gut and help prevent your immune system from attacking things that it shouldn't, like food, good bacteria, or your intestinal lining. As we've discussed, there is a delicate balance with bacteria. We want to let good bacteria grow and live, but we don't want to let good bacteria (or fungus) overgrow. Exercise might make your immune system less aggressive in cleaning out good bacteria, which may be why we see the rugby players have improved diversity in their gut microbiotas.

It has been shown that hormones released during exercise, like noradrenaline, stimulate the growth of healthy bacteria.[44] E. coli is often stereotyped as being a bad guy; however, there are many types of E. coli, and several are good guys.[45] In fact, some E. coli probiotics have shown impressive results for treating IBD and IBS.[46]

Was this the only study that showed being fit and exercising can cause you to have a healthy microbiota? No. Another study found that your level of cardiovascular fitness *predicts* microbiotal diversity,[47] meaning level of fitness appeared to be causing the healthy microbiota. However, just because some exercise is good does not mean more is better. It has been shown that those who perform extreme levels of exercise are at increased risk for infection.[48] Too much exercise may also cause leaky gut.[49] This is likely because too much exercise can cause immune suppression. This again hints at the importance of balance. For example, other studies have shown moderate exercise may reduce risk of colon cancer, while excessive amounts may be damaging to your gut.[50]

## HOW SHOULD YOU EXERCISE TO INCREASE OR OPTIMIZE YOUR MICROBIOTAL HEALTH?

Today, there are no studies that directly answer this question. However, based on what we do know, there are a few assumptions we can make:

- Too much or too little exercise can be problematic.
- Exercise is a stressor, a healthy stressor, but a stressor nonetheless.
- The more stress you have in your life, the less exercise you can likely tolerate.
  - » Examples of stress include illness, lack of sleep, poor diet, psychological/emotional stress, injury.
- Conversely, the healthier you are, the more exercise you can tolerate.
- Exercising without a break may be the most stressful on your body; for example, circuits with no rest or prolonged cardiovascular exercise (such as aerobics classes) with no rest may be a problem for those trying to recover from burnout or illness.[51]
- You must ensure you are exercising enough but not too much.
  - » Signs of exercising too much include not sleeping well, chronic sore muscles or muscle pulls or injuries in general, fatigue after workouts, increased fatigue during the day, lack of motivation during workouts, depressed mood or depressed libido.

If you are ill or trying to recover from burnout, I recommend

- doing a light activity (such as walking) outside (ideally in a forest-like environment) and preferably with a friend;
- starting by exercising one or two days a week, around twenty to thirty minutes each time, and pushing yourself hard enough to break a light sweat;
- pay attention to the signs of overtraining; if you do not experience any, you can slowly ramp up your amount of exercise.

If you need some sort of test or measurement to tell you you're overdoing it, HRV (heart rate variability) is a simple and very inexpensive way to monitor yourself. Learn more about HRV on my website: http://drruscio.com/hrv-novel-tool-assessing-stress-levels-podcast-28/.

What if you are so fatigued that you feel exercise causes you to feel worse or to crash? This is often reported by people with chronic fatigue syndrome. A Cochrane Database systematic review has found exercise to be an effective treatment in improving chronic fatigue.[52] Exercise seems to be helpful even in the case of chronic fatigue syndrome, so do your best to slowly start a program and to stick with it. For those wondering about exercising with adrenal fatigue, physiologist Dr. Mike T. Nelson and I recently discussed the topic: http://drruscio.com/hrv-novel-tool-assessing-stress-levels-podcast-28/. In another conversation, we offer ideas about how to determine your ideal level of exercise if you have adrenal fatigue (see the website for more information: http://drruscio.com/exercise-adrenal-fatigue-mike-t-nelson-episode-29/).

There is no one-size-fits-all recommendation here. If you're working a low-stress job, have lots of free time, eat perfectly, sleep a lot, and have no other stress in your life—you can likely exercise hard five to seven days a week with no problem. If you are a parent, work fifty hours a week, don't sleep enough, and are stressed about money—you will likely burn out if you try exercising hard five to seven days a week. Start with a conservative plan, and gradually increase the amount you exercise to find your ideal level.

As we age, it's important that we maintain muscle mass for both metabolic health and to maintain functionality. I recommend that you incorporate at least one—ideally two—day(s) of strength training into your exercise routine for every day of cardio-type exercise. So, for every one day of cardio, you should perform one to two days of strength training. This will ensure you maintain adequate muscle mass and maintain functionality.

Maintaining adequate muscle mass is an excellent predictor of your overall health. Weight-bearing exercise and adequate protein intake are two of the most important factors for maintaining your muscle.[53] Recent nutritional recommendations call for increased protein intake compared to previous recommendations, especially for those who are ill or aging. The recommendation is 1.2 g to 1.5 g of protein for every 1 kg (2.2 lb.) of body weight. You can use this protein calculator to easily determine how much protein you should strive for every day: www.bodybuilding.com/fun/caltp.htm. For now, though, I wouldn't recommend being overly fastidious about calculating this and would simply recommend that you follow our dietary guidelines in part 3.

Finally, I should mention that walking is the foundation of fitness. It is the most important form of exercise you can obtain. If you can do nothing else, you should walk. If you are performing other types of exercise, you should make sure that you are also walking. Walking was a fundamental part of our evolution—we walked everywhere. We evolved under conditions of constant movement. Sitting all day and then exercising like a maniac for thirty minutes isn't what our bodies

evolved to do. Do your best to walk every day and as often as you can. On days when I work from my home office and spend most of the day in front of a computer, I set an alarm to sound every forty-five minutes. I then get up and take a short walk. If you work in an office, you might want to take a short walk around the office or to the bathroom and back every forty-five minutes or so. Definitely take a walk during your lunch break—outside if weather permits. I've interviewed many top experts in fitness, and they are all in agreement: walking is foundational to your health and fitness. So, if you're not sure how to get started with exercise, simply start walking as much as you can.

Exercise is an example of how we can modulate our internal environment to make our bodies a hospitable place for healthy bacteria to grow. By obtaining the appropriate amount of exercise, you will modulate your immune system to allow more good bacteria to grow, thus optimizing your microbiota and overall health.

## CONCEPT SUMMARY

- Sun exposure confers cancer-protective effects that have nothing to do with vitamin D levels.

- Sun exposure may help prevent cancers that are more common and more dangerous than skin cancer.

- The more exposure you have to a natural environment, the more bacteria from that environment you are exposed to, which then has a beneficial impact on your microbiota and immune system.

- Low vitamin D status is more likely to be a marker of ill health than a cause of disease.

- Use vitamin D supplementation as a fallback and supplement reasonably, not excessively. Try to obtain your vitamin D from the sun.

- Vitamin D supplementation can be beneficial for those with IBS and those with thyroid autoimmunity.

- It has been shown that the health improvements from nature may be independent of exercise.

- Exercise improves your internal environment, and this internal environment allows healthy bacteria (your microbiota) to flourish.

- Exercise may improve your gut microbiota's bacterial diversity.

- Too little or too much exercise can be problematic. Balance is key.

- Walking is the foundation of fitness. It is the most important form of exercise you can obtain.

1   Michael A. Conlon and Anthony R. Bird, "The Impact of Diet and Lifestyle on Gut Microbiota and Human Health," *Nutrients*, 2015, doi:10.3390/nu7010017.

2   Jane L. Benjamin et al., "Smokers with Active Crohn's Disease Have a Clinically Relevant Dysbiosis of the Gastrointestinal Microbiota," *Inflammatory Bowel Diseases* 18, no. 6 (2012): 1092–1100, doi:10.1002/ibd.21864.

3   Luc Biedermann et al., "Smoking Cessation Induces Profound Changes in the Composition of the Intestinal Microbiota in Humans," *PLoS ONE* 8, no. 3 (2013), doi:10.1371/journal.pone.0059260.

4   Leigh A. Beamish et al., "Air Pollution: An Environmental Factor Contributing to Intestinal Disease," *Journal of Crohn's and Colitis*, 2011, doi:10.1016/j.crohns.2011.02.017.

5   Saad Y. Salim et al., "Air Pollution Effects on the Gut Microbiota," *Gut Microbes* 5, no. 2 (2013): 215–19, doi:10.4161/gmic.27251.

6   Lillias H. Maguire et al., "Association of Geographic and Seasonal Variation with Diverticulitis Admissions," *JAMA Surgery* 150, no. 1 (2015): 74–77, doi:10.1001/jamasurg.2014.2049; B. N. Limketkai et al., "Lower Regional and Temporal Ultraviolet Exposure Is Associated with Increased Rates and Severity of Inflammatory Bowel Disease Hospitalisation," *Alimentary Pharmacology and Therapeutics* 40, no. 5 (2014): 508–17, doi:10.1111/apt.12845.

7   Andrew Stewart Kemp et al., "The Influence of Sun Exposure in Childhood and Adolescence on Atopic Disease at Adolescence," *Pediatric Allergy and Immunology* 24, no. 5 (2013): 493–500, doi:10.1111/pai.12085.

8   Han van der Rhee et al., "Is Prevention of Cancer by Sun Exposure More Than Just the Effect of Vitamin D? A Systematic Review of Epidemiological Studies," *European Journal of Cancer (Oxford, England : 1990)* 49, no. 6 (2012): 1422–36, doi:10.1016/j.ejca.2012.11.001.

9   Simon Cotterill, "What Is Cancer ? | Medical Terminology for Cancer," last modified February 1, 2014, www.cancerindex.org/medterm/medtm2.htm; "Kentucky Cancer Registry," last modified December 14, 2016, accessed October 10, 2017, www.kcr.uky.edu/; "Cancer Facts for Demographic Groups," *Cancer Prevention and Control*, last modified June 5, 2017, www.cdc.gov/cancer/dcpc/data/women.htm; "Common Cancer Types—National Cancer Institute," last modified February 13, 2017, www.cancer.gov/types/common-cancers.

10  Alan B. Fleischer and Sarah E. Fleischer, "Solar Radiation and the Incidence and Mortality of Leading Invasive Cancers in the United States," *Dermato-Endocrinology* 8, no. 1 (2016), doi:10.1080/19381980.2016.1162366.

11  P. G. Lindqvist et al., "Avoidance of Sun Exposure Is a Risk Factor for All-Cause Mortality: Results from the Melanoma in Southern Sweden Cohort," *Journal of Internal Medicine* 276, no. 1 (2014): 77–86, doi:10.1111/joim.12251.

12   Ling Yang et al., "Ultraviolet Exposure and Mortality among Women in Sweden," *Cancer Epidemiology Biomarkers and Prevention* 20, no. 4 (2011): 683–90, doi:10.1158/1055-9965.EPI-10-0982; Carole A. Baggerly et al., "Sunlight and Vitamin D: Necessary for Public Health," *Journal of the American College of Nutrition*, 2015, doi:10.1080/07315724.2015.1039866; Ben Schöttker et al., "Vitamin D and Mortality: Meta-Analysis of Individual Participant Data from a Large Consortium of Cohort Studies from Europe and the United States," *BMJ (Clinical Research Ed.)* 348, no. June (2014): g3656, doi:10.1136/bmj.g3656.

13   Julia A. Newton-Bishop et al., "Serum 25-Hydroxyvitamin D3 Levels Are Associated with Breslow Thickness at Presentation and Survival from Melanoma," *Journal of Clinical Oncology* 27, no. 32 (2009): 5439–44, doi:10.1200/JCO.2009.22.1135.

14   Michael F. Holick, "Shedding New Light on the Role of the Sunshine Vitamin D for Skin Health: The lncRNA-Skin Cancer Connection," *Experimental Dermatology* 23, no. 6 (2014): 391–92, doi:10.1111/exd.12386.

15   Martine F. Luxwolda et al., "Traditionally Living Populations in East Africa Have a Mean Serum 25-Hydroxyvitamin D Concentration of 115 Nmol/l," *British Journal of Nutrition* 108, no. 9 (2012): 1557–61, doi:10.1017/S0007114511007161.

16   Carole A. Baggerly et al., "Sunlight and Vitamin D: Necessary for Public Health," *Journal of the American College of Nutrition*, 2015, doi:10.1080/07315724.2015.1039866.

17   Michael F. Holick et al., "Evaluation, Treatment, and Prevention of Vitamin D Deficiency: An Endocrine Society Clinical Practice Guideline," *Journal of Clinical Endocrinology and Metabolism* 96, no. 7 (2011): 1911–30, doi:10.1210/jc.2011-0385.

18   E. Hypponen et al., "Intake of Vitamin D and Risk of Type 1 Diabetes: A Birth Cohort Study," *Lancet* 358 (2001): 1500–1503, doi:10.1016/S0140-6736(01)06580-1.

19   E. Theodoratou et al., "Vitamin D and Multiple Health Outcomes: Umbrella Review of Systematic Reviews," *Annals of Plastic Surgery* 75, no. 3 (2015): 353–57.

20   Philippe Autier et al., "Vitamin D Status and Ill Health: A Systematic Review," *Lancet Diabetes & Endocrinology* 2, no. 1 (2014): 76–89, doi:10.1016/S2213-8587(13)70165-7.

21   R. Chowdhury et al., "Vitamin D and Risk of Cause Specific Death: Systematic Review and Meta-Analysis of Observational Cohort and Randomised Intervention Studies," *BMJ* 348, no. apr01 2 (2014): g1903–g1903, doi:10.1136/bmj.g1903.

22   A. Abbasnezhad et al., "Effect of Vitamin D on Gastrointestinal Symptoms and Health-Related Quality of Life in Irritable Bowel Syndrome Patients: A Randomized Double-Blind Clinical Trial," *Neurogastroenterology and Motility: The Official Journal of the European Gastrointestinal Motility Society* 28, no. 10 (2016): 1533–44, doi:10.1111/nmo.12851.

23   Elias E. Mazokopakis et al., "Is Vitamin D Related to Pathogenesis and Treatment of Hashimoto's Thyroiditis?," *Hellenic Journal of Nuclear Medicine* 18, no. 3 (2015): 222–27.

24   Greg P. Blaney et al., "Vitamin D Metabolites as Clinical Markers in Autoimmune and Chronic Disease," *Annals of the New York Academy of Sciences*, 1173:384–90, 2009, doi:10.1111/j.1749-6632.2009.04875.x.

25   Tea Skaaby, "The Relationship of Vitamin D Status to Risk of Cardiovascular Disease and Mortality," *Danish Medical Journal* 62, no. 2 (2015).

26   Norimasa Takayama et al., "Emotional, Restorative, and Vitalizing Effects of Forest and Urban Environments at Four Sites in Japan," *International Journal of Environmental Research and Public Health* 11, no. 7 (2014): 7207–30, doi:10.3390/ijerph110707207.

27   G. A. Rook, "Regulation of the Immune System by Biodiversity from the Natural Environment: An Ecosystem Service Essential to Health," *Proceedings of the National Academy of Sciences* 110, no. 46 (2013): 18360–67, doi:10.1073/pnas.1313731110.

28   T. Takano, "Urban Residential Environments and Senior Citizens' Longevity in Megacity Areas: The Importance of Walkable Green Spaces," *Journal of Epidemiology & Community Health* 56, no. 12 (2002): 913–18, doi:10.1136/jech.56.12.913.

29   Qing Li et al., "Visiting a Forest, but Not a City, Increases Human Natural Killer Activity and Expression of Anticancer Proteins," *International Journal of Immunopathology and Pharmacology* 21, no. 1 (2008): 117–27, doi:13 [pii].

30   Gregory N. Bratman et al., "Nature Experience Reduces Rumination and Subgenual Prefrontal Cortex Activation," *Proceedings of the National Academy of Sciences* 112, no. 28 (2015): 8567–72, doi:10.1073/pnas.1510459112.

31   S. J. MacNeill et al., "Asthma and Allergies: Is the Farming Environment (Still) Protective in Poland? The GABRIEL Advanced Studies," *Allergy: European Journal of Allergy and Clinical Immunology* 68, no. 6 (2013): 771–79, doi:10.1111/all.12141; N. Nicolaou et al., "Allergic Disease in Urban and Rural Populations: Increasing Prevalence with Increasing Urbanization," *Allergy: European Journal of Allergy and Clinical Immunology*, 2005, doi:10.1111/j.1398-9995.2005.00961.x.

32    J. K. Hou et al., "Distribution and Manifestations of Inflammatory Bowel Disease in Asians, Hispanics, and African Americans: A Systematic Review," *American Journal of Gastroenterology* 104, no. 8 (2009): 2100–2109, doi:10.1038/ajg.2009.190.

33    G. W. Lowis, "The Social Epidemiology of Multiple Sclerosis," *Science of the Total Environment* 90 (1990): 163–90.

34    J. Peen et al., "The Current Status of Urban-Rural Differences in Psychiatric Disorders," *Acta Psychiatrica Scandinavica*, 2010, doi:10.1111/j.1600-0447.2009.01438.x.

35    E. Morita et al., "Psychological Effects of Forest Environments on Healthy Adults: Shinrin-Yoku (Forest-Air Bathing, Walking) as a Possible Method of Stress Reduction," *Public Health* 121, no. 1 (2007): 54–63, doi:10.1016/j.puhe.2006.05.024; Terry Hartig et al., "Tracking Restoration in Natural and Urban Field Settings," *Journal of Environmental Psychology* 23, no. 2 (2003): 109–23, doi:10.1016/S0272-4944(02)00109-3; Richard M. Ryan et al., "Vitalizing Effects of Being Outdoors and in Nature," *Journal of Environmental Psychology* 30, no. 2 (2010): 159–68, doi:10.1016/j.jenvp.2009.10.009; Richard Mitchell and Frank Popham, "Effect of Exposure to Natural Environment on Health Inequalities: An Observational Population Study," *Lancet* 372, no. 9650 (2008): 1655–60, doi:10.1016/S0140-6736(08)61689-X; Jenny Roe and Peter Aspinall, "The Restorative Benefits of Walking in Urban and Rural Settings in Adults with Good and Poor Mental Health," *Health and Place* 17, no. 1 (2011): 103–13, doi:10.1016/j.healthplace.2010.09.003; J. Maas et al., "Green Space, Urbanity, and Health: How Strong Is the Relation?," *Journal of Epidemiology & Community Health* 60, no. 7 (2006): 587–92, doi:10.1136/jech.2005.043125; Bum Jin Park et al., "The Physiological Effects of Shinrin-Yoku (Taking in the Forest Atmosphere or Forest Bathing): Evidence from Field Experiments in 24 Forests across Japan," *Environmental Health and Preventive Medicine*, 2010, doi:10.1007/s12199-009-0086-9; Masahiro Toda et al., "Effects of Woodland Walking on Salivary Stress Markers Cortisol and Chromogranin A," *Complementary Therapies in Medicine* 21, no. 1 (2013): 29–34, doi:10.1016/j.ctim.2012.11.004; Gen-Xiang Mao et al., "Therapeutic Effect of Forest Bathing on Human Hypertension in the Elderly," *Journal of Cardiology* 60, no. 6 (2012): 495–502, doi:10.1016/j.jjcc.2012.08.003.

36    Kate Lachowycz and Andy P. Jones, "Does Walking Explain Associations between Access to Greenspace and Lower Mortality?," *Social Science and Medicine* 107 (2014): 9–17, doi:10.1016/j.socscimed.2014.02.023.

37    G. A. Rook, "Regulation of the Immune System by Biodiversity from the Natural Environment: An Ecosystem Service Essential to Health," *Proceedings of the National Academy of Sciences* 110, no. 46 (2013): 18360–67, doi:10.1073/pnas.1313731110.

38    I. Hanski et al., "Environmental Biodiversity, Human Microbiota, and Allergy Are Interrelated," *Proceedings of the National Academy of Sciences* 109, no. 21 (2012): 8334–39, doi:10.1073/pnas.1205624109.

39    Richard A. Fuller et al., "Psychological Benefits of Greenspace Increase with Biodiversity," *Biology Letters* 3, no. 4 (2007): 390–94, doi:10.1098/rsbl.2007.0149.

40    Kohei Kawakami et al., "Effects of Phytoncides on Blood Pressure under Restraint Stress in SHRSP," *Clinical and Experimental Pharmacology and Physiology* 31, no. SUPPL. 2 (2004), doi:10.1111/j.1440-1681.2004.04102.x.

41    Vanessa Perez et al., "Air Ions and Mood Outcomes: A Review and Meta-Analysis," *BMC Psychiatry* 13, no. 1 (2013): 29, doi:10.1186/1471-244X-13-29.

42    Siobhan F. Clarke et al., "Exercise and Associated Dietary Extremes Impact on Gut Microbial Diversity," *Gut* 63, no. 12 (2014): 1913–20, doi:10.1136/gutjnl-2013-306541.

43    Stéphane Bermon et al., "The Microbiota: An Exercise Immunology Perspective," *Exercise Immunology Review*, 2015; Michael Gleeson et al., "Exercise and Toll-like Receptors," *Exercise Immunology Review*, 2006.

44    Mark Lyte and Sharon Ernst, "Catecholamine Induced Growth of Gram Negative Bacteria," *Life Sciences* 50, no. 3 (1992): 203–12, doi:10.1016/0024-3205(92)90273-R; P. P. Freestone et al., "Growth Stimulation of Intestinal Commensal Escherichia Coli by Catecholamines: A Possible Contributory Factor in Trauma-Induced Sepsis," *Shock* 18, no. 5 (2002): 465–70, doi:10.1097/00024382-200211000-00014.

45    Gulietta M. Pupo et al., "Evolutionary Relationships among Pathogenic and Nonpathogenic Escherichia Coli Strains Inferred from Multilocus Enzyme Electrophoresis and Mdh Sequence Studies," *Infection and Immunity* 65, no. 7 (1997): 2685–92.

46    Wolfgang Kruis, "Maintaining Remission of Ulcerative Colitis with the Probiotic Escherichia Coli Nissle 1917 Is as Effective as with Standard Mesalazine," *Gut* 53, no. 11 (2004): 1617–23, doi:10.1136/gut.2003.037747; B. J. Rembacken et al., "Non-Pathogenic Escherichia Coli versus Mesalazine for the Treatment of Ulcerative Colitis: A Randomised Trial," *Lancet* 354, no. 9179 (1999): 635–39, doi:10.1016/S0140-6736(98)06343-0; Wolfgang Kruis et al., "A Double-Blind Placebo-Controlled Trial to Study Therapeutic Effects of Probiotic Escherichia Coli Nissle 1917 in Subgroups of Patients with Irritable Bowel Syndrome," *International Journal of Colorectal Disease* 27, no. 4 (2012): 467–74, doi:10.1007/s00384-011-1363-9; Markus Magerl et al., "Non-Pathogenic

Commensal Escherichia Coli Bacteria Can Inhibit Degranulation of Mast Cells," *Experimental Dermatology* 17, no. 5 (2008): 427–35, doi:10.1111/j.1600-0625.2008.00704.x.

47    Mehrbod Estaki et al., "Cardiorespiratory Fitness as a Predictor of Intestinal Microbial Diversity and Distinct Metagenomic Functions," *Microbiome* 4, no. 1 (2016): 42, doi:10.1186/s40168-016-0189-7.

48    David C. Nieman, "Special Feature for the Olympics: Effects of Exercise on the Immune System: Exercise Effects on Systemic Immunity," *Immunology and Cell Biology* 78, no. 5 (2000): 496–501, doi:10.1111/j.1440-1711.2000.t01-5-.x; David C. Nieman, "Risk of Upper Respiratory Tract Infection in Athletes: An Epidemiologic and Immunologic Perspective," *Journal of Athletic Training*, 1997; David C. Nieman, "Is Infection Risk Linked to Exercise Workload?," *Medicine and Science in Sports and Exercise*, 2000, doi:10.1097/00005768-200007001-00005; M. Gleeson and D. B. Pyne, "Special Feature for the Olympics: Effects of Exercise on the Immune System: Exercise Effects on Mucosal Immunity," *Immunology and Cell Biology* 78, no. 5 (2000): 536–44, doi:10.1111/j.1440-1711.2000.t01-8-.x; M. Gleeson, "Mucosal Immunity and Respiratory Illness in Elite Athletes," *International Journal of Sports Medicine* 21 Suppl. 1 (2000): S33–43, doi:10.1055/s-2000-1450.

49    Manfred Lamprecht and Anita Frauwallner, "Exercise, Intestinal Barrier Dysfunction and Probiotic Supplementation," *Medicine and Sport Science* 59 (2012): 47–56, doi:10.1159/000342169; Micah Zuhl et al., "Exercise Regulation of Intestinal Tight Junction Proteins," *British Journal of Sports Medicine* 48, no. 12 (2014): 980–86, doi:10.1136/bjsports-2012-091585.

50    H. P. Peters et al., "Potential Benefits and Hazards of Physical Activity and Exercise on the Gastrointestinal Tract," *Gut* 48, no. 3 (2001): 435–39, doi:10.1136/GUT.48.3.435.

51    K. A. Brooks and Carter J. G., "Overtraining, Exercise, and Adrenal Insufficiency," *Journal of Novel Physiotherapies* 3, no. 125 (2013): 1–10, doi:10.4172/2165-7025.1000125.Overtraining; T. K. Szivak et al., "Adrenal Cortical Responses to High-Intensity, Short Rest, Resistance Exercise in Men and Women," *Journal of Strength and Conditioning Research*, 2013, 748–60, doi:10.1519/JSC.0b013e318259e009.

52    Lillebeth Larun et al., "Exercise Therapy for Chronic Fatigue Syndrome," *Cochrane Database of Systematic Reviews*, 2016, doi:10.1002/14651858.CD003200.pub6.

53    Leigh Breen and Stuart M Phillips, "Skeletal Muscle Protein Metabolism in the Elderly: Interventions to Counteract the 'Anabolic Resistance' of Ageing," *Nutrition & Metabolism* 8, no. 1 (2011): 68, doi:10.1186/1743-7075-8-68.

# CHAPTER 12

# SLEEP: A FUNDAMENTAL FOR GUT AND OVERALL HEALTH

## IMPROVE YOUR ENVIRONMENT BY OPTIMIZING YOUR SLEEP

Sleep is another factor that affects your internal environment. The quality and quantity of your sleep alter the bacteria living in that environment. Good sleep equals a good environment, which equals good bacteria. Bad sleep equals a bad environment, which equals bad bacteria. Although it's very early in our understanding of the specific microbiota effects of sleep, there are some very important things you should know about how sleep affects your gut and your overall health.

There are three parameters that we'll look at in our discussion of sleep: duration, consistency, and intensity.

### DURATION

Very high-level scientific data suggest consistently getting too short (less than six to seven hours) or too long (more than nine hours) sleep duration is associated with poor health. Why might sleeping more than nine hours be associated with conditions such as weight gain, metabolic syndrome, and cardiovascular disease? My interpretation (and it's just speculation) is that those who are sleeping more than nine hours might be suffering from an underlying illness or imbalance that causes them to do so. Whatever the reason, we clearly see too much sleep can be as bad as not enough.

A prudent recommendation for how much sleep to get is that you should average eight hours per night, sleeping slightly more or less depending on how you feel. If you find you consistently can only get six hours (because you're wakeful) or consistently need nine or more hours, you may want to check in with your doctor. If you're not *allowing* yourself enough sleep time, it's important you work to change this.

### CONSISTENCY

Rhythm of sleep is important, too. It has been shown that maintaining the same sleep rhythm (circadian rhythm) is as important as duration. By "rhythm" we mean that you have roughly the same bedtime and rising time every night and day.

Maintaining this sleep rhythm might be more important than the amount of sleep itself. For example, night-shift workers who obtain adequate sleep duration still show an increased risk for several diseases,[1] including breast cancer,[2] likely because their rhythm is off. That is, they're not consistently going to bed at night and rising in the morning at roughly the same time every day.

## INTENSITY

Intensity refers to how soundly you sleep. The more wakeful you are, the poorer the sleep intensity.

## WHAT IF I DON'T SLEEP WELL?

Inflammatory, digestive, blood sugar, and hormonal (female and adrenal hormones) issues can interfere with your sleep. These issues can cause you to be unable to fall asleep or cause you to wake up unable to go back to sleep. If you are suffering from either of these, you should check in with your doctor or a good functional-medicine doctor. Also, sleep apnea can be a major threat to sleep. Risk factors for sleep apnea are being overweight, older, and male; having a family history of apnea; use of alcohol, sedatives, or tranquilizers; smoking; and nasal congestion. Stress is another factor that can interfere with your sleep. If you are under a lot of stress and notice you're not sleeping well, it's imperative you take steps to mitigate your stress and restore your sleep.

If you don't sleep well (can't fall asleep or stay asleep) or if you consistently need more than nine hours, it's likely you have some internal problem that needs to be investigated. Are sleep problems hard to fix? In my experience, no. One of the most common improvements I see in my patients is improved sleep. What do we do? Focus on the underlying problems listed above: often digestive, but also hormonal and blood sugar issues. As you work through our action steps in part 5, you will likely see dramatic improvements in your sleep.

Is sleep really that important? Yes! We have far better data that supports the importance of sleep than any supplement or herbs. Let's have a quick look at how poor sleep affects health outcomes.

## SLEEP AND OVERALL CHANCE OF DISEASE OR DEATH

Two systematic reviews with meta-analyses have shown that consistently sleeping less than seven hours or more than nine hours per night is associated with an increased risk of disease or death.[3] And while not all the data agree on this,[4] the majority of the evidence supports this finding.

## SLEEP AND YOUR HEART

My good friend Robb Wolf, who has been developing a cardiovascular risk-assessment program, remarked on how impactful sleep is for lab markers of cardiovascular disease. You can read his observations on my website: http://drruscio.com/podcast-robb-wolf-heart-disease-gut-health-medical-politics/#respond.

Robb's observations are certainly in alignment with the science.

Two different systematic reviews with meta-analyses have shown both long and short sleep duration are associated with high blood pressure.[5] Two other systematic reviews with meta-analyses have found short or long sleep duration associated with increased cardiovascular disease.[6] But remember it's not just about the duration of sleep. The quality is also important. It has been shown poor sleep quality worsens hypertension.[7]

Here are a few additional fun facts that exemplify how poor sleep is bad for your heart and cardiovascular system:

- Moderate sleep restriction causes arterial endothelial (blood vessel lining) dysfunction.[8]
- Snoring is associated with increased risk of heart attack, and inadequate sleep is associated with increased risk of heart attack.[9]
- Insomnia increases your risk of cardiovascular disease.[10]
- Untreated sleep apnea increases chance of death and cardiovascular disease.[11]
- Poor sleep has a negative effect on lipoproteins.[12]

## SLEEP, WEIGHT, AND METABOLISM

As with cardiovascular disease, we see extremely high-level scientific data supporting the association of poor sleep with weight gain, obesity, and metabolic syndrome.

Here is what we know:

- A meta-analysis has shown short and long sleep duration associated with increased type 2 diabetes.[13]
- A systematic review with meta-analysis has shown short and long sleep duration associated with increased risk of metabolic syndrome.[14]
- A systematic review with meta-analysis has shown short sleep duration associated with obesity in children.[15]
- Sleeping less leads to increased sugary-food intake.[16]
- Sleep deprivation may increase fat mass.[17]
- Blue light exposure at night (for example, television) suppresses metabolism the next morning.[18]
- Healthy timing of light exposure favorably affects obesity.[19]

And while there has been some criticism that the sleep studies are not perfect,[20] it still appears there is a strong and incontrovertible trend in the data showing poor sleep associated with weight gain, obesity, and metabolic syndrome.

It's not just about the sleep duration, the quality is important. Studies have shown

- sleep disruption has a negative impact on metabolic health;[21]
- poor sleep quality may contribute to obesity;[22]
- poor sleep quality is an independent risk factor for obesity—even after controlling for other factors, like exercise;[23]
- sleep disruption is a risk factor for metabolic syndrome.[24]

## SLEEP AND YOUR BRAIN

Here are a few fun facts connecting sleep and your brain:

- Poor-quality sleep means poorer cognitive performance.[25]
- Poor sleep in children decreases psychological health and increases health complaints.[26]
- Sleep helps your brain repair, rewire, and remove toxins.[27]
- Improved sleep patterns help with ADHD.[28]

## SLEEP AND YOUR IMMUNE SYSTEM

You've probably realized that poor sleep doesn't help anything. To pile on one more way poor sleep harms your health, researchers have found that sleep disorders increase risk of autoimmune conditions[29] and that the less sleep you get, the higher the risk of catching a cold.

We can clearly see that problems with sleep cause problems with health, but what is happening with the gut and microbiota?

## SLEEP AND YOUR GUT

After covering all the ways in which poor sleep can detract from your health, you are likely motivated to sleep more and better. But what if you're saying to yourself, "I try to sleep, but I just can't!" Well, there is good news: by improving your gut health, your sleep can dramatically improve. In the next chapter, we'll cover specific strategies for testing and treating a gut problem. By treating the problem, your sleep should improve. But, first, let's discuss the sleep–gut connection.

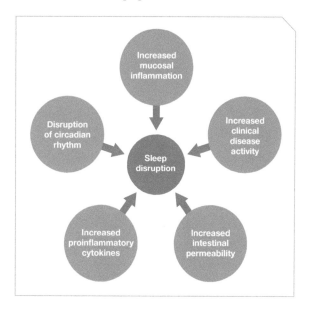

It has been shown that digestive tract inflammation decreases sleep quality.[30] Another study provides a great visual to help you see the connection between your gut and sleep.[31]

As the diagram illustrates, inflammation (cytokines), leaky gut (intestinal damage and permeability), disease activity, mucous membrane inflammation (inflammation in the lining of your intestines), and disrupted sleep rhythm (day/night rhythm) can all interfere with sleep.

### The IBS connection

As you learned earlier, it's not only about how *much* you sleep but also the *rhythm of your sleep*— going to bed and waking at the same times. It has been shown that participation in shift work, especially rotating shift work, is associated with the development of IBS and abdominal pain. These results were independent of sleep quality— meaning even if you sleep well, you have increased risk of IBS if your sleep rhythm is off.[32]

### The melatonin connection

Melatonin is a hormone released by your body when you sleep. Usually, the better you sleep, the more melatonin you release. This hormone might be the major connection between sleep and your gut. Supplementing with melatonin is typically done at bedtime to aid with sleep; supplementing with melatonin has also been shown helpful in IBS.[33]

It has been shown that poor sleep leads to lower melatonin, which then directly correlates to gut damage (leaky gut).[34] And, conversely, higher melatonin levels correlated with less leaky gut.[35] So, as melatonin goes up, leaky gut appears to go down.

**Better Sleep** = ⬆ **Melatonin** ⇒ ⬇ **Leaky Gut**

Now that we are learning how absolutely critical gut health is for overall health, it's interesting to ponder—maybe the reason we see so many diseases associated with poor sleep is because poor sleep negatively affects your gut, and the gut can negatively affect any other system in the body. In any case, gut problems can definitely cause problems with sleep. It has happened to me, I see it daily in my patients, and we see it supported in the literature. If you are suffering with a sleep problem, improving your gut health should help.

## SLEEP AND YOUR MICROBIOTA

Although there are only a couple of studies that specifically examine sleep's connection to the microbiota, the results are very interesting.

In 2014, a paper was published in the journal *Cell*. It examined the effects of jet lag on humans and mice. Jet lag would be an example of sleep-rhythm disruption and potentially an example of sleep loss as well. When the researchers tracked a group of humans before and after experiencing jet lag, they observed a noticeable shift in these subjects' microbiota. Was this a good or bad change, though? In an attempt to answer this question, the researchers performed a fecal transplant from the human subjects to mice, essentially transplanting the microbiota from the jet-lagged humans into mice. These mice then gained weight and experienced elevations of their blood sugar. When the microbiota from non-jet-lagged humans was transplanted into other mice, there was no change! This suggests the microbiotal changes that occur from jet lag caused weight gain and high blood sugar. This study does *not* tell us if the effects occurred as a result of flying or the time zone change, which disrupted the subjects' sleep rhythms, or if it was a combined result.

In this same study, we see an interesting example of how poor sleep can amplify the effects of an unhealthy diet. When mice who had their sleep rhythms disrupted, via jet lag, were fed an unhealthy diet (for mice, this means a high-fat diet), they gained weight. There was no weight gain in the other mice fed this same unhealthy diet who maintained a normal sleep cycle.[36] Similar mouse results have been published by others.[37] So, yes, poor sleep may amplify the effects of an unhealthy diet.

## TIPS AND STRATEGIES FOR OPTIMUM SLEEP

- Reduce blue light at night: use blue-light filters (which can be downloaded for computers, tablets, and phones), or use blue-light-filtering glasses.
- Keep your sleeping environment cool.
- Keep your bedroom quiet.[38]
- Avoid stressful prebed activities: no arguments, fight scenes on TV, news, or anything that will stress you out or stimulate you.
- Strive to be in bed by ten or eleven and then sleep seven to nine hours, but if you consistently find you can't get seven hours or need more than nine, consult a doctor—something might be off.

- For those with sleep apnea, sleeping on your stomach, with the aid of a special pillow and mattress, may improve sleep quality. This may eliminate the need for your CPAP mask.[39]
- If you can't sleep, nap. Napping helps protect against negative effects of sleep deprivation.[40]
- Try music therapy. It can help with sleep quality.[41]

### HERE ARE SOME THINGS TO INVESTIGATE IF YOU'RE HAVING SLEEP PROBLEMS

Hormonal imbalances
· Female hormones—hot flashes can cause insomnia. Sometimes women have very subtle hot flashes that are not enough to wake them up feeling super hot and sweaty but are still enough to wake them up. We will cover how to know if you have female hormone imbalances and treatment options in part 5.
· Adrenal hormones—problems here can cause the inability to fall asleep or the inability to stay asleep. Taking an adrenal-support supplement may help. Having frequent meals during the day and having a snack when you wake up may also help. We will cover adrenal supplement options in part 5.

Inflammatory or digestive issues
· More on this in part 5 also.

If you are serious about being healthy, sleep must be a priority. You cannot achieve your optimum health if you are not sleeping well. I rarely make such strong statements, but the research here is clear. You must make this a priority if you want to feel your best.

# CONCEPT SUMMARY

- Sleep is another factor that affects your internal environment and can impact your microbiota negatively or positively.

- Very high-level scientific data suggest consistently getting sleep of short (less than six to seven hours) or long (more than nine hours) duration is associated with poor health.

- It has been shown that maintaining the same sleep rhythm (circadian rhythm) is as important as duration.

- High-level scientific data show poor sleep contributes to weight gain, obesity, and metabolic syndrome.

- Sleep helps your brain repair, rewire, and remove toxins.

- Sleep disorders increase your risk for autoimmune disease.

- It has been shown that participation in shift work, especially rotating shift work, is associated with the development of IBS.

- The reason we see so many diseases associated with poor sleep might be because poor sleep negatively affects the gut, and the gut can negatively affect any other system.

1   E. F. Chernikova, "The Influence of Shift Work on Worker's Health Status (Review)," [In Russian.] *Gigiena I Sanitariia* 94, no. 3 (2015): 44–48, http://europepmc.org/abstract/med/26302558.

2   J. C. Benabu et al., "Night Work, Shift Work: Breast Cancer Risk Factor?," [In French.] *Gynecologie, Obstetrique & Fertilite* 43, no. 12 (2015): 791–99, doi:10.1016/j.gyobfe.2015.10.004.

3   Lisa Gallicchio and Bindu Kalesan, "Sleep Duration and Mortality: A Systematic Review and Meta-Analysis," *Journal of Sleep Research* 18, no. 2 (2009): 148–58, doi:10.1111/j.1365-2869.2008.00732.x; Francesco P. Cappuccio et al., "Sleep Duration and All-Cause Mortality: A Systematic Review and Meta-Analysis of Prospective Studies," *Sleep* 33, no. 5 (2010): 585–92, doi:10.1093/sleep/33.5.585.

4   Lianne M. Kurina et al., "Sleep Duration and All-Cause Mortality: A Critical Review of Measurement and Associations," *Annals of Epidemiology* 23, no. 6 (2013): 361–70, doi:10.1016/j.annepidem.2013.03.015.

5   Qijuan Wang et al., "Short Sleep Duration Is Associated with Hypertension Risk among Adults: A Systematic Review and Meta-Analysis," *Hypertension Research: Official Journal of the Japanese Society of Hypertension* 35, no. 44 (2012): 1012–18, doi:10.1038/hr.2012.91; Xiaofan Guo et al., "Epidemiological Evidence for the Link between Sleep Duration and High Blood Pressure: A Systematic Review and Meta-Analysis," *Sleep Medicine* 14, no. 4 (2013): 324–32, doi:10.1016/j.sleep.2012.12.001.

6   Xiaorong Yang et al., "Association of Sleep Duration with the Morbidity and Mortality of Coronary Artery Disease: A Meta-Analysis of Prospective Studies," *Heart, Lung & Circulation* 24, no. 12 (2015): 1180–90, doi:10.1016/j.hlc.2015.08.005; Francesco P. Cappuccio et al., "Sleep Duration Predicts Cardiovascular Outcomes: A Systematic Review and Meta-Analysis of Prospective Studies," *European Heart Journal*, 2011, doi:10.1093/eurheartj/ehr007.

7   Kai Lu et al., "Interaction of Sleep Duration and Sleep Quality on Hypertension Prevalence in Adult Chinese Males," *Journal of Epidemiology* 25, no. 6 (2015): 415–22, doi:10.2188/jea.JE20140139.

8   Andrew D. Calvin et al., "Experimental Sleep Restriction Causes Endothelial Dysfunction in Healthy Humans," *Journal of the American Heart Association* 3, no. 6 (2014), doi:10.1161/JAHA.114.001143.

9   Dongfang Xie et al., "Sleep Duration, Snoring Habits, and Risk of Acute Myocardial Infarction in China Population: Results of the INTERHEART Study," *BMC Public Health* 14, no. 1 (2014): 531, doi:10.1186/1471-2458-14-531.

10  A. Silva-Costa et al., "Disentangling the Effects of Insomnia and Night Work on Cardiovascular Diseases: A Study in Nursing Professionals," *Brazilian Journal of Medical and Biological Research* 48, no. 2 (2015): 120–27, doi:10.1590/1414-431X20143965.

11   Maria Inês Pires Fonseca et al., "Death and Disability in Patients with Sleep Apnea—A Meta-Analysis," *Arquivos Brasileiros de Cardiologia*, 2014, 58–65, doi:10.5935/abc.20140172.

12   A. Knutson, "Serum Lipoproteins in Day and Shift Workers: A Prospective Study," *British Journal of Industrial Medicine* 47, no. 2 (1990): 132–34, doi:10.1136/oem.47.2.132.

13   Zhilei Shan et al., "Sleep Duration and Risk of Type 2 Diabetes: A Meta-Analysis of Prospective Studies," *Diabetes Care* 38, no. 3 (2015): 529–37, doi:10.2337/dc14-2073.

14   Bo Xi et al., "Short Sleep Duration Predicts Risk of Metabolic Syndrome: A Systematic Review and Meta-Analysis," *Sleep Medicine Reviews* 18, no. 4 (2014): 293–97, doi:10.1016/j.smrv.2013.06.001.

15   Y. Fatima et al., "Longitudinal Impact of Sleep on Overweight and Obesity in Children and Adolescents: A Systematic Review and Bias-Adjusted Meta-Analysis," *Obesity Reviews* 16, no. 2 (2015): 137–49, doi:10.1111/obr.12245.

16   M. F. Hjorth et al., "Change in Sleep Duration and Proposed Dietary Risk Factors for Obesity in Danish School Children," *Pediatric Obesity* 9, no. 6 (2014): e156–59, doi:10.1111/ijpo.264.

17   Julie D. Shlisky et al., "Partial Sleep Deprivation and Energy Balance in Adults: An Emerging Issue for Consideration by Dietetics Practitioners," *Journal of the Academy of Nutrition and Dietetics* 112, no. 11 (2012): 1785–97, doi:10.1016/j.jand.2012.07.032.

18   Momoko Kayaba et al., "The Effect of Nocturnal Blue Light Exposure from Light-Emitting Diodes on Wakefulness and Energy Metabolism the Following Morning," *Environmental Health and Preventive Medicine* 19, no. 5 (2014): 354–61, doi:10.1007/s12199-014-0402-x.

19   Kathryn J. Reid et al., "Timing and Intensity of Light Correlate with Body Weight in Adults," *PLoS ONE* 9, no. 4 (2014), doi:10.1371/journal.pone.0092251.

20   Matthew Guidolin and Michael Gradisar, "Is Shortened Sleep Duration a Risk Factor for Overweight and Obesity during Adolescence? A Review of the Empirical Literature," *Sleep Medicine*, 2012, doi:10.1016/j.sleep.2012.03.016; Sanjay R. Patel and Frank B. Hu, "Short Sleep Duration and Weight Gain: A Systematic Review," *Obesity (Silver Spring, Md.)* 16, no. 3 (2008): 643–53, doi:10.1038/oby.2007.118.

21   Arlet V. Nedeltcheva and Frank A. J. L. Scheer, "Metabolic Effects of Sleep Disruption, Links to Obesity and Diabetes," *Current Opinion in Endocrinology, Diabetes, and Obesity* 21, no. 4 (2014): 293–98, doi:10.1097/MED.0000000000000082.

22   Alison L. Miller et al., "Sleep Patterns and Obesity in Childhood," *Current Opinion in Endocrinology, Diabetes, and Obesity* 22, no. 1 (2015): 41–47, doi:10.1097/MED.0000000000000125.

23   Miji Kim, "Association between Objectively Measured Sleep Quality and Obesity in Community-Dwelling Adults Aged Eighty Years or Older: A Cross-Sectional Study," *Journal of Korean Medical Science* 30, no. 2 (2015): 199–206, doi:10.3346/jkms.2015.30.2.199.

24   Mae Sheikh-Ali and Jaisri Maharaj, "Circadian Clock Desynchronisation and Metabolic Syndrome," *Postgraduate Medical Journal* 90, no. 1066 (2014): 461–66, doi:10.1136/postgradmedj-2013-132366.

25   Yeonsu Song et al., "Relationships between Sleep Stages and Changes in Cognitive Function in Older Men: The MrOS Sleep Study," *SLEEP*, 2015, doi:10.5665/sleep.4500.

26   Victor Segura-Jiménez et al., "Association of Sleep Patterns with Psychological Positive Health and Health Complaints in Children and Adolescents," *Quality of Life Research : An International Journal of Quality of Life Aspects of Treatment, Care and Rehabilitation* 24, no. 4 (2015): 885–95, doi:10.1007/s11136-014-0827-0.

27   Henna-Kaisa Wigren and Tarja Stenberg, "How Does Sleeping Restore Our Brain?," [In Finnish.] *Duodecim; Laaketieteellinen Aikakauskirja* 131, no. 2 (2015): 151–56, http://europepmc.org/abstract/med/26237917.

28   Zahra Keshavarzi et al., "In a Randomized Case–Control Trial with Ten-Year-Olds Suffering from Attention Deficit/Hyperactivity Disorder (ADHD) Sleep and Psychological Functioning Improved during a Twelve-Week Sleep-Training Program," *World Journal of Biological Psychiatry* 15, no. 8 (2014): 609–19, doi:10.3109/15622975.2014.922698.

29   Y. H. Hsiao et al., "Sleep Disorders and Increased Risk of Autoimmune Diseases in Individuals without Sleep Apnea," *Sleep* 38, no. 4 (2015): 581–86, doi:10.5665/sleep.4574; Jiunn-Horng Kang and Herng-Ching Lin, "Obstructive Sleep Apnea and the Risk of Autoimmune Diseases: A Longitudinal Population-Based Study," *Sleep Medicine* 13, no. 6 (2012): 583–88, doi:10.1016/j.sleep.2012.03.002.

30   Robin G. Wilson et al., "High C-Reactive Protein Is Associated with Poor Sleep Quality Independent of Nocturnal Symptoms in Patients with Inflammatory Bowel Disease," *Digestive Diseases and Sciences* 60, no. 7 (2015): 2136–43, doi:10.1007/s10620-015-3580-5.

31    Garth R. Swanson et al., "Sleep Disturbances and Inflammatory Bowel Disease: A Potential Trigger for Disease Flare?," *Expert Review of Clinical Immunology* 7, no. 1 (2011): 29–36, doi:10.1586/eci.10.83.

32    Hye In Kim et al., "Impact of Shiftwork on Irritable Bowel Syndrome and Functional Dyspepsia," *Journal of Korean Medical Science* 28, no. 3 (2013): 431–37, doi:10.3346/jkms.2013.28.3.431; Borko Nojkov et al., "The Impact of Rotating Shift Work on the Prevalence of Irritable Bowel Syndrome in Nurses," *American Journal of Gastroenterology* 105, no. 4 (2010): 842–47, doi:10.1038/ajg.2010.48; Garth R. Swanson et al., "Sleep Disturbances and Inflammatory Bowel Disease: A Potential Trigger for Disease Flare?," *Expert Review of Clinical Immunology* 7, no. 1 (2011): 29–36, doi:10.1586/eci.10.83.

33    Kewin Tien Ho Siah et al., "Melatonin for the Treatment of Irritable Bowel Syndrome," *World Journal of Gastroenterology* 20, no. 10 (2014): 2492–98, doi:10.3748/wjg.v20.i10.2492.

34    Garth R. Swanson et al., "Decreased Melatonin Secretion Is Associated with Increased Intestinal Permeability and Marker of Endotoxemia in Alcoholics," *American Journal of Physiology—Gastrointestinal and Liver Physiology* 308, no. 12 (2015): G1004–11, doi:10.1152/ajpgi.00002.2015.

35    Tomoyuki Kawada, "Sleep Parameters by Actigraphy and Relationship between Plasma Melatonin and Intestinal Permeability in Alcoholics," *American Journal of Physiology—Gastrointestinal and Liver Physiology* 309, no. 4 (August 15, 2015): G279, doi:10.1152/ajpgi.00153.2015.

36    Christoph A. Thaiss et al., "Transkingdom Control of Microbiota Diurnal Oscillations Promotes Metabolic Homeostasis," *Cell* 159, no. 3 (2014): 514–29, doi:10.1016/j.cell.2014.09.048.

37    Robin M. Voigt et al., "Circadian Disorganization Alters Intestinal Microbiota," *PLoS ONE* 9, no. 5 (2014), doi:10.1371/journal.pone.0097500.

38    Frank Schmidt et al., "Nighttime Aircraft Noise Impairs Endothelial Function and Increases Blood Pressure in Patients with or at High Risk for Coronary Artery Disease," *Clinical Research in Cardiology: Official Journal of the German Cardiac Society* 104, no. 1 (2015): 23–30, doi:10.1007/s00392-014-0751-x.

39    Armin Bidarian-Moniri et al., "Mattress and Pillow for Prone Positioning for Treatment of Obstructive Sleep Apnoea," *Acta Oto-Laryngologica* 135, no. 3 (2015): 271–76, doi:10.3109/00016489.2014.968674.

40    Ken Tokizawa et al., "Effects of Partial Sleep Restriction and Subsequent Daytime Napping on Prolonged Exertional Heat Strain," *Occupational and Environmental Medicine* 72, no. 7 (2015): 521–28, doi:10.1136/oemed-2014-102548.

41    Chun-Fang Wang et al., "Music Therapy Improves Sleep Quality in Acute and Chronic Sleep Disorders: A Meta-Analysis of Ten Randomized Studies," *International Journal of Nursing Studies* 51, no. 1 (2014): 51–62, doi:10.1016/j.ijnurstu.2013.03.008.

# CHAPTER 13

# STRESS AND ADRENAL FATIGUE

## IMPROVE YOUR ENVIRONMENT BY REMOVING STRESS

It probably won't surprise you to learn that stress can negatively affect your gut and microbiota. Excessive stress appears to negatively affect virtually every part of the body. Stress has been shown to cause

- gut damage (leaky gut);[1]
- enhanced gut immunity, short-term;[2]
- decreased gut immunity (immunosuppression), long-term, which correlates with increased risk of infection;[3]
- decreased intestinal mucous membrane,[4] which is likely why stress causes decreased immunity and leaky gut;
- decreased blood flow to the intestinal tract;
- suppression of stomach acid secretion;[5]
- slowing of stomach and small-intestinal motility;[6]
- delayed wound healing.[7]

None of these are particularly problematic if the stress is short-term, but these can be very problematic in the long term. When we look at how the gut responds to stress, we see long-term stress creates the perfect storm for gut problems.

### SUE: A REAL-WORLD EXAMPLE OF THE STRESS–GUT CONNECTION

Sue is in her early thirties and has been living a high-stress lifestyle for years. In rapid succession, she finished her master's degree, got married, and moved to a suburb, which gave her a lengthy commute every day. Sue is unwilling to give up her six-day-a-week exercise routine but finds it hard to make time for exercise after work, her commute, and spending time with her husband. She decides to sleep a little less to be able to fit it all in.

The additional stress of her commute, combined with less sleep, now makes her six-days-per-week exercise routine too much for her body. Sue doesn't realize it, but her body is now under too much stress. Soon, she starts noticing she is not sleeping well, tossing and turning and waking up one hour before her alarm goes off, unable to fall back to sleep. She is tired during the day and notices her coffee consumption is steadily increasing. Her muscles are sore more frequently, and she notices nagging muscle pulls and joint pain she never had before. She also starts craving sugary foods.

A few months later, Sue starts to feel bloated all the time and notices she is not going to the bathroom every day. Sue notices food reactions— some foods now make her feel tired and give her brain fog. She decides to clean up her diet and start taking a probiotic. This helps, but she still does not feel anywhere close to how she used to. What is happening internally to Sue?

First, the long-term stress causes Sue's stomach to release less acid. Normally, the highly acidic environment of the stomach does not allow bacteria to grow in the small intestine,[8] which is food's next stop after the stomach. Because Sue has less acid, more bacteria are able to grow. The stress impairs the motility of her small intestine, which worsens bacterial overgrowth and weakens the immune system of her intestine. When intestinal motility slows, it's like water that becomes stagnant; stagnant water fosters bacterial growth, while running water does not. Stagnant intestinal motility encourages bacterial growth; good intestinal motility does not.

So, there is increased bacteria in Sue's small intestine, and the bacteria are just sitting there because of the impaired motility. At the same time, Sue's immune system is weak, and the protective mucous membrane in her intestine has become worn and thin because of it.

What does all this mean? It means Sue now has SIBO and leaky gut. The SIBO is causing the constipation and bloating. The leaky gut is causing the fatigue and brain fog. And her overtraining is causing burnout/adrenal fatigue, which is causing her to have insomnia, fatigue, and cravings. Her muscles can't repair themselves because of the overtraining, and this is causing chronic soreness and muscle pulls.

Sue reads an article online that leads her to think she has an adrenal problem—essentially a decline in the level of energy-providing stress hormones like cortisol, known as adrenal fatigue. She tries some adrenal supplements to fix her adrenal problem. She feels better for a while but then feels lousy again a few months later. This is because Sue is not treating the problem; she is treating a symptom—the problem is not her adrenal hormones; her adrenal hormone imbalances are a symptom of the actual problem. What Sue should do is adjust her lifestyle so she is not in a chronic stress response. This would entail exercising one or two days less and getting more sleep. She needs the proper diagnosis and treatment of SIBO— which can take even more stress off her system. She can use adrenal support to help give her a little boost and support recovery, but this will not fix the cause of her problem. This is a mistake I see patients make quite often.

Is what happened to Sue rare? No, not at all. Sue has SIBO, and SIBO often manifests with the symptoms of IBS: gas, bloating, constipation, and diarrhea. Although it's a controversial assertion, some researchers now believe most cases of IBS are actually caused by SIBO. IBS is estimated to effect 15% of the United States population[9] and 11% of the world.[10] However, 75% of IBS may go undiagnosed, because patients with IBS don't see their doctors for a diagnosis.[11] This means the actual percentage of people with IBS might be much, much higher.

How does stress factor into this? It has been well documented that stress makes IBS worse.[12] And we just detailed Sue's case, in which stress caused SIBO, which then manifested as IBS. So, what happened in Sue's case can be quite common. Connecting the dots, here is how this may play out: stress damages the gut, this causes SIBO, and SIBO then manifests as a bunch of symptoms known as IBS, fatigue, and insomnia.

We've looked at how stress affects your gut and what a real-world example of this looks like. Let's now look more specifically at stress's effect on the microbiota.

## STRESS AND YOUR MICROBIOTA

Stress has been documented to worsen IBS and IBD.[13] Stress has been shown to cause us to make poor food choices,[14] which leads to craving foods high in fat and carbs.

Stress might first negatively affect your microbiota, which then causes the worsening of digestive symptoms and diseases. For example, it has been shown that college students have decreased levels of the healthy bacteria lactobacilli during periods of exam stress when compared to their nonstressed peers.[15] These findings have been affirmed by other researchers as well.[16] This is especially interesting to consider because numerous clinical trial have shown IBS, IBD, and digestive symptoms in general improve after taking lactobacillus-based probiotics.

We've learned a lot about how stress negatively affects your gut microbiota via animal studies. I try to focus on human studies; however, it would be unethical to conduct some experiments on humans, so we're limited to animal studies. Let's discuss a few findings from these animal studies that are worth mentioning.

When mice were exposed to just two hours of social stress, their microbiotas shifted, a shift that included a reduction in lactobacilli.[17] The hormones released as part of stress might be a key reason for its negative effects. It has even been shown that stress hormones can fuel the growth of potentially dangerous bacteria in the gut.[18]

The most practical and important data here is that physiological stress has been shown to impede wound healing in both animals and humans[19] and

that social stress has been shown to impede wound healing as well.[20]

## STRESS, MOTILITY, AND AN INFLAMMATORY MICROBIOTA

A fascinating mouse study has shown once more that stress negatively affects the microbiota. After exposure to social stress, mice experienced a shift in their microbiotas that increased inflammation. So, stress caused an inflammatory microbiota. Here is the fascinating part: if these mice were exposed to stress again, more inflammation occurred. However, if these mice were treated with antibiotics *before* being exposed to stress again—no inflammation![21] Similar findings have been documented by others.[22]

This helps validate much of what has already been observed clinically and that we've been discussing. Interventions that "prune" the microbiota or decrease bacterial overgrowth may be helpful for those with gut imbalances. Examples of approaches that prune bacterial overgrowths are eating a low-carb or low-FODMAP diet and using herbal antimicrobials and, in select cases, antibiotics.

Does this mean we want *no* bacteria or that we should focus exclusively on killing bacteria in our guts? No. More isn't always better. Mice that have no bacteria in their guts (known as germ-free mice) have been shown to be more sensitive to stress; specifically, compared to normal mice, their HPA axis responds more to stress.[23] "HPA axis" is just a fancy way of saying your brain and your hormonal glands respond to stress together.

The bacteria in your gut are also needed for healthy motility (movement). Intestinal motility is important, because it ensures food moves through your intestinal tract. If movement/motility slows, bacteria can overgrow and cause problems.

Germ-free mice (mice with no bacteria in their guts) do not have healthy intestinal motility, but when we add bacteria back into the guts of these mice, we see their motility improve.[24] So, it appears a healthy microbiota is important for motility (Gut Geeks, specifically, the migratory motor complex). In fact, researchers are even starting to find that fractions of a bacterium known as LPS bind to receptors known as toll-like receptors (TLR4s), which then stimulate motility via the nerves of your gut.[25] It's almost as if bacteria flip the switch in your gut to stimulate motility.[26]

It's also worth mentioning that simple and free interventions for stress, such as breathing, movement, and meditation, have been shown to decrease inflammation and improve quality of life in those with IBD.[27] The basics go a long way.

## BACTERIAL STRESS RELIEF

We discussed how mice with no bacteria in their guts (germ-free mice) are more sensitive to stress. Does this mean probiotics might be able to help with stress? Yes! Randomized control trials have found probiotics can alleviate depression, anger, hostility, and anxiety, while also decreasing stress-hormone levels.[28] In fact, a systematic review with meta-analysis of clinical trials has found probiotics lead to a significant reduction in depression.[29]

## STRESS AND LIFESTYLE

Dan Buettner wrote a book titled *Thrive: Finding Happiness the Blue Zones Way*. He embarked on a study of the happiest societies around the world in an attempt to find commonalities among happy people. He observed a few interesting things:

Income did not correlate with happiness, nor did power. However, the time people spent with their friends and family seemed to be directly proportional to their happiness. Also, the longer someone's commute, the less happy he or she was. Some of the people Dan examines in his book provide striking illustrations of how imbalanced our lifestyles have become in Westernized societies.

For example, an Asian real-estate tycoon worth millions is miserable, while a village woman in Argentina who doesn't even have a bank account feels joyous every day.[30]

Buettner's observations are powerful, but has anyone taken the next step to examine them more scientifically? Yes. Research has shown the quality of your relationships may have a significant impact on your ability to heal. If you're reading this, you likely fit into one of two categories: someone who is healthy and looking to feel even better; or someone who is sick and looking to improve his or her health. If you're healthy, more social time will likely increase your happiness. If you're sick, healthy relationships can help you heal.

How do relationships aid in healing? Healthy relationships may help balance stress hormones, and balanced stress hormones allow you to heal more quickly. Research has shown that the wounds of isolated hamsters heal more slowly than nonisolated hamsters. Not only that, but if the adrenal glands of these isolated hamsters are removed, their healing time normalizes! This implies that stress hormones, which are produced by the adrenal glands, are the reason poor-quality relationships can impede healing.[31] The *problem* is the imbalanced levels of stress hormones, but the *cause* of this is the stress.

In humans, it has been shown that women with healthy relationships experience less stress-hormone release after a stressful event.[32] You may have heard of the "fight or flight" reaction to stress, but researcher Shelly Taylor has proposed another equally important reaction to stress: "tend and befriend."[33]

Taylor's work suggests that in times of stress, we become more dependent upon our partners, friends, family, and social groups. In other words, stress may bring us together as a means of coping. Stress stimulating togetherness has a strong evolutionary benefit, because those who come together and support each other during stress have an increased chance of survival. You need a modern-day tribe to cope with modern-day stress.

The hormone oxytocin may be an important part of this "tend and befriend" response. Oxytocin appears to foster trust and the desire for social contact. Again, oxytocin may also blunt the release of stress hormones. High levels of stress hormones can be damaging to the body. Interestingly, women may be more sensitive to the effects of oxytocin than men since estrogen enhances the effects of oxytocin. So, to put it simply, women may need more tending and befriending in response to stress than men.

Spending time with loved ones is a great method of stress relief. Time in nature, as we discussed, is another powerful method for decreasing stress and increasing well-being. Unfortunately, TV and the Internet have taken us away from both of these. It has been documented that people are spending less time in nature *because* they are spending more time watching TV and on the Internet.[34] There is evidence that increased time on the Internet correlates with poor health:

- The more time people spend on Internet media, the more depressed and anxious they become.[35]
- The more time people spend on Facebook specifically, the more distressed they become and the lower their self-esteem.[36]
- Online chatting correlates with depression and loneliness.[37]

Clearly, getting away from the computer and getting into nature can yield impressive results. Time in nature has also been shown to make people

- more caring;[38]
- less impulsive;[39]
- kinder.[40]

Stepping away from the computer and spending time in nature can help you improve your social relationships *and* improve your health. If you don't have much nature close by, or if harsh winters or scorching summers prevent enjoying time in nature, that's OK. Don't forget how powerful it can be to sit in a cozy room and chat with friends or family.

## STRESS RELIEF, DANISH-STYLE

There is an entire philosophy that encompasses this: *hygge*. Hygge (pronounced *hew-guh*) is a philosophy for happy living that comes from the Danish, who consistently rank as having one of the world's happiest societies. A major tenet of the happy hygge lifestyle is good conversation in a cozy atmosphere, often dimly lit by candle. So, if going outdoors doesn't work, shut off the lights, light some candles, and nestle in to enjoy some good conversation with a friend or loved one.

Let's zoom way out for a second. As I write this, I'm picturing people who are struggling with their health. They spend hours a day in front of the computer doing research about their health. They obsess over what to eat. They obsess over what tests to get. They've given up on hobbies, exercise, and social time. The sad truth here is they could inadvertently be making their health *worse* by not being in nature and not taking time for friends and hobbies. They're increasing their stress, depression, and anxiety levels *because* they're obsessing over their diet and spending more time on the Internet.

This is not to say that you shouldn't perform your research and take steps to improve your diet—you certainly should. However, there is a point at which the time and energy invested in improving your health becomes a negative

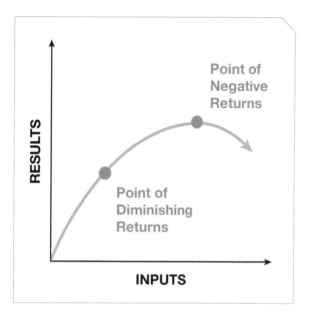

Point of Negative Returns

Point of Diminishing Returns

RESULTS

INPUTS

summarize many of these concepts.[41] Remember, we don't want to blindly replicate our ancestors' environment—some of their practices might make us sick. We're filtering these recommendations through modern clinical findings.

investment. This is illustrated by the law of diminishing returns. Initial investment has high yields. Further investment still has positive yield, but not as much. But even more investment starts to have a negative yield.

Don't sacrifice your friends, hobbies, and time in nature—proven tools for improving your health and well-being—to do research about your health. I know it's tough; I've been there—but don't lose your grip on these important fundamentals of good health. Make sure you don't neglect the life you're trying to improve in an attempt to become healthier.

## Don't make yourself miserable in your attempt to be healthy.

Consider this: Is a healthy person with a neglected life any better off than an ill person with a rich and fulfilling life?

Our goal in examining the impact of our environment on our health and making changes to it is to try to replicate the environment of our ancestors. To a certain extent, this new microbiota information is just another way of reinforcing why it's so important to do so. Recent publications

### OUR ANCESTORS ROUTINELY EXPERIENCED:

- **Natural olfactory stimulants; phytoncides**

- **Natural light (daytime blue in particular)**

- **Contact with non-pathogenic microbial diversity**

- **Darkness at night**

- **Physical activity in natural environments**

- **Opportunity for privacy and solitude**

- **Intake of relatively unprocessed foods; phytochemicals**

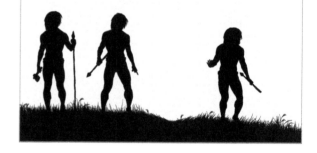

# IMPROVING YOUR ENVIRONMENT BY ADDRESSING ADRENAL FATIGUE

When people are under high amounts of stress for a prolonged period of time, they can start to become fatigued. Often, this is described as adrenal fatigue.

Adrenal fatigue is a condition in which your body becomes hormonally imbalanced due to chronic stress. I'm not a big fan of this term because it tends to take the focus off the problem—the cause of stress—and places it on the symptom, which is altered hormonal production. I'll use the term, though, to keep things simple. In adrenal fatigue, the ability of your adrenal glands to produce adrenal hormones becomes diminished.

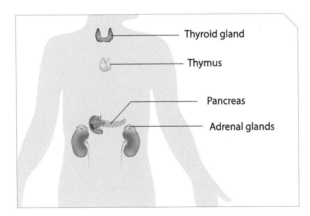

Thyroid gland

Thymus

Pancreas

Adrenal glands

What are adrenal hormones? There are many, but some of the most relevant are cortisol, adrenaline, DHEA, testosterone, estrogen, and progesterone. We don't need to define these hormones one by one, but let's organize them into two general categories: stress hormones and antiaging hormones. Cortisol and adrenaline are stress hormones. You need the right level of these to feel your best—not too much but not too little. DHEA, testosterone, estrogen, and progesterone are antiaging hormones (in fact, many antiaging doctors give these hormones to patients).

When the levels of these adrenal hormones are off, you might experience any number of the following symptoms:

- Fatigue
- Insomnia
- Sugar cravings
- Depression
- Caffeine dependence
- Dizziness when standing up quickly
- A weakened immune system
- Low libido
- Brain fog or impaired cognition

Because of the wide variety of symptoms adrenal fatigue can cause, pretty much everyone who has heard of it thinks they have it. This has spawned a dizzying amount of information and treatments on the topic: adrenal diets, adrenal testing, adrenal supplements, and so on. But here is a very important fact that is not often mentioned:

*the adrenal glands malfunction as a direct result of stress; therefore, the solution to adrenal fatigue is fixing the source of the stress.*

Why does this matter? Because I want you to feel better as fast as possible. I want to prevent you from doing what I did when I was ill and what many of my patients do before they see me: wasting time and money chasing down adrenal symptoms, adrenal tests, and trying various adrenal support programs while at the same time completely overlooking the root cause of the adrenal problem. Following that path will result in symptoms that never fully go away and quickly creep back. Not only did I learn this with my own experience as a patient, but I learned it clinically with the patients I treat. In the clinic, I spent several years testing the adrenals of my patients and then a few years *not* testing the adrenals but rather focusing on finding and fixing the source of stress. I obtain much better results with adrenal fatigue when ***I stop treating the adrenal test results and start treating the patient***. And guess what? Working through our Great-in-8 is a way to treat yourself that's very similar to how I treat my patients. As I do with my patients, we will use adrenal support as part of the Great-in-8. However, it's very important for you to understand adrenal support is not some magical cure-all but rather one of many treatments that work synergistically as part of our Great-in-8 plan to help you restore your health.

### GUT GEEKS

*A recent systematic review of fifty-eight high-quality studies found adrenal-fatigue testing to be highly inaccurate. Various types of adrenal tests were evaluated in attempts to find a correlation between adrenal testing and fatigue. What was found? To put it simply, over 50% of the time there was no correlation between fatigue and adrenal test results. Adrenal testing is tempting in theory, but sadly it does not deliver in practice.*[42]

To summarize, when your body has been under prolonged stress, you can experience adrenal fatigue and subsequently adrenal-fatigue symptoms. Treating the cause of stress is the only way to truly recover from adrenal fatigue. Stress can have many forms. Some are obvious: relationship stress, financial stress, lack of sleep. Others are not as apparent. There is one type of stress that is often overlooked. This stressor is a major cause of adrenal fatigue, and overlooking it prevents people from recovering from all their symptoms. Can you guess what type of stress this is? Digestive stress!

## THE GUT–ADRENAL FATIGUE CONNECTION— WHY YOU MUST HEAL YOUR GUT TO RECOVER

After diet and lifestyle, the most common cause of stress on the body is the gut. There have been countless patients who have come into my office complaining of chronic adrenal fatigue. They might be experiencing chronic insomnia, fatigue, or depression that has never fully responded to fancy adrenal-support programs. For the majority of these patients, the problem isn't the adrenals, it's a problem in the gut. Fixing this problem finally provides relief to their insomnia, fatigue, depression, or [insert troubling symptom here]. This again illustrates the far-reaching influence of the gut. Is healing the gut a 100% guarantee for fixing adrenal fatigue? No. But most of the time, it will, which is why addressing gut health is so crucial.

Debbie is a great example of how pivotal the health of your gut is to the health of your adrenals.

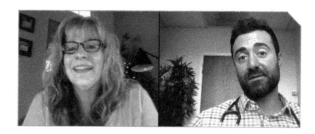

She was plagued with insomnia, fatigue, anxiety, poor mental clarity, and weight gain. These are all symptoms that can be associated with adrenal fatigue. Did we test her adrenals? No. Did these symptoms go away? Yes. Debbie did great. We supported her adrenals while we treated her for intestinal infections and imbalances. Addressing this is what really allowed Debbie to respond and feel better. Treating her with adrenal support without addressing her gut's health would have done very little. All of Debbie's adrenal symptoms went away without any adrenal testing. Omitting the adrenal testing saved her at least a few hundred dollars. Again, this conservative thinking, applied consistently, can be the difference between saving or spending thousands of dollars, when all is said and done.

Why are gut problems such a major source of stress for the body? Probably because problems in the gut can easily cause:

- inflammation—which can occur because of eating inflammatory foods or from bacterial/fungal imbalances or infections;
- autoimmunity—brought about by problems with the small intestine, where most of the immune system resides;
- nutrient malabsorption—damage to the gut can result in malabsorption of vital nutrients.

All of these can cause chronic internal stress, can lead to adrenal fatigue, and can thwart recovery from fatigue, insomnia, cravings, or any of the other adrenal fatigue symptoms. Imagine this: every time you eat, you inadvertently are feeding SIBO, which damages the lining of your intestines, causes inflammation, and makes your immune system to go haywire. If you're eating three or four times a day, can you imagine the *impact*? Imagine if you got into three to four fights per day with your boss or spouse? You would be drained, right? The equivalent of this can happen in your gut and *is* happening for many people. If you did nothing to address this, how could testing and adrenal supplements possibly help you recover? This is why the health of the gut is such a pivotal piece of recovering from adrenal fatigue.

As we work through our Great-in-8, you'll improve the health of your gut and, therefore, the health of your adrenals. However, it is important to mention that some adrenal support may also help with the healing of your gut.

## THE ADRENAL FATIGUE–GUT CONNECTION—HOW ADRENAL SUPPORT CAN HELP HEAL YOUR GUT

You must heal your gut to recover from adrenal fatigue, but does this mean we should discard adrenal support completely? No. Adrenal support might actually be able to help the gut heal, which is part of the reason why adrenal support is included in our Great-in-8. Adrenal support can also be used in the short term to reduce the symptoms of adrenal fatigue. It's fine to use adrenal support as long as we are treating the underlying cause of the adrenal fatigue at the same time.

Earlier, we covered the numerous ways in which stress can negatively affect your gut and your microbiota. Remember how college students under exam stress experienced a negative shift of intestinal bacteria? There are some herbal medicines that actually help your body cope with stress and also help to balance stress-hormone levels. This class of herbs is known as adaptogens or adaptogenic herbs. What's interesting about this class of herbal medicines is they work to *correct* adrenal hormonal imbalances, whether high or low. If someone's stress/adrenal hormones are high, adaptogenic herbs help lower them. If someone's stress hormones are low, adaptogenic herbs help to increase them.

The herb ginseng works as an adaptogen. Recently, a study showed that ginseng promoted the growth of healthy intestinal bacteria like bifidobacterium and lactobacillus and prevented the growth of harmful bacteria.[43] These results were from rat and cell studies, so we have to be cautious with how much we infer from them, but they're interesting findings nonetheless.

Adaptogenic herbs have been used in numerous human clinical trials and have been shown to be very safe and provide various benefits like improved mood, fatigue, cortisol levels, memory, immune function, and endurance.[44] None of these studies used adrenal testing to guide the treatment—more reinforcement for the recommendation to skip the test and try the treatment. Adaptogenic herbs also have a long history of use in traditional Chinese medicine and Ayurvedic (traditional Indian) medicine and have been used by these cultures as natural ways to increase energy, stamina, and mood.

Adrenal glandulars are another type of adrenal support. These are extracts of adrenal glands, usually from cows or pigs. Studies that look at glandulars are extremely sparse, but I've been using glandulars with patients for years, and they are safe and seem to provide benefit. How do glandulars work? Adrenal glandulars may provide nutrients your adrenal glands need for repair. This may be why some hunter-gatherer cultures ate the adrenal glands of the animals they killed and valued them greatly. Glandulars may also contain a small amount of adrenal hormones. This can give your adrenal glands a break from needing to produce all the hormones on their own. This may be similar to thyroid glandular extracts like Armour Thyroid, but adrenal glandulars contain far less of the hormones. There is also a theory that consuming glandulars can help to dampen autoimmunity. There have been a few animal studies that supported this, but nothing definitive as of yet, and nothing in humans.[45]

Is there good clinical trial data showing adrenal glandulars help? No. The studies just haven't been done. So, this is a case where we will be evidence *based* but not evidence *limited*. Adrenal glandulars are usually inexpensive, appear to be very safe, and seem to provide some benefit—so using them fits within our conservative model, if we aim to use them for a short period.

Now that we have covered the important topics related to lifestyle, let's move on to part 4. In part 4, we will discuss direct gut treatments, like probiotics, supplemental prebiotics, and antimicrobial herbs.

## CONCEPT SUMMARY

- Stress can negatively affect your microbiota, which then causes the worsening of digestive symptoms and diseases.

- Simple and free interventions, like breathing, movement, and meditation, have been shown to decrease inflammation and improve quality of life in those with IBD.

- Healthy relationships may help balance stress hormones, and balanced stress hormones allow you to heal more quickly.

- Don't get your body healthier at the expense of your quality of life. Don't make yourself miserable in your attempt to be healthy.

- You must heal your gut to overcome adrenal fatigue.

- Adrenal support may help to buffer the negative effects of stress and may aid in gut healing.

1    Tim Vanuytsel et al., "Psychological Stress and Corticotropin-Releasing Hormone Increase Intestinal Permeability in Humans by a Mast Cell-Dependent Mechanism," *Gut* 63, no. 8 (2014): 1293–99, doi:10.1136/gutjnl-2013-305690.

2    Rebecca G. Allen et al., "Stressor-Induced Increase in Microbicidal Activity of Splenic Macrophages Is Dependent upon Peroxynitrite Production," *Infection and Immunity* 80, no. 10 (2012): 3429–37, doi:10.1128/IAI.00714-12.

3   Gillian D. Pullinger et al., "Norepinephrine Augments Salmonella Enterica–Induced Enteritis in a Manner Associated with Increased Net Replication but Independent of the Putative Adrenergic Sensor Kinases QseC and QseE," *Infection and Immunity* 78, no. 1 (2010): 372–80, doi:10.1128/IAI.01203-09.

4   Adriana Jarillo-Luna et al., "Effect of Repeated Restraint Stress on the Levels of Intestinal IgA in Mice," *Psychoneuroendocrinology* 32, no. 6 (2007): 681–92, doi:10.1016/j.psyneuen.2007.04.009.

5   K. Shichijo et al., "The Role of Sympathetic Neurons for Low Susceptibility to Stress in Gastric Lesions," *Life Sciences* 53, no. 3 (1993): 261–67, doi:10.1016/0024-3205(93)90677-U.

6   Yukiomi Nakade et al., "Restraint Stress Delays Solid Gastric Emptying via a Central CRF and Peripheral Sympathetic Neuron in Rats," *American Journal of Physiology—Regulatory, Integrative and Comparative Physiology* 288, no. 2 (2005): R427–32, doi:10.1152/ajpregu.00499.2004.

7   Jean Philippe Gouin and Janice K. Kiecolt-Glaser, "The Impact of Psychological Stress on Wound Healing: Methods and Mechanisms," *Immunology and Allergy Clinics of North America*, 2011, doi:10.1016/j.iac.2010.09.010.

8   B. S. Drasar and Margot Shiner, "Studies on the Intestinal Flora 1," *Gut* 10, no. 10 (1969): 812–19, doi:10.1016/S0016-5085(69)80067-3.

9   N. J. Talley et al., "Epidemiology of Colonic Symptoms and the Irritable Bowel Syndrome," *Gastroenterology* 101, no. 4 (1991): 927–34, doi:S0016508591003505 [pii].

10  Caroline Canavan et al., "The Epidemiology of Irritable Bowel Syndrome," *Clinical Epidemiology*, 2014, doi:10.2147/CLEP.S40245.

11  F. A. Luscombe, "Health-Related Quality of Life and Associated Psychosocial Factors in Irritable Bowel Syndrome: A Review," *Quality of Life Research: An International Journal of Quality of Life Aspects of Treatment, Care and Rehabilitation* 9, no. 2 (2000): 161–76, www.ncbi.nlm.nih.gov/pubmed/10983480.

12  Hong-Yan Qin et al., "Impact of Psychological Stress on Irritable Bowel Syndrome," *World Journal of Gastroenterology* 20, no. 39 (2014): 14126–31, doi:10.3748/wjg.v20.i39.14126.

13  Charles N. Bernstein et al., "A Prospective Population-Based Study of Triggers of Symptomatic Flares in IBD," *American Journal of Gastroenterology* 105, no. 9 (2010): 1994–2002, doi:10.1038/ajg.2010.140; Hong-Yan Qin et al., "Impact of Psychological Stress on Irritable Bowel Syndrome," *World Journal of Gastroenterology* 20, no. 39 (2014): 14126–31, doi:10.3748/wjg.v20.i39.14126.

14  Clifford J. Roberts et al., "Increases in Weight during Chronic Stress Are Partially Associated with a Switch in Food Choice toward Increased Carbohydrate and Saturated Fat Intake," *European Eating Disorders Review* 22, no. 1 (2014): 77–82, doi:10.1002/erv.2264.

15  Simon R. Knowles et al., "Investigating the Role of Perceived Stress on Bacterial Flora Activity and Salivary Cortisol Secretion: A Possible Mechanism Underlying Susceptibility to Illness," *Biological Psychology* 77, no. 2 (2008): 132–37, doi:10.1016/j.biopsycho.2007.09.010.

16  Michael T. Bailey, "Influence of Stressor-Induced Nervous System Activation on the Intestinal Microbiota and the Importance for Immunomodulation," *Advances in Experimental Medicine and Biology* 817 (2014): 255–76, doi:10.1007/978-1-4939-0897-4_12.

17  Michael T. Bailey et al., "Exposure to a Social Stressor Alters the Structure of the Intestinal Microbiota: Implications for Stressor-Induced Immunomodulation," *Brain, Behavior, and Immunity* 25, no. 3 (2011): 397–407, doi:10.1016/j.bbi.2010.10.023.

18  Gillian D. Pullinger et al., "Norepinephrine Augments Salmonella Enterica–Induced Enteritis in a Manner Associated with Increased Net Replication but Independent of the Putative Adrenergic Sensor Kinases QseC and QseE," *Infection and Immunity* 78, no. 1 (2010): 372–80, doi:10.1128/IAI.01203-09; Michael T. Bailey et al., "In Vivo Adaptation of Attenuated Salmonella Typhimurium Results in Increased Growth upon Exposure to Norepinephrine," *Physiology and Behavior* 67, no. 3 (1999): 359–64, doi:10.1016/S0031-9384(99)00087-6.

19  Jean Philippe Gouin and Janice K. Kiecolt-Glaser, "The Impact of Psychological Stress on Wound Healing: Methods and Mechanisms," *Immunology and Allergy Clinics of North America*, 2011, doi:10.1016/j.iac.2010.09.010.

20  Linglan Yang et al., "Social Isolation Impairs Oral Palatal Wound Healing in Sprague-Dawley Rats: A Role for miR-29 and miR-203 via VEGF Suppression," *PLoS ONE* 8, no. 8 (2013), doi:10.1371/journal.pone.0072359.

21  Michael T. Bailey et al., "Exposure to a Social Stressor Alters the Structure of the Intestinal Microbiota: Implications for Stressor-Induced Immunomodulation," *Brain, Behavior, and Immunity* 25, no. 3 (2011): 397–407, doi:10.1016/j.bbi.2010.10.023.

22  Thomas Maslanik et al., "Commensal Bacteria and MAMPs Are Necessary for Stress-Induced Increases in IL-1 and IL-18 but Not IL-6, IL-10 or MCP-1," *PLoS ONE* 7, no. 12 (2012), doi:10.1371/journal.pone.0050636.

23  Nobuyuki Sudo et al., "Postnatal Microbial Colonization Programs the Hypothalamic-Pituitary-Adrenal System for Stress Response in Mice," *Journal of Physiology* 558, no. 1 (2004): 263–75, doi:10.1113/jphysiol.2004.063388.

24    P. Caenepeel et al., "Interdigestive Myoelectric Complex in Germ-Free Rats," *Digestive Diseases and Sciences* 34, no. 8 (1989): 1180–84, doi:10.1007/BF01537265.

25    Mallappa Anitha et al., "Gut Microbial Products Regulate Murine Gastrointestinal Motility via Toll-like Receptor 4 Signaling," *Gastroenterology* 143, no. 4 (2012), doi:10.1053/j.gastro.2012.06.034.

26    Andrés Uribe et al., "Microflora Modulates Endocrine Cells in the Gastrointestinal Mucosa of the Rat," *Gastroenterology* 107, no. 5 (1994): 1259–69, doi:10.1016/0016-5085(94)90526-6.

27    Patricia L. Gerbarg et al., "The Effect of Breathing, Movement, and Meditation on Psychological and Physical Symptoms and Inflammatory Biomarkers in Inflammatory Bowel Disease," *Inflammatory Bowel Diseases* 21, no. 12 (2015): 2886–96, doi:10.1097 /MIB.0000000000000568.

28    Michaël Messaoudi et al., "Beneficial Psychological Effects of a Probiotic Formulation (Lactobacillus Helveticus R0052 and Bifidobacterium Longum R0175) in Healthy Human Volunteers," *Gut Microbes* 2, no. 4 (2011): 256–61, doi:10.4161/gmic.2.4.16108; Laura Steenbergen et al., "A Randomized Controlled Trial to Test the Effect of Multispecies Probiotics on Cognitive Reactivity to Sad Mood," *Brain, Behavior, and Immunity* 48 (2015): 258–64, doi:10.1016/j.bbi.2015.04.003; Michaël Messaoudi et al., "Assessment of Psychotropic-Like Properties of a Probiotic Formulation (Lactobacillus Helveticus R0052 and Bifidobacterium Longum R0175) in Rats and Human Subjects," *British Journal of Nutrition* 105, no. 5 (2011): 755–64, doi:10.1017/S0007114510004319.

29    Ruixue Huang et al., "Effect of Probiotics on Depression: A Systematic Review and Meta-Analysis of Randomized Controlled Trials," *Nutrients*, 2016, doi:10.3390/nu8080483.

30    Dan Buettner, *Thrive: Finding Happiness the Blue Zones Way* (Washington, DC: National Geographic Society, 2010).

31    Courtney E. Detillion et al., "Social Facilitation of Wound Healing," *Psychoneuroendocrinology* 29, no. 8 (2004): 1004–11, doi:10.1016 /j.psyneuen.2003.10.003.

32    Shelley E. Taylor et al., "Relation of Oxytocin to Psychological Stress Responses and Hypothalamic-Pituitary-Adrenocortical Axis Activity in Older Women," *Psychosomatic Medicine* 68, no. 2 (2006): 238–45, doi:10.1097/01.psy.0000203242.95990.74.

33    Shelley E. Taylor et al., "Biobehavioral Responses to Stress in Females: Tend-and-Befriend, Not Fight-or-Flight," *Psychological Review* 107, no. 3 (2000): 411–29, doi:10.1037/0033-295X.107.3.411.

34    O. R. W. Pergams and P. A. Zaradic, "Is Love of Nature in the US Becoming Love of Electronic Media?," *Journal of Environmental Management* 80 (2006): 387–93.

35    Mark W. Becker et al., "Media Multitasking Is Associated with Symptoms of Depression and Social Anxiety," *Cyberpsychology, Behavior, and Social Networking* 16, no. 2 (2013): 132–35, doi:10.1089/cyber.2012.0291.

36    Wenhong Chen and Kye-Hyoung Lee, "Sharing, Liking, Commenting, and Distressed? The Pathway between Facebook Interaction and Psychological Distress," *Cyberpsychology, Behavior, and Social Networking* 16, no. 10 (2013): 728–34, doi:10.1089/cyber.2012.0272.

37    Marisa Salanova et al., "The Dark Side of Technologies: Technostress among Users of Information and Communication Technologies," *International Journal of Psychology* 48, no. 3 (2013): 422–36, doi:10.1080/00207594.2012.680460; Regina J. J. M. van den Eijnden et al., "Online Communication, Compulsive Internet Use, and Psychosocial Well-Being among Adolescents: A Longitudinal Study," *Developmental Psychology* 44, no. 3 (2008): 655–65, doi:10.1037/0012-1649.44.3.655.

38    Netta Weinstein et al., "Can Nature Make Us More Caring? Effects of Immersion in Nature on Intrinsic Aspirations and Generosity," *Personality and Social Psychology Bulletin* 35, no. 10 (2009): 1315–29, doi:10.1177/0146167209341649.

39    Meredith S. Berry et al., "The Nature of Impulsivity: Visual Exposure to Natural Environments Decreases Impulsive Decision-Making in a Delay Discounting Task," *PLoS ONE* 9, no. 5 (2014), doi:10.1371/journal.pone.0097915.

40    A. J. van der Wal et al., "Do Natural Landscapes Reduce Future Discounting in Humans?," *Proceedings of the Royal Society B: Biological Sciences* 280, no. 1773 (2013), doi:10.1098/rspb.2013.2295.

41    Alan C. Logan et al., "Natural Environments, Ancestral Diets, and Microbial Ecology: Is There a Modern 'Paleo-Deficit Disorder'? Part II," *Journal of Physiological Anthropology* 34, no. 1 (March 10, 2015): 9, doi:10.1186/s40101-014-0040-4.

42    F. A. Cadegiani and C. E. Kater, "Adrenal Fatigue Does Not Exist: A Systematic Review," *BMC Endocrine Disorders* 16 (August 24, 2016): 48, doi: 10.1186/s12902-016-0128-4.

43    Mingzhang Guo et al., "Red Ginseng and Semen Coicis Can Improve the Structure of Gut Microbiota and Relieve the Symptoms of Ulcerative Colitis," *Journal of Ethnopharmacology* 162 (2015): 7–13, doi:10.1016/j.jep.2014.12.029.

44    Alexander Panossian and Georg Wikman, "Evidence-Based Efficacy of Adaptogens in Fatigue, and Molecular Mechanisms Related to Their Stress-Protective Activity," *Current Clinical Pharmacology* 4, no. 3 (2009): 198–219, doi:10.2174/157488409789375311; Jerome

Sarris et al., "Herbal Medicine for Depression, Anxiety and Insomnia: A Review of Psychopharmacology and Clinical Evidence," *European Neuropsychopharmacology*, 2011, doi:10.1016/j.euroneuro.2011.04.002; Y. J. Cho et al., "A Fourteen-Week Randomized, Placebo-Controlled, Double-Blind Clinical Trial to Evaluate the Efficacy and Safety of Ginseng Polysaccharide (Y-75)," *Journal of Translational Medicine* 12, no. 1 (2014): 283, doi:10.1186/s12967-014-0283-1; Erik M. G. Olsson et al., "A Randomised, Double-Blind, Placebo-Controlled, Parallel-Group Study of the Standardised Extract SHR-5 of the Roots of Rhodiola Rosea in the Treatment of Subjects with Stress-Related Fatigue," *Planta Medica* 75, no. 2 (2009): 105–12, doi:10.1055/s-0028-1088346; K. J. Lee and G. E. Ji, "The Effect of Fermented Red Ginseng on Depression Is Mediated by Lipids," *Nutritional Neuroscience* 17, no. 1 (2014): 7–15, doi:10.1179/1476830513Y.0000000059; Anastasia Ossoukhova et al., "Improved Working Memory Performance Following Administration of a Single Dose of American Ginseng (Panax Quinquefolius L.) to Healthy Middle-Age Adults," *Human Psychopharmacology* 30, no. 2 (2015): 108–22, doi:10.1002/hup.2463; Jun J. Mao et al., "Rhodiola Rosea versus Sertraline for Major Depressive Disorder: A Randomized Placebo-Controlled Trial," *Phytomedicine* 22, no. 3 (2015): 394–99, doi:10.1016/j.phymed.2015.01.010; Sana Ishaque et al., "Rhodiola Rosea for Physical and Mental Fatigue: A Systematic Review," *BMC Complementary and Alternative Medicine* 12, no. 1 (2012): 1208, doi:10.1186/1472-6882-12-70; Mohammad Kaleem Ahmad et al., "Withania Somnifera Improves Semen Quality by Regulating Reproductive Hormone Levels and Oxidative Stress in Seminal Plasma of Infertile Males," *Fertility and Sterility* 94, no. 3 (2010): 989–96, doi:10.1016/j.fertnstert.2009.04.046; Sarah Benson et al., "An Acute, Double-Blind, Placebo-Controlled Crossover Study of 320 Mg and 640 Mg Doses of Bacopa Monnieri (CDRI 08) on Multitasking Stress Reactivity and Mood," *Phytotherapy Research* 28, no. 4 (2014): 551–59, doi:10.1002/ptr.5029.

45  V. C. Guimaraes et al., "Suppression of Development of Experimental Autoimmune Thyroiditis by Oral Administration of Thyroglobulin," *Endocrinology* 136, no. 8 (August 1, 1995): 3353–59, doi:10.1210/endo.136.8.7543043; C. A. Gardine et al., "Characterization of the T Lymphocyte Subsets and Lymphoid Populations Involved in the Induction of Low-Dose Oral Tolerance to Human Thyroglobulin," *Cellular Immunology* 212, no. 1 (2001): 1–15, doi:10.1006/cimm.2001.1840.

# PART 4

---

# TOOLS FOR HEALING
# YOUR GUT

# CHAPTER 14

# PROBIOTICS

## ARE PROBIOTICS THE RIGHT TREATMENT?

*"Could a missing bacteria in your gut be making you overweight? Does a bacteria hold the key to your constipation? Find out about the anti-inflammatory bacteria that can cure Crohn's disease!"*

This part of the book will help you cut through media claims like this. As we discussed earlier, claims like these are often based on questionable science and are usually more concerned with marketing than making factual health claims. However, there are also some gut treatments that can vastly improve your health. Here in part 4, we'll cover common gut and microbiota treatments and give you an idea of what you can reasonably expect—no hype, no speculation, no bandwagon to jump on or off. We will review interventions that will directly influence your gut and microbiota, including prebiotics, fiber, probiotics, antimicrobial herbs, antibiotics, elemental diets, and fecal microbiota transplants. We'll examine what the high-level clinical science tells

us for each one of these interventions and look at the evidence for their impact on

- obesity and being overweight;
- diabetes, insulin resistance, and metabolic syndrome (metabolism);
- IBS—irritable bowel syndrome (gas, bloating, constipation/diarrhea, abdominal pain);
- IBD—inflammatory bowel disease (Crohn's and ulcerative colitis);
- celiac disease;
- autoimmunity, mood, and fatigue.

How does this tie into our Great-in-8 Action Plan? If you find that your symptoms aren't responding to dietary and lifestyle changes, the next step will be incorporating the available gut treatments into your plan. These gut treatments are the focus of part 4.

Part 4 will be your definitive resource for fact-checking claims you hear or read elsewhere. For example, if you hear prebiotics can cause weight loss, reference this section to understand if this is true and how much weight loss you can expect.

In this section, the levels of evidence are important. As you know, not all studies are created equal. So, here is a quick reminder regarding the types of studies and why they are important:

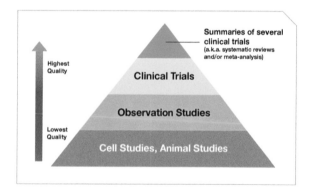

- RCTs—randomized clinical trials (also known as randomized control trials)—these are human studies that control for the placebo effect and usually look at health outcomes like prolonged life, weight loss, improved blood sugar, less inflammation, and less bloating. These studies are arguably the highest level of scientific evidence.
- Systematic reviews—these studies review many RCTs and other data. Systematic reviews are like a summary of what thirty people had to say about a café. Just remember it's a review of all the data.
- Meta-analyses—these studies are the equivalent of taking the reviews of thirty people eating at a café and then using math to give the café a numeric score. For example, when you ask people what they think about the café, you ask them to rate it on a scale of one to one hundred. Then, you calculate the average of all the scores. The average score of this café might be twenty-five out of one hundred. Or you might ask just one person, and that person might have rated the café as a ninety-five. If the average score was a twenty-five out of one hundred, the chances of you having a ninety-five-out-of-one-hundred experience is very slim. Simple, right? "Meta" means "big picture." So, a meta-analysis is just a big-picture analysis or summary.

- **IBS/SIBO**—Preliminary data show probiotics to be effective in treating SIBO, both in improving symptoms and in improving lab values. One study has shown probiotics to be more effective when compared directly to the antibiotic metronidazole. Both lactobacilli/bifidobacteria probiotics and soil-based probiotics (specifically bacillus) have been shown to be effective. Lactobacilli/bifidobacteria may be more effective, however. The dosage used was anywhere from 33 million to 6.5 billion CFUs.
- **IBD**—Three different types of probiotics have been shown to be helpful in IBD, according to RCTs and systematic-review papers: Lactobacillus/Bifidobacterium mixtures, Saccharomyces boulardii, and E. coli Nissle 1917. Herbal anti-inflammatories have been shown to be equally as effective as some IBD drugs, according to two meta-analyses and one systematic review. Note, the best and most natural approach may be probiotics used in conjunction with herbal anti-inflammatory medicines.
- Dosage for Lactobacillus/Bifidobacterium mixtures are anywhere from a hundred billion to nine hundred billion colony-forming units daily. Dosage of S. boulardii is one gram per day, which equals twenty billion colony-forming units. Dosage of E. coli Nissle is usually one to two capsules per day.
- **Weight loss**—The best results using probiotics for weight loss over several weeks have shown between 2.2–3.7 pounds lost in obese/overweight subjects. Lactobacillus probiotics were used in both studies. The dosages used were 100 billion CFUs per day of Lactobacillus gasseri and 320 million CFUs per day of Lactobacillus rhamnosus CGMCC1.3724.
- **Celiac disease**—One study has shown probiotics decrease symptoms in those with celiac disease, using a lactobacilli mixture at 4 billion CFUs per day. Another study showed children with celiac disease who take a Bifidobacterium longum probiotic achieve better height (no pun intended ☺).
- **Diabetes**—A five-point and sixteen-point reduction in blood sugar from probiotics was the average effect found in two recent systematic reviews with meta-analyses. Prebiotics are more effective in treating diabetes than probiotics.
- **Mood and fatigue**—A systematic review also found probiotics to be an effective treatment for depression. A small number of RCTs have shown probiotics can help with depression, anxiety, hostility, anger, sadness, and stress-hormone levels—using Lactobacillus and Bifidobacterium mixtures. Chronic fatigue and fibromyalgia may also improve after a gut-healing diet and nutritional support.

That is our summary of probiotics, which provides an overview of the type of benefit you can expect by using them. We'll cover the details that support this summary a little later. Before we do, however, let's briefly discuss some of the basics of probiotics in case you are new to this topic.

Probiotics are defined as microorganisms that provide health benefit to their host. You have likely heard that yogurt contains probiotics. But there is much more to the world of these beneficial bacteria (microorganisms) than just yogurt. For example, most people have around a thousand different species occupying their gut; yogurt may contain five to ten species. So, what are the important types of probiotics, and how do they make us healthier?

## PROBIOTIC TYPES AND FUNCTIONS

### Lactic acid producers

Many probiotic bacteria belong to the genus of Lactobacillus or the genus of Bifidobacterium. Within these genera, there are likely some probiotic species you have heard of before, like

Lactobacillus acidophilus or Bifidobacterium infantis.

Lactobacillus
- Most lactobacilli are transient but important; there are over a hundred species.
- Lactobacillus acidophilus is not a normal member of the gut-bacteria community, while other types of probiotics, like Lactobacillus gasseri and reuteri, are normal residents.
- Some lactobacilli are known as homofermentative, while others are known as heterofermentative.

For those of you who are wondering, the prefix "homo" means "the same," while "hetero" means "different." "Fermentative" means to break down one thing and produce something else. So, homofermenters produce one type of stuff, while heterofermenters produce multiple types of stuff. OK, why does this matter? Homofermenters produce lactic acid, but heterofermenters produce lactic acid and can produce gases, like carbon dioxide. People with SIBO often report gas and bloating. This might be because they have overgrowths of heterofermentative bacteria, which are producing too much gas.

Bifidobacterium
- Bifidobacteria typically reside in the large intestine; there are over thirty species.
- They are established by breastfeeding.
- They exhibit numerous health benefits, from intestinal-barrier function to protecting from colon cancer.

Lactobacillus- and Bifidobacterium-species probiotics are the most well studied of all probiotics. They have many impressive health benefits for those with IBS (which causes diarrhea, constipation, bloating, gas, and pain) and SIBO, as well as for brain fog, depression, weight loss, blood sugar

reduction, treatment of infection, improved skin, and more. We will detail when and how to use these types of probiotics later in the next chapter.

Here are a few other genera of probiotics:

Escherichia
- Escherichia coli (E. coli) is a normal inhabitant of your gut and one of the most commonly found bacterial species upon stool testing. This means the presence of E. coli on stool tests is normal.
- Certain E. coli have been associated with food poisoning, and, therefore, E. coli is often stereotyped as a bad guy. For some types of E. coli, like E. coli O157:H7, this is certainly true. However, E. coli appears to only become damaging after undergoing changes, specifically after acquiring certain genetic material.[1]
- An E. coli probiotic known as E. coli Nissle 1917 is nonpathogenic, like many other forms of E. coli. As we will discuss, there have been some impressive clinical trials in diarrhea and IBD using E. coli Nissle 1917 probiotics.
- E. coli also produces lactic acid, and E. coli Nissle is a normal member of your microbiota.[2]

Streptococcus
- Streptococcus are usually pathogenic (harmful); however, Streptococcus thermophiles promotes health and is found in yogurt cultures, along with Lactobacillus bulgaricus.

Enterococcus
- Although Enterococcus faecium has health benefits, it has also become highly antibiotic resistant and is responsible for hospital-acquired infections; it is not advised for use.

Pediococcus
- These may also have some health benefits.
- They are reparative to intestines and may help balance the immune system.

There are a few other types (genera) of probiotics that are defined as non–lactic acid producing.

## NON–LACTIC ACID PRODUCERS

### Bacillus
- These are also known as spore-forming bacteria or soil-based organisms. This is because they are ubiquitous in soil and water, and they often spend part of their life cycle in the dormant "spore" state. These may be an important type of probiotic to include in supplemental programs, because they may help replace what we are missing due to our reduced contact with soil and natural environments.
- A number of species show health benefits, including Bacillus coagulans and Bacillus subtilis. This type of probiotic, like many others, has been shown to improve/balance the microbiota.[3]
- Some bacilli are harmful, so use well-labeled and tested strains. These types of probiotics should be avoided in critically ill patients but otherwise are very safe.[4]

### Propionibacterium
- These are commonly found on the skin.
- They stimulate the growth of bifidobacteria and have other health benefits.

## PHAGES

Phages are a new player in the probiotic world. Phages are viruses that inhabit and influence your gut bacteria. They have been used successfully for treating certain types of infections. However, the types of phages that have been used in clinical research don't appear to be commercially available. There are a few important unanswered questions regarding the currently available phages that warrant caution with their use until answered. Namely, what effect do the non-studied but commercially available phages have?

## FUNGAL (YEAST) PROBIOTICS

### Saccharomyces boulardii
- S. boulardii is not a normal part of human microbiota, meaning it does not colonize us. It also does not appear to be affected by stomach acid or bile, but it does produce lactic acid.
- It has been used successfully to treat diarrhea, to treat C. difficile infection, to prevent relapse of Crohn's disease, and as a treatment for IBD.[5] It also has antifungal (candida) effects and disrupts fungal biofilm.[6] This means S. boulardii can help fight fungal (candida) overgrowths in your intestines and can do so in part by breaking down the protective layer (biofilm) that forms over fungus.
- S. boulardii has been shown effective in treating digestive tract parasites such as entamoebas, giardia, and Blastocystis hominis.[7] When antibiotics are coadministered with S. boulardii, it increases success compared to antibiotics alone.[8]
- Even more exciting, S. boulardii has been shown to be as effective as the antibiotic metronidazole (Flagyl) in treating Blastocystis hominis (a potential gut pathogen/infection).[9]
- S. boulardii has also shown the ability to increase clearance of H. pylori infections, according to systematic reviews with meta-analyses[10] and according to clinical trials.[11]
- Although S. boulardii does not appear to colonize,[12] it has shown some pretty impressive results, including the ability to correct dysbiosis (imbalances in your microbiota).[13]

This last fact about S. boulardii is a good transition to an important point.

We have discussed how these probiotics can cause dramatic improvement in your gut and microbiota health, but there is one additional point here we should cover. Most of these probiotics have shown benefit, but they do not colonize you. In fact, many of these probiotics seem to exert antibacterial effects, working like antibiotics to clear infections and correct dysbiosis. Let's now expand on the idea that much of the benefit from probiotics might actually come from their antibacterial actions.

## PROBIOTICS AS TRANSIENT, ANTIBACTERIAL AGENTS

I hate to be a party pooper, but most probiotics don't appear to colonize you! Does this mean you shouldn't use probiotics? Absolutely not. Probiotics cause transient and substantial benefits; the effects may even be long-term, even though the bacteria will only be around for a few weeks at best.

In her article in *Nature*, Catherine A. Lozupone states, "The gut microbiota generally shows colonization resistance, in which the native microbiota prohibits harmful [pathogenic] and potentially beneficial [probiotic] microbes from establishing."[14] This is actually a good thing. This means your gut microbiota is resistant to colonization from bad guys, but it also means you can't take probiotics and expect them to "stick." But remember probiotics still have many positive effects, many of which you've probably already heard about. So, the fact that they don't stick doesn't really matter.

In your intestinal tract, the more densely populated with bacteria an area is, the harder it is for probiotics to have an effect. Think of it this way: the more densely populated a city is, the harder it is to find an apartment, right? Try to find an apartment in downtown Manhattan compared to the countryside of Kentucky. The more populated (colonized), the harder it is to move in (have an effect). Because of this, it has been suggested that probiotics may exert more of an effect on the small intestine than the large intestine. The small intestine is colonized at a density of around $10^5$ (100,000), whereas the large intestine is colonized

at a density of around $10^{14}$ (100,000,000,000,000).[15] So, because there are fewer bacteria in the small intestine, probiotics may have more of an impact there.

Additional support of the finding that probiotics aren't able to colonize you can be found in a review paper published in 2008: "all probiotics appear to have a short life span within the gut and need repeated dosing to keep a constant level . . . it is apparent that a week after stopping oral intake, they largely disappear from the stool."[16]

This is supported by other papers that have found evidence that probiotics can only be seen in the stool for one to four weeks after discontinuation.[17] There is some data showing probiotics may colonize you, but, again, the majority of the data suggest they do not.

Further evidence for probiotics not colonizing comes from studies using what's called "heat-killed" probiotics. As the name implies, heat-killed probiotics have been heated to death. If a dead probiotic shows benefit, it supports the thinking that benefit from probiotics is not due to colonization or reseeding or repopulation or whatever you want to call it. Here are a few highlights regarding the benefits of heat-killed probiotics:

- A multicenter RCT found that heat-killed Lactobacillus was more effective than living Lactobacillus in treating diarrhea.[18]
- Another RCT found heat-killed probiotics improved IBS symptoms.[19]
- Heat-killed Lactobacillus was shown to be a successful treatment for skin allergy (atopic dermatitis) in adults.[20]
- Heat-killed Lactobacillus decreased the incidence of colds in the elderly.[21]
- Heat-killed probiotics enhanced immune function in the elderly.[22]
- Heat-killed probiotics have anticandida effects in mice.[23]

Does this mean using live probiotics is unnecessary? I don't believe so. Most of the probiotic studies use live probiotics, so I recommend we use them clinically. The positive effect of the heat-killed probiotics is merely meant to illustrate that even dead probiotics, which of course can't colonize you, can still have a positive effect. Again, this supports the idea that the benefits from probiotics are not from recolonization.

So, probiotics are transient but still appear to have beneficial effects. In part, their effects help nudge the ecosystem of bacteria and fungi back into balance. This is a very good thing, because once the ecosystem is nudged back into balance, it may stay in balance all on its own, even after you discontinue a probiotic—this might be how probiotics exert their longer-term effects. When my patients learn probiotics don't colonize, they sometimes get frustrated and ask, "Well, why even bother taking a probiotic after antibiotics if the probiotics don't add back the good bacteria?" Well, it's important to note that when taking antibiotics to clear an infection, the antibiotics give the microbiota a push, shifting them out of balance. Probiotics have been shown to help nudge the microbiota back into balance more quickly.[24] Just remember this is not achieved by recolonizing. Probiotics can help edge the ecosystem back into balance. Once balance is achieved, and as long as a healthy internal environment is present, the ecosystem should remain in balance.

What about probiotics being antibacterial agents? Probiotics have been shown to be an effective treatment for SIBO. We also have evidence showing that some probiotics are as effective as antifungal drugs in treating fungi[25] and that probiotics are as effective as antiparasitic medications in treating parasites.[26] The antibacterial effect of probiotics can help to reduce bacterial overgrowths, correct imbalances, and clear infections. Perhaps this is why probiotics seem to work better than prebiotics in improving overall gut health.

### Other functions of probiotics

Probiotics don't appear to colonize but rather have transient and often antibacterial benefits. So, how do probiotics improve your health? What are they doing while they are in your gut?

The *Journal of Clinical Gastroenterology* offers some answers regarding how probiotics exert their health benefits. Probiotics can

- increase microbiota diversity and numbers of phylotypes (bacterial groups);
- decrease pathogens and their toxins;
- alter bacterial-community structure to enhance evenness, stabilize bacterial communities when "nudged" (for example with antibiotics), or promote a more rapid recovery from imbalance;
- directly inhibit harmful microbes through multiple mechanisms, like the production of inhibitory compounds (like antibacterial compounds) and by promoting immune responses against specific microbes;
- influence harmful microbes by inhibiting attachment through stimulating intestinal mucus production, reinforcing gut-barrier effects, and reducing gut inflammation; all this encourages microbes that are associated with a healthier gut environment.[27]

The journal *Trends in Microbiology* offers some other interesting notes:

- Ingested probiotics can temporarily support resident bacterial communities as part of our transient microbiome.
- Ingested probiotics can cause major shifts in the composition of the microbiome of the small intestine, whereas alterations in the large intestine are limited.[28]

# CONCEPT REVIEW

- Probiotics are bacterial species of organisms that provide benefit to the host.
- Probiotics are not all the same: some produce acids, some produce gas, and some are found in soil.
- Probiotics do not appear to colonize you (they are transient), but they do provide substantial benefits.
- Probiotics can help clear infections from the gut and resolve imbalances (dysbioses).
- Probiotics can enhance the effectiveness of antibiotics and, in some cases, are as effective as antibiotics in treating infections. They also return the gut microbiota to normal after antibiotics.
- Probiotics have more of an impact on your small intestine than they do on the large intestine.
- Probiotics rebalance the gut microbiota and help increase diversity and the amount of good bacteria.
- Probiotics stimulate the immune system and enhance your gut's protective mucous membrane.

We've covered a brief summary of the clinical benefits of probiotics. Then we covered some basics regarding the types of probiotics and how they function in our bodies. Let's now return to our discussion of clinical benefits. What really matters are the types of health benefits probiotics can provide and the types of improvements we see in clinical trials. If you have condition *X*, what benefits do we see when we give probiotic *Y* to people who also have condition *X*? We have already mentioned some of the general health benefits, but let's now detail how probiotics can help specific health conditions.

# PROBIOTICS FOR SPECIFIC CONDITIONS

## IBS, SIBO, AND PROBIOTICS— SHOULD YOU TAKE PROBIOTICS WITH THESE CONDITIONS?

Two meta-analyses have shown probiotics significantly improve symptoms in those with IBS and have no side effects.[29]

There is no strong consensus as to which probiotic strains are best for IBS, but a trend does emerge suggesting multiple-strain probiotics are best. Some evidence suggests that a multistrain probiotic that also includes Bifidobacterium infantis is best.[30]

Clinically, I have found multispecies strains are best, but I'm not convinced the B. infantis makes a large difference. A dose of anywhere from 100 billion CFUs to 900 billion CFUs per day can be used. It's usually best to start around 100 billion and slowly work your way up. There is no need to increase beyond a dose that causes desired improvement.

You may have heard that probiotics can help with diarrhea, but what about constipation? Can probiotics also help with constipation and constipation-type IBS? Two clinical trials have found that, yes, probiotics can help with IBS.[31]

Since IBS can be caused by small-intestinal bacterial overgrowth, should you take a probiotic if you have or suspect you have SIBO? This is a controversial question. Some feel you should not, because with SIBO, you already have too much bacteria. However, looking at the studies, we see probiotics actually help with SIBO and may even be effective as a stand-alone treatment. Thank you to Dr. Allison Siebecker for making me aware of some of the early research here.

How can probiotics help decrease bacteria in the small intestine? We have already outlined how probiotics can actually be antibacterial. And probiotics don't colonize you, which is probably why they don't increase bacteria in the small intestine—they don't stick. To put it simply, we are using bacteria to treat bacteria. Here are a few specific reasons probiotics may help treat SIBO:

- Probiotics transiently compete with SIBO bacteria for food and may help starve SIBO.
- Probiotics help stimulate intestinal motility, which helps to sweep out SIBO.
- Probiotics enhance your immune system, which then helps you fight SIBO.
- Probiotics are anti-inflammatory, which helps with intestinal motility and with your immune system.
- Probiotics may help increase your intestine's protective mucous membrane.

**FINDINGS OF STUDIES USING PROBIOTICS TO TREAT SIBO INCLUDE THE FOLLOWING:**

1. A symptomatic improvement of 82% was seen when using a probiotic as the only treatment for SIBO patients (the probiotics contained 33 million CFUs Lactobacillus casei and L. plantarum, Streptococcus faecalis, and Bifidobacter brevis dosed once to twice a day). This improvement was 30% better than a group of patients being treated with the antibiotic metronidazole.[32]
2. A 64% reduction of SIBO gas levels was seen after using Lactobacillus casei Shirota as the only treatment (6.5 billion Lactobacillus casei Shirota).[33]
3. A 47% SIBO eradication rate was shown when using a dose of 6 billion spores of Bacillus clausii, a soil-based/spore-forming probiotic.[34]

This is likely why treating SIBO with probiotics and antibiotics is more effective than treating SIBO with *pre*biotics and antibiotics.[35] At least this is what preliminary studies show.

**GUT GEEKS**

*One study has shown that adding prebiotics to antibiotics for SIBO enhances the treatment effect.[36] I am certainly open to this idea, but all things considered, the addition of probiotics to SIBO treatment makes more sense than prebiotics. At least according to our current understanding and my clinical observations.*

# IBD (ULCERATIVE COLITIS AND CROHN'S DISEASE) AND PROBIOTICS

IBD is usually diagnosed as either ulcerative colitis or Crohn's disease, although there are other subsets of IBD, such as collagenous colitis, indeterminate colitis, and microscopic colitis. These are all conditions where there is a high level of inflammation in the gut. This inflammation is often caused by autoimmunity. In IBD, the autoimmunity is usually against intestinal tissue or intestinal bacteria.

**SOME COMMON SYMPTOMS OF IBD**

Ulcerative colitis
- Diarrhea, which is somewhat constant, chronic, and sometimes bloody
- Frequent smaller bowel movements
- Fever, fatigue, weight loss, anemia

Crohn's disease
- Cramping and abdominal pain
- Fatigue
- Prolonged diarrhea
- Weight loss, fever
- Rectal bleeding

There is a spectrum of severity of IBD. Some patients with very mild cases can simply improve their diets and will feel great. Other patients (those with severe cases) may require special and specific diets, probiotics, herbs, and even medications. The most severe may need surgery. Fortunately, diet and natural medicines can be highly effective for IBD.

Probiotics have been shown to be very helpful for IBD. A recent review showed that in Crohn's disease, the probiotic VSL#3 (essentially a Lactobacillus/Bifidobacterium mixture) at six grams/day (which equals 900 billion CFUs) worked as effectively as the medication mesalamine (four grams/day) in maintaining remission. But the best evidence was for the probiotic Saccharomyces boulardii at one gram/day (which equals 20 billion CFUs) used with the anti-inflammatory drug mesalamine (two grams/day).[37]

E. coli Nissle 1917 was also shown to reduce Crohn's disease relapse rates.[38] Again, this is not the type of E. coli you hear about in the news. This type of E. coli is a healthy, normal, important member of your intestinal microbiota. Another review has found E. coli Nissle 1917 effective for maintaining remission. This same paper also found the best approach for treating active ulcerative colitis was with VSL#3 combined with an anti-inflammatory drug.[39]

The typical dose of E. coli Nissle is one capsule per day for four days in a row, then two capsules per day thereafter. For higher dosages, you can increase by one capsule every four days, but do not exceed three capsules twice per day (six per day).[40]

Other reviews have found probiotics (specifically a Lactobacillus and Bifidobacterium blend such as VSL#3 or E. coli Nissle 1917) to be equally effective for ulcerative colitis as anti-inflammatory drugs like mesalamine.[41]

Do you have to use anti-inflammatory drugs? No. Herbal anti-inflammatories have been shown to be as effective as a popular and effective drug called mesalamine. It's important to note that these findings are high-level scientific findings. Two meta-analyses and one systematic review have found comparable effectiveness between mesalamine-type drugs and herbal anti-inflammatory treatments.[42]

It's my preference to use a probiotic in conjunction with an anti-inflammatory herb, selecting each based upon the type of IBD I'm treating. This is a great place to start and can prevent many patients from needing more powerful drugs that carry concerning side effects. One systematic review has found probiotics do not help maintain remission,[43] but overall the data suggest probiotics are helpful.

Well-performed studies of the microbiota in patients with IBD have found high levels of the phylum (bacterial group) Proteobacteria to be associated with IBD.[44] We discussed earlier that E. coli Nissle 1917 is one of the most helpful probiotics for IBD. E. coli Nissle 1917 is in fact a member of the Proteobacteria group. This means patients became healthier when taking a probiotic from a bacterial group already shown to be overgrown in IBD. This is a powerful example of why we can't and shouldn't extrapolate microbiota-association findings to make clinical recommendations. Clinical recommendations should be based on clinical trials when available. Imagine all the patients who would miss out on the IBD-quelling aid of E. coli Nissle 1917 if they were following advice derived from this type of erroneous assumption, the kind we warned against in chapter 3.

## WEIGHT LOSS AND PROBIOTICS

Studies show you can lose a statistically significant amount of weight from taking a probiotic. However, there is a difference between "statistically significant" and "meaningful." Statistically significant means that it's not a mathematic coincidence. But this doesn't mean a given result would be meaningful to *you* in a real-world sense. Probiotics as a treatment for weight loss is a good example of the difference between statistically significant results and meaningful results. Of all the studies performed, the best results using probiotics for weight loss were between 2.2 and 3.7 pounds of weight loss in obese subjects. This was statistically significant, yes, but losing three pounds if you are one hundred pounds over a healthy weight is not really meaningful.

Below is a summary of the best results for using probiotics for weight loss in human RCTs:

- Subjects lost 2.2 lb. with Lactobacillus gasseri (100 billion CFUs per day).[45]
- Subjects lost 3.7 lb. with Lactobacillus rhamnosus CGMCC1.3724 (320 million CFUs per day).[46]

So, while there is some weight-loss effect from probiotics, the effect appears to be minimal.

## CELIAC DISEASE AND PROBIOTICS

One RCT using Bifidobacterium infantis showed probiotics improve symptoms in celiac disease.[47] This same study also showed less intestinal inflammation, improved indigestion, and reduced constipation in celiac patients taking probiotics. Another RCT examined children with celiac disease who were given probiotics (Bifidobacterium longum CECT 7347). The children on the probiotics achieved better height than the children on a placebo, possibly from increased absorption of nutrients.[48]

Perhaps part of the reason we see these findings is because probiotics can help treat SIBO. Patients with celiac disease have an increased likelihood of SIBO, which we know can be treated with probiotics. So, maybe this is why we see celiac symptoms (which are very similar to SIBO symptoms) and height improve after probiotics—because the probiotics are helping rebalance gut bacteria in those with celiac disease. Of course, the probiotics are likely providing other benefits, too, as we discussed earlier.

One RCT using the probiotic VLS#3 found it helped to break down gluten. These findings appear to be dependent upon synergy of many strains and did not occur when using one strain.[49]

Should you get superanalytical and detailed and try to select the one perfect species of probiotics bacteria that matches your particular condition? Or should you focus on a well-rounded probiotic with a blend of many important species? Based on our discussion so far, what do you think? It's my opinion, based on the research and as this study supports, your best bet is to aim for a blend or mixture of highly effective strains. Don't go crazy trying to custom match one species for one disease. In our Great-in-8 plan, we'll cover how to easily get the right mix of probiotic species.

## INSULIN RESISTANCE AND PROBIOTICS

Systematic reviews of placebo-controlled trials (again, possibly the highest level of scientific evidence) have shown probiotics have a significant favorable effect on blood sugar levels.[50] What type of real-world effect does this translate to though? A systematic review with meta-analysis shows probiotics reduce fasting blood glucose by around sixteen points (mg/dL) and are best when multiple-species mixtures are used over the course of eight weeks.[51] Another systematic review with meta-analysis showed an average 5.5-point reduction in fasting blood glucose.[52] Of all the studies, the best results achieved were found in a study of diabetics eating probiotic yogurt. This caused a thirty-point reduction in fasting blood glucose compared to the placebo group, which I would consider meaningful.[53] The total body of evidence, however, suggests a five-to-sixteen-point reduction is most likely, which is a marginal change.

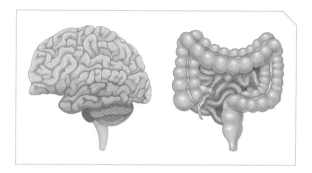

How can something that improves the health of your gut, like probiotics, aid with mood problems like depression and anxiety? This happens through what's known as the gut–brain connection. We know when there is inflammation in the intestines, it can also cause inflammation in the brain. Think of it this way: your intestines are like your second brain (in fact, that's a nickname for the enteric nervous system, which is contained in your gut). If you think about it, your intestines even resemble your brain. This might be because during early fetal development, your gut and your brain both develop from the same clump of cells.[54]

We know that inflammation can interfere with neurotransmitters, which are happy-mood and focus-brain hormones. Where does inflammation come from? You guessed it. One of the most common sources of inflammation is your gut.

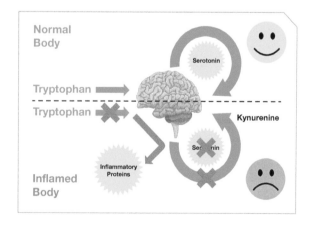

How does gut inflammation affect your neurotransmitters? This diagram will help you visualize what happens. Normally, your body will take dietary protein and break it down into amino acids. One of these amino acids is tryptophan. Tryptophan is converted into your happy-mood chemical—serotonin (this is depicted by the top half of this diagram). But when high levels of inflammation are present, you get robbed of your happy-mood chemical. Instead of making your happy-mood serotonin, the body uses serotonin to make inflammatory proteins. This is known as the kynurenine pathway (this is depicted by the bottom half of this diagram).[55]

Inflammation robs your brain of the stuff it needs to produce the neurotransmitters that make you happy.

Bacteria also play a role in making the gut a major source of inflammation. It has been shown that leaky gut correlates with depression. When you have leaky gut, too much stuff gets through your gut lining—including bacteria. When these bacteria leak through your gut, they then cause your immune system to attack (with inflammation), which fuels depression.[56]

These are all interesting mechanisms and concepts, but do you remember our rule to prevent being misled by health claims? Demand human outcome studies, preferably clinical trials. It's one thing to talk about an interesting mechanism, but the clinical trials help us see if there is actually a solution.

An RCT has shown depression, anger, hostility, anxiety, and stress-hormone levels all improved after taking probiotics.[57] Another RCT has shown probiotics make you happier, with fewer negative thoughts and sadness.[58] Both studies used a mixture of Lactobacillus and Bifidobacterium probiotics. These results have been replicated by other studies in humans.[59] In fact, a systematic review with meta-analysis of clinical trials has found probiotics lead to a significant reduction in depression.[60]

As we have discussed throughout this book, the beneficial effects of improving your gut health are far-reaching. A fascinating study shows how improving gut health can even improve chronic fatigue syndrome and fibromyalgia. In this study, levels of bacteria in the subjects' blood were tracked before and after undergoing a treatment meant to repair the gut. In this study, levels of six bacteria were tracked in the subjects: Hafnia alvei, Pseudomonas aeruginosa, Morganella morganii, Pseudomonas putida, Citrobacter koseri, and Klebsiella pneumoniae.

These bacteria were tracked both before and after intake of natural anti-inflammatory substances (glutamine, N-acetyl cysteine, and zinc), and in conjunction with an anti-inflammatory diet.

OK, so what happened? Over half of the patients experienced marked improvement in their symptoms, which correlated with decreased bacteria in the blood.[61] This is great—it illustrates how the root cause of your fatigue might be a problem in your gut. But why didn't everyone improve? This illustrates another important principle: if diet and nutritional supports don't fix your gut, there is likely an infection or bacterial imbalance that must be addressed. In our Great-in-8 plan, we take this into account: we start with diet, nutrition, and lifestyle and then reevaluate. For many, changes to diet, nutrition, and lifestyle fix all their problems. For the ones whose problems haven't been fixed, we move on to more advanced methods for gut healing.

1    H. Brussow et al., "Phages and the Evolution of Bacterial Pathogens: From Genomic Rearrangements to Lysogenic Conversion," *Microbiology and Molecular Biology Reviews* 68, no. 3 (2004): 560–602, doi:10.1128/MMBR.68.3.560-602.2004.

2    Rosalie Maltby et al., "Nutritional Basis for Colonization Resistance by Human Commensal Escherichia Coli Strains HS and Nissle 1917 against E. Coli O157:H7 in the Mouse Intestine," *PLoS ONE* 8, no. 1 (2013), doi:10.1371/journal.pone.0053957.

3    Edna P. Nyangale et al., "Bacillus Coagulans GBI-30, 6086 Modulates Faecalibacterium Prausnitzii in Older Men and Women," *Journal of Nutrition* 145, no. 7 (2015): 1446–52, doi:10.3945/jn.114.199802.

4    David R. Snydman, "The Safety of Probiotics," *Clinical Infectious Diseases* 46, no. s2 (2008): S104–11, doi:10.1086/523331.

5    Samir Jawhara and Daniel Poulain, "Saccharomyces Boulardii Decreases Inflammation and Intestinal Colonization by Candida Albicans in a Mouse Model of Chemically-Induced Colitis," *Medical Mycology* 45, no. 8 (2007): 691–700, doi:10.1080/13693780701523013; Charlotte Hedin et al., "Evidence for the Use of Probiotics and Prebiotics in Inflammatory Bowel Disease: A Review of Clinical Trials," *Proceedings of the Nutrition Society* 66, no. 3 (2007): 307–15, doi:10.1017/S0029665107005563; E. B. Avalueva et al., "[Use of Saccharomyces Boulardii in Treating Patients Inflammatory Bowel Diseases (Clinical Trial)]," *Experimental & Clinical Gastroenterology*, no. 7 (2010): 103–11.

6    Anna Krasowska et al., "The Antagonistic Effect of Saccharomyces Boulardii on Candida Albicans Filamentation, Adhesion and Biofilm Formation," *FEMS Yeast Research* 9, no. 8 (2009): 1312–21, doi:10.1111/j.1567-1364.2009.00559.x.

7    Bulent Besirbellioglu et al., "Saccharomyces Boulardii and Infection due to Giardia Lamblia," *Scandinavian Journal of Infectious Diseases* 38, no. 6–7 (2006): 479–81, doi:10.1080/00365540600561769.

8    Makbule Eren et al., "Clinical Efficacy Comparison of Saccharomyces Boulardii and Yogurt Fluid in Acute Non-Bloody Diarrhea in Children: A Randomized, Controlled, Open Label Study," *American Journal of Tropical Medicine and Hygiene* 82, no. 3 (2010): 488–91, doi:10.4269/ajtmh.2010.09-0529.

9    Ener Cagri Dinleyici et al., "Clinical Efficacy of Saccharomyces Boulardii or Metronidazole in Symptomatic Children with Blastocystis Hominis Infection," *Parasitology Research* 108, no. 3 (2011): 541–45, doi:10.1007/s00436-010-2095-4.

10   H. Szajewska et al., "Systematic Review with Meta-Analysis: Saccharomyces Boulardii Supplementation and Eradication of Helicobacter Pylori Infection," *Alimentary Pharmacology & Therapeutics* 41, no. 12 (2015): 1237–45, doi:10.1111/apt.13214; Ener Cagri

Dinleyici et al., "Saccharomyces Boulardii CNCM I-745 in Different Clinical Conditions," *Expert Opinion on Biological Therapy*, July (2014): 1–17, doi:10.1517/14712598.2014.937419.

11    Peter Malfertheiner et al., "Management of *Helicobacter Pylori* Infection—the Maastricht IV/Florence Consensus Report," *Gut* 61, no. 5 (2012): 646–64, doi:10.1136/gutjnl-2012-302084; Mehmet Cindoruk et al., "Efficacy and Safety of Saccharomyces Boulardii in the Fourteen-Day Triple Anti-Helicobacter Pylori Therapy: A Prospective Randomized Placebo-Controlled Double-Blind Study," *Helicobacter* 12, no. 4 (2007): 309–16, doi:10.1111/j.1523-5378.2007.00516.x.

12    Gianluca Ianiro et al., "Role of Yeasts in Healthy and Impaired Gut Microbiota: The Gut Mycome," *Current Pharmaceutical Design*, 2013, 1–5, doi:10.2174/13816128113196660723.

13    Margret I. Moré and Alexander Swidsinski, "Saccharomyces Boulardii CNCM I-745 Supports Regeneration of the Intestinal Microbiota after Diarrheic Dysbiosis—A Review," *Clinical and Experimental Gastroenterology*, 2015, doi:10.2147/CEG.S85574.

14    Catherine A. Lozupone et al., "Diversity, Stability and Resilience of the Human Gut Microbiota," *Nature* 489, no. 7415 (2012): 220–30, doi:10.1038/nature11550.

15    Sahar el Aidy et al., "The Small Intestine Microbiota, Nutritional Modulation and Relevance for Health," *Current Opinion in Biotechnology*, 2015, doi:10.1016/j.copbio.2014.09.005.

16    R. Spiller, "Review Article: Probiotics and Prebiotics in Irritable Bowel Syndrome," *Alimentary Pharmacology and Therapeutics*, 2008, doi:10.1111/j.1365-2036.2008.03750.x.

17    Mary Ellen Sanders, "Impact of Probiotics on Colonizing Microbiota of the Gut," *Journal of Clinical Gastroenterology* 45 Suppl., November (2011): S115–9, doi:10.1097/MCG.0b013e318227414a.

18    Shu Dong Xiao et al., "Multicenter Randomized Controlled Trial of Heat-Killed Lactobacillus Acidophilus LB in Patients with Chronic Diarrhea," *Chinese Journal of Digestive Diseases* 3, no. 4 (2002): 167–71, doi:10.1046/j.1443-9573.2002.00095.x.

19    G. M. Halpern et al., "Treatment of Irritable Bowel Syndrome with Lacteol Fort: A Randomized, Double-Blind, Crossover Trial," *American Journal of Gastroenterology* 91, no. 8 (1996): 1579–85, www.ncbi.nlm.nih.gov/pubmed/8759665.

20    Yusuku Inoue et al., "Effects of Oral Administration of Lactobacillus Acidophilus L-92 on the Symptoms and Serum Cytokines of Atopic Dermatitis in Japanese Adults: A Double-Blind, Randomized, Clinical Trial," *International Archives of Allergy and Immunology* 165, no. 4 (2014): 247–54, doi:10.1159/000369806.

21    Shoji Shinkai et al., "Immunoprotective Effects of Oral Intake of Heat-Killed Lactobacillus Pentosus Strain b240 in Elderly Adults: A Randomised, Double-Blind, Placebo-Controlled Trial," *British Journal of Nutrition* 109, no. 10 (2013): 1856–65, doi:10.1017/S0007114512003753.

22    K. Miyazawa et al., "Heat-Killed Lactobacillus Gasseri Can Enhance Immunity in the Elderly in a Double-Blind, Placebo-Controlled Clinical Study," *Beneficial Microbes* 6, no. 4 (2015): 441–49, doi:10.3920/BM2014.0108.

23    Kazumi Hayama et al., "Protective Activity of S-PT84, a Heat-Killed Preparation of Lactobacillus Pentosus, against Oral and Gastric Candidiasis in an Experimental Murine Model," *Japanese Journal of Medical Mycology* 55, no. 3 (2014): J123–29, doi:10.3314/mmj.55.J123.

24    Mary Ellen Sanders, "Impact of Probiotics on Colonizing Microbiota of the Gut," *Journal of Clinical Gastroenterology* 45 Suppl. November (2011): S115–9, doi:10.1097/MCG.0b013e318227414a.

25    Gamze Demirel et al., "Prophylactic Saccharomyces Boulardii versus Nystatin for the Prevention of Fungal Colonization and Invasive Fungal Infection in Premature Infants," *European Journal of Pediatrics* 172, no. 10 (2013): 1321–26, doi:10.1007/s00431-013-2041-4.

26    Bulent Besirbellioglu et al., "Saccharomyces Boulardii and Infection due to Giardia Lamblia," *Scandinavian Journal of Infectious Diseases* 38, no. 6–7 (2006): 479–81, doi:10.1080/00365540600561769; Ener Cagri Dinleyici et al., "Clinical Efficacy of Saccharomyces Boulardii or Metronidazole in Symptomatic Children with Blastocystis Hominis Infection," *Parasitology Research* 108, no. 3 (2011): 541–45, doi:10.1007/s00436-010-2095-4.

27    Mary Ellen Sanders, "Impact of Probiotics on Colonizing Microbiota of the Gut," *Journal of Clinical Gastroenterology* 45 Suppl., November (2011): S115–9, doi:10.1097/MCG.0b013e318227414a.

28    Muriel Derrien and Johan E. T. van Hylckama Vlieg, "Fate, Activity, and Impact of Ingested Bacteria within the Human Gut Microbiota," *Trends in Microbiology*, 2015, doi:10.1016/j.tim.2015.03.002.

29    Lynne V. McFarland and Sascha Dublin, "Meta-Analysis of Probiotics for the Treatment of Irritable Bowel Syndrome," *World Journal of Gastroenterology: WJG* 14, no. 17 (2008): 2650–61, doi:10.3748/wjg.14.2650; María Ortiz-Lucas et al., "Effect of Probiotic Species on

Irritable Bowel Syndrome Symptoms: A Bring Up-To-Date Meta-Analysis," *Revista Española de Enfermedades Digestivas: Organo Oficial de La Sociedad Española de Patología Digestiva* 105 (2013): 19–36, doi:10.4321/S1130-01082013000100005.

30    R. Spiller, "Review Article: Probiotics and Prebiotics in Irritable Bowel Syndrome," *Alimentary Pharmacology and Therapeutics*, 2008, doi:10.1111/j.1365-2036.2008.03750.x.

31    V. Ojetti et al., "Effect of Lactobacillus Reuteri (DSM 17938) on Methane Production in Patients Affected by Functional Constipation: A Retrospective Study," *European Review for Medical and Pharmacological Sciences* 21, no. 7 (2017): 1702–8; Valerio Mezzasalma et al., "A Randomized, Double-Blind, Placebo-Controlled Trial: The Efficacy of Multispecies Probiotic Supplementation in Alleviating Symptoms of Irritable Bowel Syndrome Associated with Constipation," *BioMed Research International*, 2016, doi:10.1155/2016/4740907.

32    Luis Oscar Soifer et al., "Comparative Clinical Efficacy of a Probiotic vs. an Antibiotic in the Treatment of Patients with Intestinal Bacterial Overgrowth and Chronic Abdominal Functional Distension: A Pilot Study," *Acta Gastroenterologica Latinoamericana* 40, no. 4 (2010): 323–27, www.ncbi.nlm.nih.gov/pubmed/21381407.

33    Jacqueline S. Barrett et al., "Probiotic Effects on Intestinal Fermentation Patterns in Patients with Irritable Bowel Syndrome," *World Journal of Gastroenterology* 14, no. 32 (2008): 5020–24, doi:10.3748/wjg.14.5020.

34    Maurizio Gabrielli et al., "Bacillus Clausii as a Treatment of Small Intestinal Bacterial Overgrowth," *American Journal of Gastroenterology* 104, no. 5 (2009): 1327–28, doi:10.1038/ajg.2009.91.

35    Rosa Rosania et al., "Effect of Probiotic or Prebiotic Supplementation on Antibiotic Therapy in the Small Intestinal Bacterial Overgrowth: A Comparative Evaluation," *Current Clinical Pharmacology* 8, no. 2 (2013): 169–72, doi:10.2174/15748847113089990048.

36    M. Furnari et al., "Clinical Trial: The Combination of Rifaximin with Partially Hydrolysed Guar Gum Is More Effective than Rifaximin Alone in Eradicating Small Intestinal Bacterial Overgrowth," *Alimentary Pharmacology and Therapeutics* 32, no. 8 (2010): 1000–1006, doi:10.1111/j.1365-2036.2010.04436.x.

37    Charlotte Hedin et al., "Evidence for the Use of Probiotics and Prebiotics in Inflammatory Bowel Disease: A Review of Clinical Trials," *Proceedings of the Nutrition Society* 66, no. 3 (2007): 307–15, doi:10.1017/S0029665107005563.

38    H. A. Malchow, "Crohn's Disease and Escherichia Coli. A New Approach in Therapy to Maintain Remission of Colonic Crohn's Disease?," *Journal of Clinical Gastroenterology* 25, no. 4 (1997): 653–58, doi:10.1097/00004836-199712000-00021.

39    Charlotte Hedin et al., "Evidence for the Use of Probiotics and Prebiotics in Inflammatory Bowel Disease: A Review of Clinical Trials," *Proceedings of the Nutrition Society* 66, no. 3 (2007): 307–15, doi:10.1017/S0029665107005563.

40    Jobst Henker et al., "Probiotic Escherichia Coli Nissle 1917 (EcN) for Successful Remission Maintenance of Ulcerative Colitis in Children and Adolescents: An Open-Label Pilot Study," *Zeitschrift Fur Gastroenterologie* 46, no. 9 (2008): 874–75, doi:10.1055/s-2008-1027463; Wolfgang Kruis et al., "Maintaining Remission of Ulcerative Colitis with the Probiotic Escherichia Coli Nissle 1917 Is as Effective as with Standard Mesalazine," *Gut* 53, no. 11 (2004): 1617–23, doi:10.1136/gut.2003.037747; Wolfgang Kruis et al., "A Double-Blind Placebo-Controlled Trial to Study Therapeutic Effects of Probiotic Escherichia Coli Nissle 1917 in Subgroups of Patients with Irritable Bowel Syndrome," *International Journal of Colorectal Disease* 27, no. 4 (2012): 467–74, doi:10.1007/s00384-011-1363-9; Wolfgang Kruis et al., "Double-Blind Comparison of an Oral Escherichia Coli Preparation and Mesalazine in Maintaining Remission of Ulcerative Colitis," *Alimentary Pharmacology & Therapeutics* 11, no. 5 (1997): 853–58, doi:10.1046/j.1365-2036.1997.00225.x.

41    Wolfgang Kruis et al., "Maintaining Remission of Ulcerative Colitis with the Probiotic Escherichia Coli Nissle 1917 Is as Effective as with Standard Mesalazine," *Gut* 53, no. 11 (2004): 1617–23, doi:10.1136/gut.2003.037747; Matthew A. Ciorba, "A Gastroenterologist's Guide to Probiotics." *Clinical Gastroenterology and Hepatology*, 2012, doi:10.1016/j.cgh.2012.03.024.

42    Roja Rahimi et al., "Comparison of the Efficacy and Tolerability of Herbal Medicines with 5-Aminosalisylates in Inflammatory Bowel Disease: A Meta-Analysis of Placebo Controlled Clinical Trials Involving 812 Patients," *International Journal of Pharmacology* 9, no. 4 (2013): 227–44, doi:10.3923/ijp.2013.227.244; S. C. Ng et al., "Systematic Review: The Efficacy of Herbal Therapy in Inflammatory Bowel Disease," *Alimentary Pharmacology and Therapeutics*, 2013, doi:10.1111/apt.12464; Roja Rahimi et al., "Induction of Clinical Response and Remission of Inflammatory Bowel Disease by Use of Herbal Medicines: A Meta-Analysis," *World Journal of Gastroenterology* 19, no. 34 (2013): 5738–49, doi:10.3748/wjg.v19.i34.5738.

43    Khimara Naidoo et al., "Probiotics for Maintenance of Remission in Ulcerative Colitis," in *Cochrane Database of Systematic Reviews*, 2011, doi:10.1002/14651858.CD007443.pub2.

44    William A. Walters et al., "Meta-Analyses of Human Gut Microbes Associated with Obesity and IBD," *FEBS Letters* 588, no. 22 (2014): 4223–33, doi:10.1016/j.febslet.2014.09.039.

45    Y. Kadooka et al., "Regulation of Abdominal Adiposity by Probiotics (Lactobacillus Gasseri SBT2055) in Adults with Obese Tendencies in a Randomized Controlled Trial," *European Journal of Clinical Nutrition* 64, no. 6 (2010): 636–43, doi:10.1038/ejcn.2010.19.

46    Marina Sanchez et al., "Effect of Lactobacillus Rhamnosus CGMCC1.3724 Supplementation on Weight Loss and Maintenance in Obese Men and Women," *British Journal of Nutrition* 111, no. 8 (2014): 1507–19, doi:10.1017/S0007114513003875.

47    Edgardo Smecuol et al., "Exploratory, Randomized, Double-Blind, Placebo-Controlled Study on the Effects of Bifidobacterium Infantis Natren Life Start Strain Super Strain in Active Celiac Disease," *Journal of Clinical Gastroenterology* 47, no. 2 (2013): 139–47, doi:10.1097/MCG.0b013e31827759ac.

48    Marta Olivares et al., "Double-Blind, Randomised, Placebo-Controlled Intervention Trial to Evaluate the Effects of Bifidobacterium Longum CECT 7347 in Children with Newly Diagnosed Coeliac Disease," *British Journal of Nutrition* 112, no. 1 (2014): 30–40, doi:10.1017/S0007114514000609.

49    Maria De Angelis et al., "VSL#3 Probiotic Preparation Has the Capacity to Hydrolyze Gliadin Polypeptides Responsible for Celiac Sprue," *Biochimica et Biophysica Acta—Molecular Basis of Disease* 1762, no. 1 (2006): 80–93, doi:10.1016/j.bbadis.2005.09.008.

50    Yuting Ruan et al., "Effect of Probiotics on Glycemic Control: A Systematic Review and Meta-Analysis of Randomized, Controlled Trials," *PLoS ONE* 10, no. 7 (2015), doi:10.1371/journal.pone.0132121.

51    Qingqing Zhang et al., "Effect of Probiotics on Glucose Metabolism in Patients with Type 2 Diabetes Mellitus: A Meta-Analysis of Randomized Controlled Trials," *Medicina* 52, no. 1 (2015): 28–34, doi:10.1016/j.medici.2015.11.008.

52    Yuting Ruan et al., "Effect of Probiotics on Glycemic Control: A Systematic Review and Meta-Analysis of Randomized, Controlled Trials," *PLoS ONE* 10, no. 7 (2015), doi:10.1371/journal.pone.0132121.

53    Majid Mohamadshahi et al., "Effects of Probiotic Yogurt Consumption on Inflammatory Biomarkers in Patients with Type 2 Diabetes," *BioImpacts* 4, no. 2 (2014): 83–88, doi:10.5681/bi.2014.007.

54    Laura McDaniel, "What Is the Gut-Brain Connection? | Developmental Disabilities Resources and Information, Minnesota," *Connect WC*, 2017, accessed October 10, 2017, www.connectwc.org/what-is-the-gut-brain-connection.html.

55    M. P. Heyes et al., "Quinolinic Acid and Kynurenine Pathway Metabolism in Inflammatory and Non-Inflammatory Neurological Disease," *Brain* 115, no. 5 (1992): 1249–73, doi:10.1093/brain/115.5.1249; Michael Maes et al., "The Immune Effects of TRYCATs (Tryptophan Catabolites along the IDO Pathway): Relevance for Depression—and Other Conditions Characterized by Tryptophan Depletion Induced by Inflammation," *Neuroendocrinology Letters* 28, no. 6 (2007): 826–31, doi:NEL280607A11 [pii].

56    Michael Maes et al., "Increased IgA and IgM Responses against Gut Commensals in Chronic Depression: Further Evidence for Increased Bacterial Translocation or Leaky Gut," *Journal of Affective Disorders* 141, no. 1 (2012): 55–62, doi:10.1016/j.jad.2012.02.023; Michael Maes et al., "The Gut-Brain Barrier in Major Depression: Intestinal Mucosal Dysfunction with an Increased Translocation of LPS from Gram Negative Enterobacteria (Leaky Gut) Plays a Role in the Inflammatory Pathophysiology of Depression," *Neuroendocrinology Letters* 29, no. 1 (2008): 117–24, doi:NEL290108A12 [pii].

57    Michaël Messaoudi et al., "Assessment of Psychotropic-Like Properties of a Probiotic Formulation (Lactobacillus Helveticus R0052 and Bifidobacterium Longum R0175) in Rats and Human Subjects," *British Journal of Nutrition* 105, no. 5 (2011): 755–64, doi:10.1017/S0007114510004319.

58    Laura Steenbergen et al., "A Randomized Controlled Trial to Test the Effect of Multispecies Probiotics on Cognitive Reactivity to Sad Mood," *Brain, Behavior, and Immunity* 48 (2015): 258–64, doi:10.1016/j.bbi.2015.04.003.

59    Michaël Messaoudi et al., "Beneficial Psychological Effects of a Probiotic Formulation (*Lactobacillus Helveticus* R0052 and *Bifidobacterium Longum* R0175) in Healthy Human Volunteers," *Gut Microbes* 2, no. 4 (2011): 256–61, doi:10.4161/gmic.2.4.16108; A. Venket Rao et al., "A Randomized, Double-Blind, Placebo-Controlled Pilot Study of a Probiotic in Emotional Symptoms of Chronic Fatigue Syndrome," *Gut Pathogens* 1, no. 1 (2009): 6, doi:10.1186/1757-4749-1-6.

60    Ruixue Huang et al., "Effect of Probiotics on Depression: A Systematic Review and Meta-Analysis of Randomized Controlled Trials," *Nutrients*, 2016, doi:10.3390/nu8080483.

61    Michaël Maes and Jean Claude Leunis, "Normalization of Leaky Gut in Chronic Fatigue Syndrome (CFS) Is Accompanied by a Clinical Improvement: Effects of Age, Duration of Illness and the Translocation of LPS from Gram-Negative Bacteria," *Neuroendocrinology Letters* 29, no. 6 (2008): 902–10, doi:NEL290608A08 [pii].

# CHAPTER 15

# THE STOMACH AND DIGESTIVE ACID

## HOW THE STOMACH WORKS

If diet and lifestyle don't provide adequate relief, two of the first gut treatments we add in are probiotics and digestive acid/enzymes. We just discussed probiotics; let's now discuss stomach acid and digestive enzymes.

These are some common symptoms that can be aided by addressing stomach acid and digestive enzymes:

- Indigestion
- Reflux
- Burping/belching
- Gas
- Bloating or feeling excessively full after eating
- Loose stools
- Anemia and malabsorption
- Floating stools, fat in stool

But what are digestive enzymes and stomach acid, and how do they work? Sorry to torture you with an anatomy diagram, but it will help you understand what's going on. The first main point

of digestion occurs in the stomach, so let's start there.

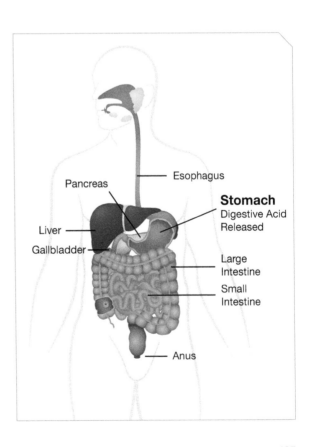

## STOMACH ACID

When food arrives in your stomach, your stomach produces acid to help start the digestive process. This is called stomach acid or hydrochloric acid (HCl). Stomach acid is important for a few reasons: digestion of proteins, absorption of minerals, control of parasites/bacteria/fungi, and because it signals to other parts of the digestive tract that food is on its way.

Inadequate stomach-acid production can cause malabsorption of nutrients like protein and calcium. It can also increase risk for things like SIBO and problems with digestive function in the esophagus and small intestine. Too much stomach acid can irritate the stomach lining and even cause ulcers. Some people have too much acid, and others have too little.

Typical symptoms of too little stomach acid include
- burping/belching;
- feeling excessively full after eating/feeling like food just sits in your stomach;
- feeling bloated;
- reflux, heartburn, indigestion.

Typical symptoms of too much stomach acid include
- burping/belching;
- feeling excessively full after eating/feeling like food just sits in your stomach;
- feeling bloated;
- reflux, heartburn, indigestion;
- upper abdominal pain or discomfort;
- fatty-food intolerance;
- nausea and occasional vomiting.

As you can see, there's a lot of overlap, which is why we have to work through a process to sort this out. That's exactly what we'll do when we work through our Great-in-8. We will ensure you have the correct levels of acid in your stomach and then work to resolve any of your symptoms.

If you're looking for the short story on acid, that's it. We'll go into more detail in the next two sections ("Stomach Acid—Reflux, Heartburn, Ulcers, and Indigestion" and "Stomach Acid, Autoimmunity, and Vitamin $B_{12}$"). If you're not interested in that much detail, skip ahead to the section on digestive enzymes ("Digestive Enzymes and Bile").

# STOMACH ACID—REFLUX, HEARTBURN, ULCERS, AND INDIGESTION

In many cases, reflux, heartburn, and indigestion clear after we achieve appropriate levels of stomach acid. Because both low and high acid levels can result in many of the same symptoms, this issue can be confusing. It's also a bit controversial.

***What do the clinical studies show regarding supplements or medications that decrease digestive acid?***
Let's start our discussion with medications that lower or block stomach acid. It's important to mention when acid-lowering/blocking medications are used for long periods, they carry risk of side effects and can cause significant problems. These are problems associated with low levels of stomach acid. The most likely result of acid levels getting too low is an increased risk of fungal overgrowth and SIBO. Nutrient malabsorption (calcium, magnesium, iron, $B_{12}$) and subsequent osteoporosis or even increased hip-fracture risk are also possible. There is also the possibility of increased growth of stomach tumors, although it's unclear whether these tumors are harmful.[1]

If prolonged acid lowering is bad, does this mean supplementing with extra acid could be good? This is a good question, and there is a good answer. But before we leave the topic of acid lowering, let's discuss when and how acid lowering can help you.

## TOO MUCH STOMACH ACID AND ULCERS

As with many things, when it comes to stomach acid, not everyone is the same. Some people have too much acid, which can be caused by food or bacteria. Have you ever heard someone say, "When I stopped eating [fill in a food], my heartburn went away"? Perhaps you've already experienced this yourself after trying some of the dietary recommendations we discussed earlier. When we eat foods that we have an intolerance of or are allergic to, it can cause the release of too much acid. You might have already heard of histamines and antihistamines. When people have seasonal allergies, they have high levels of histamine and find relief by taking antihistamines. Allergens cause your body to release histamine as part of the allergic response. When you eat foods you have an intolerance of or are allergic to, the same histamine release can take place.

How does this affect stomach acid? Histamine actually signals your stomach to produce acid. Lots of histamine equals lots of acid. There is even a drug class that lowers stomach acid by blocking histamine in your stomach, known as H2 blockers (Pepcid, Zantac, and Tagamet are H2 blockers). So, by eating fewer allergens, you can lower histamine and improve the heartburn or reflux caused by high acid.

Acid-blocking medications are often criticized in functional and alternative medicine circles, and for understandable reasons. As we discussed, when acid-blocking medications are used for long periods, they may carry risk of side effects and may cause significant problems, such as fungal overgrowths, SIBO, nutrient malabsorption, osteoporosis, hip fractures, and stomach tumors. Because of this, long-term use of acid-blocking drugs is starting to be seriously questioned. However, we

shouldn't throw the baby out with the bathwater, either. For those who have stomach or small-intestinal ulcers, these medications have shown an impressive ability to allow ulcer healing in as little as four to eight weeks.[2]

What is an ulcer? It's essentially a sore spot in your stomach or intestinal lining. How would you know if you had an ulcer? Here are some common symptoms that can be present with ulcers:

- Upper abdominal pain or discomfort
- Belching
- Fullness or bloating
- Early satiety/fullness
- Fatty-food intolerance
- Nausea and occasional vomiting

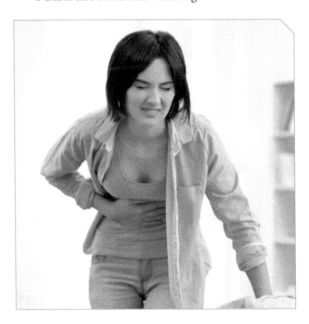

These symptoms may get better or worse after eating.

Ulcers develop from irritation and can be healed by reducing irritation. The most common irritants are

- foods—we discussed irritating and inflammatory foods earlier, and we'll discuss them again in part 5;
- lifestyle—stress may be an irritant; alcohol, caffeine, and NSAIDs (painkillers like Advil) are also irritants;
- bacteria—specifically, the stomach bacteria H. pylori;
- stomach acid—when an ulcer is present, stomach acid is an irritant; once the ulcer is healed, proper levels of stomach acid are necessary for healthy digestion.

Fortunately, there is a very high likelihood that by improving your lifestyle and diet and addressing any unwanted bacteria, your ulcers will heal. If someone has done all this and still needs additional support for healing an ulcer, a short course (four to eight weeks) of an acid-blocking medication has been shown to be highly effective and seems reasonable.

**GUT GEEKS**

*There are natural treatments available that lower stomach acid and help with ulcer healing. One landmark study has been published showing that a nutritional supplement outperformed the acid-lowering drug omeprazole in treating heartburn, reflux, and GERD. In the supplement group, 100% of patients' symptoms improved; in the drug group, 65% of patients improved. Ulcer healing was also documented in another study as well.[3] You can see a nice diagram of this supplements' ingredients, published by Pereira in 2016, here:[4]*

**Daily Dosage of Melatonin/Nutrient Supplement**

| | |
|---|---|
| Melatonin | 6 mg |
| L-Tryptophan | 200 mg |
| Vitamin B12 | 50 µg |
| Methionine | 100 mg |
| Betaine | 100 mg |
| Folic acid | 10 mg |
| Vitamin B6 | 25 mg |

Pereira RS. Regression of gastroesophageal reflux disease symptoms using dietary supplementation with melatonin, vitamins and amino acids: comparison with omeprazole. *J Pineal Res* 2006;41:195-200.

*This supplement mixture might be a treatment consideration for those who can't get their acid under control via lifestyle, diet, discontinuing NSAIDs, and addressing bacteria. However, there is the possibility that long-term use of natural agents that lower acid could have the same side effects as acid-lowering pharmaceutical drugs. At this point, we really don't know, so the goal should be short-term use.*

What if ulcers aren't your problem, but you're struggling with reflux, heartburn, or indigestion? We just discussed one natural treatment option that might work well for your symptoms. There is another natural treatment that is very well studied for indigestion ("indigestion" is simply a catchall term for any of the following: reflux, heartburn, burping, abdominal pain, bloating, fullness). The herbal blend Iberogast has been shown to be as effective as the drug cisapride in the treatment of indigestion.[5] The effectiveness of Iberogast as a successful treatment for indigestion has been reinforced by other RCTs,[6] systematic reviews,[7] and even a meta-analysis.[8]

It's important that you treat chronic heartburn or reflux because they can eventually turn into esophageal cancer. If you've been struggling with these symptoms, our Great-in-8 plan may very well resolve them. However, be sure to adhere to whatever follow-up your doctor has recommended.

We mentioned bacteria being a cause of too much acid. The prime suspect here is a bacterium called H. pylori. H. pylori bacteria should be ruled out in any case of ulcers, reflux, or indigestion. Eradication of this bacteria ensures a very high likelihood that these problems will clear. As we discussed, H. pylori may even play a role in autoimmunity: preliminary evidence shows treating this bacteria may help with thyroid autoimmunity. In step 3 of the Great-in-8, we'll use herbal medicines that can clear H. pylori if it's present.

In a small number of people, the cause of their reflux and heartburn can be traced to a faulty valve—the lower esophageal sphincter, located between your esophagus and your stomach. Iberogast appears to improve the function of this valve. Although this problem is rare, we address it in our Great-in-8 plan.

### How to know if you should supplement with stomach acid

We've covered how prolonged lowering of acid can be harmful. We've also covered how some may need a short-term acid-lowering intervention. Now, let's come back to the question: "If prolonged lowering of stomach acid is bad, does this mean supplementing with extra acid might be good?"

First, let's cover what you should *not* do. Some have recommended that to establish your ideal dose of supplemental acid (HCl), you increase your dose until you feel a burning sensation and then decrease your dose slightly. For example, if you felt a burning sensation in your stomach when you took seven pills of HCl per meal, your ideal dose is six pills. In my opinion, this is a bad idea. By the time you're feeling burning, damage may be occurring. Also, those with a healthy stomach lining may never feel burning. Very high intake of supplemental acid may lead to increased risk of stomach and small-intestinal ulcers. A high dose of supplemental acid can be as much as fifteen capsules of acid with each meal. Again, I do not recommend this.

Supplementing with acid can help or harm you, so it's important that we get this right. Let's start with what the research shows.

### What the research on supplemental acid shows

After an extensive review of the literature, I was shocked to find almost nothing supporting supplementing with digestive acid. The only references available are a handful of studies from the 1960s, most of which can't be located to fact-check. Authors funded by supplement companies have written papers recently, but all the claims made in these papers reference these older and unverifiable studies. Does this mean supplemental acid is a bad idea? Not necessarily. This may be an area where good studies just haven't been performed yet. We want to use the research to *guide* our decisions but not to *limit* them. If the research shows something doesn't work, we're not going to recommend it. But, as in this case, what if there is almost no research? We have to use whatever other information is available.

We can use clinical experience, for example. I have noticed that supplemental acid certainly seems to help *some* people, but megadosing is not needed. We can also examine what percentage of people have been documented to have low stomach acid. Of course, the higher this percentage, the higher the percentage of people who will benefit from supplemental acid. We can also use information regarding what conditions low stomach acid is associated with, which can help us determine who is at the highest risk for low stomach acid. If low stomach acid is associated with SIBO, then stomach-acid supplementation is more likely to be helpful for those with SIBO.

Who is at the highest risk for low stomach acid?

- Only 2% of the US population have documented low stomach acid[9] (as opposed to the 6.5% who have ulcers, which indicates too much acid[10])
- Any of the following factors increases the likelihood that you have low stomach acid and, therefore, could benefit from supplementation:
  » Autoimmune conditions
  » Anemia
  » Being over sixty-five
  » Chronic use of painkillers and other stomach irritants

### Autoimmune conditions and anemia

Although 2% isn't a lot, there are certain conditions that greatly increase the likelihood of someone having low stomach acid. If you have anemia or an autoimmune condition, the chances you have low stomach acid range anywhere from 5% up through 50%. Autoimmune conditions are common—they affect almost as many people as cancer, which is the second most common cause of death in the United States. To quote the National Institutes of Health's Autoimmune Diseases Coordinating Committee regarding autoimmune disease: "collectively [autoimmune diseases] are thought to affect approximately 5 to 8 percent of the United States population—14 to 22 million persons."[11]

This suggests that low stomach acid might be more common than previously thought. This corresponds with what I see in the clinic: a subset of patients seem to benefit from supplemental acid. Here are some autoimmune conditions that have been associated with low stomach acid:[12]

- Rheumatoid arthritis
- Type 1 diabetes
- Celiac disease
- Crohn's disease
- Thyroid disease—Hashimoto's and Graves'
- Sjögren's syndrome

If you have one of these autoimmune conditions and/or anemia, there is a 5%–50% chance you have low stomach acid.

## WHAT IS ANEMIA?

This is a condition of malabsorption of iron and/or B vitamins that can then affect red blood cell production. This can easily be diagnosed via a standard blood test known as a CBC with differential. Fatigue is the most common symptom of anemia.

Why does having an autoimmune condition increase the likelihood of having low stomach acid? If someone has one autoimmune condition, that person is at higher risk of having another. If this other type of autoimmunity is stomach autoimmunity, it might cause the person to have low stomach acid because certain autoimmune conditions attack the acid-making cells in the stomach.

### Age

Another risk factor for low stomach acid is age. As a general rule, the older you are the more likely it is you will do better with some digestive-acid and enzyme support because digestive secretions tend to slow with age, as our organs incur wear and tear.[13]

For example, if you have reflux at twenty-three years old, it's more likely that food or bacteria are the cause. If you have reflux at age sixty-three, it might be due to low stomach acid.

## STOMACH IRRITANTS—COFFEE, CAFFEINE, AND PAINKILLERS

### Coffee and caffeine

Are coffee and caffeine bad for your stomach? Coffee and caffeine are known to irritate the stomach lining, and chronic irritation may do damage. This can then lead to decreased stomach-acid production. Does this mean you should give up coffee? Yikes. For some, this may be a very unappealing idea. Let's take a practical look at what we know regarding coffee's and caffeine's impact on your stomach and stomach acid so we can make a reasonable recommendation.

Let's start with how coffee affects your health overall. A systematic review was published in 2016 that examined this issue.[14] Here is what the authors of this study concluded: "This qualitative assessment has shown that the health benefits clearly outweigh the risks of moderate coffee consumption in adult consumers for the majority of health outcomes considered."

To translate, overall, coffee has either no effect or a beneficial effect on your health. Here is a breakdown of specific conditions and how they relate to coffee consumption:

Coffee appears to have no effect or slight benefit for
- cancer;
- death from cardiovascular disease, triglycerides levels, and lipoprotein(a);
- metabolism, type 2 diabetes, and insulin resistance;
- neurological conditions such as Parkinson's disease, cognitive decline, and depression;
- sleep.

Coffee appears to have no effect or is slightly detrimental for
- cholesterol levels, blood pressure, and homocysteine;
- digestive conditions such as ulcers, heartburn, indigestion;
- bone health;
- fertility, pregnancy complications.

An interesting note, one study found coffee consumption increased the healthy intestinal bacteria Bifidobacterium, but not significantly.[15]

## IN SUMMARY

Overall, coffee appears to have no effect or slight benefits to your overall health. Those with digestive problems may have the highest likelihood for negative reactions, but these have not been consistently documented. Certain cardiovascular disease markers may worsen, but other markers may improve. Coffee consumption appears to have an overall protective effect (or no effect) on cardiovascular death. Those with poor bone health (osteoporosis/osteopenia) or those who are trying to get pregnant or who are pregnant may want to use coffee sparingly. Clean, fresh coffee with minimal additives can ensure you have the highest likelihood for benefit.

Now, let's examine specifics of how coffee affects your gut health. Does coffee consumption cause ulcers or reflux? A meta-analysis concluded there is no relationship between coffee consumption and typical disorders of high-acid production, specifically ulcers and reflux.[16] This has been reinforced by other studies.[17]

Does coffee consumption impact stomach acid? Interestingly, several studies have documented that coffee may actually increase acid production.[18]

What's interesting to note here is that while coffee increases stomach-acid production, it does not appear to cause the disorders associated with high stomach-acid production. However, most of the studies showing coffee increases stomach acid are looking at short-term effects. More specifically, these studies look at what happens in the stomach minutes to hours after you drink coffee but not at the effect after years of chronic consumption. Some evidence suggests that coffee *decreases* stomach-acid production when consumed chronically or long-term.[19] If this is true, it could have major implications because of all the problems that can occur secondary to low stomach-acid production.

But that's only one study. How can we more definitively answer the question of whether long-term coffee consumption leads to low stomach acid? We can look at two associated conditions known as gastritis and atrophic gastritis. Long-term irritation of the stomach usually manifests as what's known as gastritis, which literally means "stomach irritation." If gastritis continues long enough, it can become atrophic gastritis, which is essentially severe irritation. In these conditions of stomach irritation, we see decreased stomach acid. Studies on gastritis and atrophic gastritis are really the only data we have to answer our question about long-term coffee use and low stomach acid. So, if coffee consumption was found to be associated with gastritis or atrophic gastritis, coffee *could* be damaging to your stomach.

The good news, however, is that there does *not* appear to be an association between severe stomach irritation (atrophic gastritis) and coffee consumption. This implies coffee does not damage your stomach.[20]

There also does not appear to be an association with normal-acid-level stomach irritation (gastritis) and coffee consumption.[21]

## WHAT ABOUT GREEN TEA?

Not only does green tea not appear to negatively affect the stomach, a high level of green tea consumption might even protect against stomach damage.[22]

A small number of studies have shown that long-term coffee consumption is associated with stomach irritation and decreased HCl production;[23] however, it is very important to note that these results are not high quality and their findings are more likely a coincidence (for the stat geeks out there, the studies suffer from a poor P value). When we weigh all the evidence, it's fairly clear that coffee is safe.

In summary, the practical takeaway here is that coffee does not seem to cause problems with stomach-acid production. However, overuse of any stimulant can cause problems. Also, some people notice coffee simply doesn't agree with them (they may have an allergy or intolerance). And don't forget about what you put in the coffee. The more you add (sugar, cream), the greater the likelihood you might not react well. I would recommend simply taking a short break from all caffeine and coffee and seeing how you feel once you get past any withdrawal. Some may feel better. Others may notice no difference and can continue to enjoy coffee. When you reintroduce coffee, start simply, so you isolate for just the coffee's effect, and then add in cream, sugar, or other sweetener (but be careful—not too much sugar). Remember this does not have to be all or none. You may notice you feel better when you stop your daily habit and cut out coffee completely. However, after going through our Great-in-8 plan and improving your gut health, you might notice you can have coffee three or four days a week with no problem. Great! Enjoy coffee in moderation, but be careful not to overdo it.

### Painkillers

NSAIDs, like Advil, have been shown to decrease stomach-acid production,[24] so it's a good idea to use them as sparingly as possible. If you're using these for chronic pain, investigate and address the source.

### Testing your stomach-acid levels

Can you test to see if you have low or high stomach acid? Maybe you've read about a direct stomach-acid test where you swallow a sensory pill or a blood test. There may be a time and place for testing your stomach-acid levels, but initially I would advise you to simply work through our Great-in-8. There are many factors that can influence your stomach acid and many factors that can cause the symptoms associated with high or low stomach acid. As we continue to work through our steps, we'll address these factors. There is a good likelihood your symptoms will go away and there will be no need to perform testing.

To recap, food, irritants, bacteria, age, and autoimmunity affect stomach-acid levels. We already discussed how to address food and irritants. We will address bacteria in step 3. You can't change your age, but let's talk about ways you might be able to improve stomach autoimmunity.

# STOMACH ACID, STOMACH AUTOIMMUNITY, AND VITAMIN B$_{12}$

Up to 50% of those with one type of autoimmunity will also have autoimmunity against their stomach cells. Over time, this stomach autoimmunity can interfere with your stomach's ability to release the important digestive acid HCl.[25]

If you have an inadequate release of stomach acid, you can experience problems like gas, bloating, fungal or bacterial infections and overgrowths, increased parasitic infection, decreased vitamin absorption, and deficiency of iron, calcium, magnesium, and other minerals, just to name a few. If you can't absorb vitamin B$_{12}$ or iron, this can cause defective red blood cells (anemia) and may also cause a decrease in your white blood cell count. Since red blood cells carry oxygen and nutrients throughout your body, defects here can cause fatigue and poor circulation. This is one reason some thyroid patients still have fatigue even though their thyroid-hormone levels are normal; the thyroid issue has been addressed, but not the anemia. When your white blood cell count becomes low, it leaves you more susceptible to infections and colds.

Stomach autoimmunity can cause low stomach acid, which can then cause digestive problems. This stomach autoimmunity manifests in two ways: as antibodies against what is known as parietal cells or as antibodies against intrinsic factor (which is needed to absorb vitamin B$_{12}$). Remember, antibodies mean your immune system is attacking a part of your body and thus damaging it. The parietal cells are cells located in the lining of your stomach that secrete stomach acid and intrinsic factor. Studies have shown that elevation of these antibodies predicts stomach dysfunction years later.[26] The levels of these antibodies rise and fall depending on the severity of the autoimmune attack against the stomach. Although these antibodies will elevate while damage to the stomach is occurring, once most of the cells have been damaged, the antibodies decrease simply because there is nothing left for the immune system to attack.

What causes this stomach autoimmunity, and what can you do about it? Can a gluten-free diet help this stomach autoimmunity? It does not appear that a gluten-free diet will specifically help this condition. Two RCTs performed in the 1980s showed a gluten-free diet had no effect on this stomach autoimmunity.[27]

While diet may not be a key player in this specific type of autoimmunity, our friend the H.

pylori bacteria may be. We discussed earlier that this bacteria has been associated with autoimmune thyroid conditions and that treatment of this bacteria has been shown to dampen thyroid autoimmunity. A clinical trial has shown that after eradicating an H. pylori infection, stomach autoimmunity can reverse itself and disappear.[28]

Similar studies have also shown that clearing an H. pylori infection may help to normalize stomach function and stomach autoimmunity and reverse stomach damage. Interestingly, some evidence has shown Epstein-Barr virus is associated with this same type of stomach damage.[29]

Once again, not all the data agree. Some studies show no relationship between infections like H. pylori and this stomach damage.[30]

Two studies have shown that vitamin $B_{12}$ injections can stop this stomach autoimmunity,[31] so this treatment may have much potential.

How can you determine if you have this stomach autoimmunity? Ask your doctor to run the following two tests: antiparietal cell antibodies and intrinsic factor antibodies.

As you can see, there are many details and nuances regarding stomach acid. However, what we do to optimize stomach acid is fairly straightforward and is addressed when we work through our Great-in-8.

## CONCEPT SUMMARY

- Common symptoms of acid imbalance are feeling full, bloating, belching, indigestion, reflux, heartburn, and stomach pain.

- Supplemental acid can help with digestion, but it must be used in the right way because it can also make some people feel worse.

- If you have a negative reaction to supplemental acid, you probably don't need it and should not use it.

- The symptoms associated with low acid versus high acid are very similar, so your response to acid supplementation will determine if it should be used or not.

- Long-term use of acid-lowering medications carries risks, mainly of bacterial and fungal overgrowths.

- Short-term use of acid-lowering medications can be very helpful in the treatment of ulcers.

- Preliminary data suggest natural agents have shown equivalent (or better) effectiveness in treating ulcers, heartburn, reflux, and indigestion and have the ability to aid in ulcer healing.

- Those with autoimmunity and/or anemia have a higher likelihood of having low stomach acid.

- Those with ulcers should avoid supplementing with digestive acid.

- Coffee or caffeine doesn't appear to have much effect on stomach-acid production.

- Consider taking a short break from coffee and caffeine to see if this improves how you feel.

- A gluten-free diet does not appear to aid with stomach autoimmunity.

- H. pylori bacteria can cause increased or decreased stomach acid.

- Treatment of H. pylori bacteria may help with stomach autoimmunity, damage, and function.

- Treatment with $B_{12}$ injections may turn off stomach autoimmunity.

1   C. Jacobs et al., "Dysmotility and Proton Pump Inhibitor Use Are Independent Risk Factors for Small Intestinal Bacterial and/or Fungal Overgrowth," *Alimentary Pharmacology and Therapeutics* 37, no. 11 (2013): 1103–11, doi:10.1111/apt.12304; Lucio Lombardo et al., "Increased Incidence of Small Intestinal Bacterial Overgrowth during Proton Pump Inhibitor Therapy," *Clinical Gastroenterology and Hepatology* 8, no. 6 (2010): 504–8, doi:10.1016/j.cgh.2009.12.022; I. Markuljak et al., "[The Effect of Quinidine on Digoxin Plasma Levels after Discontinuation of Digoxin Therapy]," *Vnitrni Lekarstvi* 36, no. 1 (1990): 70–74; Sama Chubineh and John Birk, "Proton Pump Inhibitors: The Good, the Bad, and the Unwanted," *Southern Medical Journal* 105, no. 11 (2012): 613–18, doi:10.1097 /SMJ.0b013e31826efbea.

2   Xi Qing Ji et al., "Efficacy of Ilaprazole in the Treatment of Duodenal Ulcers: A Meta-Analysis," *World Journal of Gastroenterology* 20, no. 17 (2014): 5119–23, doi:10.3748/wjg.v20.i17.5119; N. D. Yeomans et al., "A Comparison of Omeprazole with Ranitidine for Ulcers Associated with Nonsteroidal Anti-Inflammatory Drugs. *New England Journal of Medicine* 338, no. 11 (1998): 719–26, doi:10.1056 /nejm199803123381104; Ling Wang et al., "Ilaprazole for the Treatment of Duodenal Ulcer: A Randomized, Double-Blind and Controlled Phase III Trial," *Current Medical Research and Opinion* 28, no. 1 (2012): 101–9, doi:10.1185/03007995.2011.639353.

3   Ricardo De Souza Pereira, "Regression of Gastroesophageal Reflux Disease Symptoms Using Dietary Supplementation with Melatonin, Vitamins and Amino Acids: Comparison with Omeprazole," *Journal of Pineal Research* 41, no. 3 (2006): 195–200, doi:10.1111/j.1600-079X.2006.00359.x.

4   Lyn Patrick, "Gastroesophageal Reflux Disease (GERD): A Review of Conventional and Alternative Treatments," *Alternative Medicine Review : A Journal of Clinical Therapeutic* 16, no. 2 (2011): 116–33.

5   W. Rösch et al., "A Randomised Clinical Trial Comparing the Efficacy of a Herbal Preparation STW 5 with the Prokinetic Drug Cisapride in Patients with Dysmotility Type of Functional Dyspepsia," *Zeitschrift Fur Gastroenterologie* 40, no. 6 (2002): 401–8, doi:10.1055/s-2002-32130.

6   A. Madisch et al., "A Plant Extract and Its Modified Preparation in Functional Dyspepsia. Results of a Double-Blind Placebo Controlled Comparative Study," [In German.] *Zeitschrift Fur Gastroenterologie* 39, no. 7 (2001): 511–17, doi:10.1055/s-2001-16142; Ulrike von Arnim et al., "STW 5, a Phytopharmacon for Patients with Functional Dyspepsia: Results of a Multicenter, Placebo-Controlled Double-Blind Study," *American Journal of Gastroenterology* 102, no. 6 (2007): 1268–75, doi:10.1111/j.1572-0241.2006.01183.x.

7   J. Melzer et al., "Iberis Amara L. and Iberogast—Results of a Systematic Review Concerning Functional Dyspepsia," *Journal of Herbal Pharmacotherapy* 4, no. 4 (2004): 51–59, doi:10.1300/J157v04n04_05; R. Saller et al., "Iberogast(r): Eine Moderne Phytotherapeutische Arzneimittelkombination Zur Behandlung Funktioneller Erkrankungen Des Magen-Darm-Trakts (Dyspepsie, Colon Irritabile)—von Der Pflanzenheilkunde Zur (Evidence Based Phytotherapy). Eine Systematische Übersicht," *Forschende Komplementärmedizin/Research in Complementary Medicine* 9, no. 1 (November 17, 2004): 1–20, doi:10.1159/000068645.

8   J. Melzer et al., "Meta-Analysis: Phytotherapy of Functional Dyspepsia with the Herbal Drug Preparation STW 5 (Iberogast)," *Alimentary Pharmacology and Therapeutics* 20, no. 11–12 (2004): 1279–87, doi:10.1111/j.1365-2036.2004.02275.x.

9   Andrea L. Betesh et al., "Is Achlorhydria a Cause of Iron Deficiency Anemia?," *American Journal of Clinical Nutrition*, 2015, doi:10.3945 /ajcn.114.097394.

10  "FastStats—Digestive Diseases," CDC National Center for Health Statistics, last modified May 3, 2017, accessed October 10, 2017, www.cdc.gov/nchs/fastats/digestive-diseases.htm.

11  "Autoimmune Diseases | NIH: National Institute of Allergy and Infectious Diseases," *National Institute of Allergy and Infectious Diseases*, last modified November 2012, accessed October 9, 2017, www.niaid.nih.gov/diseases-conditions/autoimmune-diseases.

12  Emanuela Miceli et al., "Common Features of Patients with Autoimmune Atrophic Gastritis," *Clinical Gastroenterology and Hepatology: The Official Clinical Practice Journal of the American Gastroenterological Association* 10, no. 7 (2012): 812–14, doi:10.1016 /j.cgh.2012.02.018; Christophe E. M. De Block et al., "Autoimmune Gastritis in Type 1 Diabetes: A Clinically Oriented Review," *Journal of Clinical Endocrinology and Metabolism*, 2008, doi:10.1210/jc.2007-2134; Christophe E. M. De Block et al., "Autoimmune Gastropathy in Type 1 Diabetic Patients with Parietal Cell Antibodies: Histological and Clinical Findings," *Diabetes Care* 26, no. 1 (2003), doi:10.2337/diacare.26.1.82; Edith Lahner and Bruno Annibale, "Pernicious Anemia: New Insights from a Gastroenterological Point of View," *World Journal of Gastroenterology*, 2009, doi:10.3748/wjg.15.5121; I. Šterzl et al., "Anti-Helicobacter Pylori, Anti-Thyroid Peroxidase, Anti-Thyroglobulin, and Anti-Gastric Parietal Cells Antibodies in Czech Population," *Physiological Research* 57, no. SUPPL. 1 (2008), www.biomed.cas.cz/physiolres/pdf/57%20Suppl%201/57_S135.pdf; R. Gillberg et al., "Gastric Morphology and Function in Dermatitis Herpetiformis and in Coeliac Disease," *Scandinavian Journal of Gastroenterology* 20, no. 2 (January 8, 1985):

133–40, doi:10.3109/00365528509089645; Mun Su Kang et al., "Bamboo Joint-Like Appearance of Stomach in Korean Patients with Crohn's Disease," [In Korean.] *Korean Journal of Gastroenterology = Taehan Sohwagi Hakhoe Chi* 48, no. 6 (December 2006): 395–400, www.ncbi.nlm.nih.gov/pubmed/17189922; Toshio Akiyama et al., "Gastric Acid Secretion, Serum Gastrin and Parietal Cell Histology in Hyperthyroidism," *Gastroenterologia Japonica* 17, no. 1: 42–49, doi:10.1007/bf02774760; T. Sugaya et al., "Atrophic Gastritis in Sjögren's Syndrome," *Nippon Rinsho. Japanese Journal of Clinical Medicine* 53, no. 10 (1995): 2540–44, www.embase .com/search/results?subaction=viewrecord&from=export&id=L126179711%5Cn.

13    James B. Carey et al., "Gastric Observations in Achlorhydria," *American Journal of Digestive Diseases* 8, no. 11 (November 1941): 401–7, doi:10.1007/BF02998244.

14    L. Kirsty Pourshahidi et al., "A Comprehensive Overview of the Risks and Benefits of Coffee Consumption," *Comprehensive Reviews in Food Science and Food Safety*, 2016, doi:10.1111/1541-4337.12206.

15    Muriel Jaquet et al., "Impact of Coffee Consumption on the Gut Microbiota: A Human Volunteer Study," *International Journal of Food Microbiology* 130, no. 2 (2009): 117–21, doi:10.1016/j.ijfoodmicro.2009.01.011.

16    Takeshi Shimamoto et al., "No Association of Coffee Consumption with Gastric Ulcer, Duodenal Ulcer, Reflux Esophagitis, and Non-Erosive Reflux Disease: A Cross-Sectional Study of 8,013 Healthy Subjects in Japan," *PLoS ONE* 8, no. 6 (2013), doi:10.1371 /journal.pone.0065996.

17    J. Boekema et al., "Coffee and Gastrointestinal Function: Facts and Fiction: A Review," *Scandinavian Journal of Gastroenterology* 34, no. 230 (1999): 35–39, doi:10.1080/003655299750025525; G. H. Elta et al., "Comparison of Coffee Intake and Coffee-Induced Symptoms in Patients with Duodenal Ulcer, Nonulcer Dyspepsia, and Normal Controls," *American Journal of Gastroenterology* 85, no. 10 (1990): 1339–42.

18    Malte Rubach et al., "A Dark Brown Roast Coffee Blend Is Less Effective at Stimulating Gastric Acid Secretion in Healthy Volunteers Compared to a Medium Roast Market Blend," *Molecular Nutrition and Food Research* 58, no. 6 (2014): 1370–73, doi:10.1002 /mnfr.201300890; Gary Van Deventer et al., "Lower Esophageal Sphincter Pressure, Acid Secretion, and Blood Gastrin after Coffee Consumption," *Digestive Diseases and Sciences* 37, no. 4 (1992): 558–69, doi:10.1007/BF01307580; K. E. McArthur and M. Feldman, "Gastric Acid Secretion, Gastrin Release, and Gastric Emptying in Humans as Affected by Liquid Meal Temperature," *American Journal of Clinical Nutrition* 49, no. 1 (1989): 51–54, http://ajcn.nutrition.org/content/49/1/51.short; R. J. Coffey et al., "The Acute Effects of Coffee and Caffeine on Human Interdigestive Exocrine Pancreatic Secretion," *Pancreas* 1, no. 1 (1986): 55–61, www.ncbi .nlm.nih.gov/pubmed/3575300; J. Boekema et al., "Coffee and Gastrointestinal Function: Facts and Fiction: A Review," *Scandinavian Journal of Gastroenterology* 34, no. 230 (1999): 35–39, doi:10.1080/003655299750025525; Mitchell L. Schubert, "Functional Anatomy and Physiology of Gastric Secretion," *Current Opinion in Gastroenterology* 31 (2015): 479–85, doi:10.1097 /MOG.0000000000000213.

19    N. Broutet, "Risk Factors for Atrophic Chronic Gastritis in a European Population: Results of the Eurohepygast Study," *Gut* 50, no. 6 (2002): 779–85, doi:10.1136/gut.50.6.779.

20    Lucy S. Ito et al., "Lifestyle Factors Associated with Atrophic Gastritis among Helicobacter Pylori-Seropositive Japanese-Brazilians in Sao Paulo," *International Journal of Clinical Oncology* 8, no. 6 (2003): 362–68, doi:10.1007/s10147-003-0355-3; K. Ohkuma et al., "Association of Helicobacter Pylori Infection with Atrophic Gastritis and Intestinal Metaplasia," *Journal of Gastroenterology and Hepatology* 15, no. 10 (2000): 1105–12, www.ncbi.nlm.nih.gov/pubmed/11106088; R. Sierra et al., "Association of Serum Pepsinogen with Atrophic Body Gastritis in Costa Rica," *Clinical and Experimental Medicine* 6, no. 2 (2006): 72–78, doi:10.1007/s10238-006 -0098-3; Adeyinka O. Laiyemo et al., "Serum Pepsinogen Level, Atrophic Gastritis and the Risk of Incident Pancreatic Cancer—A Prospective Cohort Study," *Cancer Epidemiology* 33, no. 5 (2009): 368–73, doi:10.1016/j.canep.2009.09.001.

21    J. A. Sanchez-Cuen et al., "Helicobacter Pylori Infection and Its Association with Alcohol Consumption: A Case-Control Study," [In Spanish.] *Revista de Gastroenterologia de Mexico* 78, no. 3 (2013): 144–50, doi:10.1016/j.rgmx.2013.06.003; V. Schusdziarra et al., "Effects of a Coffee-Antacid-Mixture and a Commercial Coffee with Regard to Gastrin, pH and Gastric Secretion (Author's Transl.)," [In German.] *Zeitschrift Für Gastroenterologie* 15, no. 7 (1977): 448–56, www.ncbi.nlm.nih.gov/pubmed/19888; Tarmo T. Koivisto et al., "Effect of Smoking on Gastric Histology in Helicobacter Pylori–Positive Gastritis," *Scandinavian Journal of Gastroenterology* 43, no. 10 (2008): 1177–83, doi:10.1080/00365520802116430; R. Cheli et al., "Clinical Significance of Duodenal Erosions," *Endoscopy* 16, no. 3 (May 17, 1984): 105–8, doi:10.1055/s-2007-1018547.

22    K. Shibata et al., "Green Tea Consumption and Chronic Atrophic Gastritis: A Cross-Sectional Study in a Green Tea Production Village," *Journal of Epidemiology/Japan Epidemiological Association* 10, no. 5 (2000): 310–16, http://doi.org/10.2188/jea.10.310.

23   Miyui Uno et al., "Possible Association of Interleukin 1B C-31T Polymorphism among Helicobacter Pylori Seropositive Japanese Brazilians with Susceptibility to Atrophic Gastritis," *International Journal of Molecular Medicine* 14, no. 3 (2004): 421–26; Yoshinori Ito et al., "The Risk of Helicobacter Pylori Infection and Atrophic Gastritis from Food and Drink Intake: A Cross-Sectional Study in Hokkaido, Japan," *Asian Pacific Journal of Cancer Prevention : APJCP* 1, no. 2 (2000): 147–56, www.ncbi.nlm.nih.gov/pubmed/12718682; Y. Kuwahara et al., "Relationship between Serologically Diagnosed Chronic Atrophic Gastritis, Helicobacter Pylori, and Environmental Factors in Japanese Men," *Scandinavian Journal of Gastroenterology* 35, no. 5 (2000): 476–81.

24   V. A. DeLuca, "No Acid, No Polys—No Gastritis, No Dyspepsia. A Proposal," *Journal of Clinical Gastroenterology* 11, no. 2 (April 1989): 127–31, www.ncbi.nlm.nih.gov/pubmed/2738355.

25   M. G. Whiteside et al., "The Absorption of Radioactive Vitamin B12 and the Secretion of Hydrochloric Acid in Patients with Atrophic Gastritis," *Gut* 5, no. 5 (October 1964): 385–99, www.ncbi.nlm.nih.gov/pubmed/14218551.

26   Renato Tozzoli et al., "Autoantibodies to Parietal Cells as Predictors of Atrophic Body Gastritis: A Five-Year Prospective Study in Patients with Autoimmune Thyroid Diseases," *Autoimmunity Reviews*, 2010, doi:10.1016/j.autrev.2010.08.006.

27   H. Andersson et al., "Influence of the Amount of Dietary Gluten on Gastrointestinal Morphology and Function in Dermatitis Herpetiformis," *Human Nutrition. Clinical Nutrition* 38, no. 4 (July 1984): 279–85, www.ncbi.nlm.nih.gov/pubmed/6469705; W. Kastrup et al., "Influence of Gluten-Free Diet on the Gastric Condition in Dermatitis Herpetiformis," *Scandinavian Journal of Gastroenterology* 20 (1985): 39–45, doi:10.3109/00365528509089630.

28   G. Faller et al., "Decrease of Antigastric Autoantibodies in Helicobacter Pylori Gastritis after Cure of Infection," *Pathology, Research and Practice* 195, no. 4 (1999): 243–46, doi:10.1016/S0344-0338(99)80041-7.

29   J. Arikawa et al., "Morphological Characteristics of Epstein-Barr Virus–Related Early Gastric Carcinoma: A Case-Control Study," *Pathology International* 47, no. 6 (1997): 360–67, www.ncbi.nlm.nih.gov/pubmed/9211523.

30   I. C. Kohlstadt et al., "Parietal-Cell Antibodies among Peruvians with Gastric Pathological Changes," *Scandinavian Journal of Gastroenterology* 28, no. 11 (1993): 973–77, doi:10.3109/00365529309098294; Aşkin Erdoğan and Uğur Yilmaz, "Is There a Relationship between Helicobacter Pylori and Gastric Autoimmunity?," *Turkish Journal of Gastroenterology* 22, no. 2 (2011): 134–38, doi:10.4318/tjg.2011.0181.

31   H. P. Lin et al., "Modulation of Serum Gastric Parietal Cell Antibody Level by Levamisole and Vitamin B12 in Oral Lichen Planus," *Oral Diseases* 17, no. 1 (2011): 95–101, doi:10.1111/j.1601-0825.2010.01711.x; Andy Sun et al., "Effective Vitamin B12 Treatment Can Reduce Serum Antigastric Parietal Cell Antibody Titer in Patients with Oral Mucosal Disease," *Journal of the Formosan Medical Association* 115, no. 10 (2016): 837–44, doi:10.1016/j.jfma.2016.05.003.

# CHAPTER 16

# DIGESTIVE ENZYMES

## DIGESTIVE ENZYMES

Whew, OK. We've made it through the stomach and have discussed the stomach and stomach acid in detail. Now, let's talk about digestive enzymes. After food leaves the stomach, it enters the small intestine, where most digestion occurs (part of the reason why the small intestine is such an important part of digestive health).

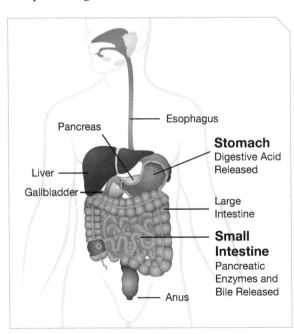

As food moves through your small intestine, your gallbladder releases bile into the small intestine and your pancreas releases pancreatic enzymes into it—these are your body's digestive enzymes. Both bile and pancreatic enzymes have a number of functions. Both are antibacterial and help to prevent SIBO. Bile chiefly aids in the digestion of fat, while pancreatic enzymes help with digestion of fats, proteins, and carbohydrates.

Deficiency in these digestive enzymes can manifest in a variety of ways, but the most common symptoms are

- bloating;
- constipation;
- diarrhea;
- smelly stools;
- fatty or floating stools;
- intolerance of fatty foods.

It's worth mentioning that SIBO can actually interfere with the ability of bile to work properly. So, someone could have healthy bile production but also have the symptoms of bile deficiency because they have SIBO, which is interfering with the bile's ability to function. This is why we give some supplemental bile in step 2 but try to wean you off it after we address any unwanted bacteria (like SIBO) in step 3.

This all sounds fairly interesting, right? The stomach releases acid, the gallbladder releases bile, and the pancreas makes pancreatic enzymes, and *all* are needed for proper digestion. But how do we know that taking a pill that contains these will have any effect? It's one thing to have mechanistic knowledge; it's another to have clinical data that shows this might be a treatment that can actually help you. What does the clinical science say here?

The research regarding enzymes and bile is more robust than digestive-acid research, and it does appear supplementing with enzymes can help with various digestive problems like gas/bloating, pain, diarrhea, malabsorption, and fat in stool.[1]

However, most of these studies are done using people with well-documented enzyme deficiencies (like lactose deficiency/lactose intolerance), who have diseases of the pancreas, or who have had intestinal surgery. As a result, it's unclear how applicable these studies are to people without these conditions. This is why yet again we'll be using a conservative approach and try to find the minimum dose needed for the minimum time.

Lab testing is not recommended for identifying the dose of enzymes someone should use.[2] Can you guess what *is* recommended? *Monitoring your response to supplementing with enzymes.* So, skip the test, and try the treatment, which is exactly how we are using enzymes in our Great-in-8.

If a little enzyme support improves your digestion, does this mean more will be better? No. Please do not make the mistake of thinking more is better with enzymes and bile. The human body is all about balance. Bile illustrates this concept well. While, yes, some supplemental bile may help with a digestive difficulty like

diarrhea, if you use too much, it can also cause diarrhea! It's well accepted that in some patients with chronic diarrhea, *excessive* bile can be the cause, and the treatment is actually bile-lowering agents.[3] And for the testing enthusiast, the recommended way to diagnose excessive bile is not testing but rather response to treatment.[4] When it comes to supplementing with enzymes and bile, we want to use the right amount. This is what we are working toward with our Great-in-8 process.

**GUT GEEKS**

*The lining of your small intestine also directly releases enzymes known as brush border enzymes. When there is inflammation, damage, overgrowth, or infection occurring in the small intestine, your ability to release these enzymes can be impaired. This can lead to poor digestion and food intolerances. However, if you can fix the underlying problem, you can restore these enzymes, improve digestion, and reduce food intolerances. This is one of the reasons people notice better digestion after following a gut-healing plan and also why some people will no longer need enzymes after gut healing.*

# CAN GLUTEN-DIGESTING ENZYMES ALLOW THE GLUTEN ALLERGIC TO INDULGE?

For those with a marked reaction to gluten, the idea of a pill that can lessen this reaction is very appealing. You're sure to hear many claims from the drug and supplement companies, who would love to get you on a few gluten-digesting pills every day for the rest of your life. To be fair, if a drug or supplement company researches and produces a product that helps you, by all means let's support this company for its good work. We want you to find what works, but we also want to prevent you from spending your money on what does not. Clinical science helps us do this. RCTs help us understand what works and to what extent. What does the science show about gluten-digesting enzymes?

Be aware that if you have celiac disease, there are currently no gluten enzymes that will allow you to eat large amounts of gluten without consequence. However, gluten-digesting enzymes may provide some aid, so let's elaborate.

We can break gluten enzymes down into two categories: pharmaceutical and dietary supplements. Let's start with the pharmaceutical enzymes.

## PHARMACEUTICAL ENZYMES

Glutenase ALV003 is a pharmaceutical enzyme that is currently being researched and will, we hope, be available as a prescription soon. The best study to date examining Glutenase ALV003 did not show any benefit to symptoms, but it did show the drug's ability to prevent intestinal damage.[5]

This study first took a group of patients with celiac disease and gave them different amounts of gluten to determine the level of gluten intake needed to elicit symptoms. They found that 1.5 grams of gluten per day or below did not cause symptoms. This study then gave everyone 2 grams per day (around one and a half pieces of bread). This was enough gluten to cause symptoms but not such severe symptoms that everyone would drop out of the study.

Along with this 2 grams of gluten per day, half the patients were given the drug Glutenase ALV003 and half were given a placebo. Those receiving the drug did not experience intestinal damage, whereas those receiving the placebo did. This is good news. However, there was no difference in symptoms in the drug group versus the placebo group. So, this drug could potentially be used to prevent intestinal damage in those with celiac disease, but it may not improve symptoms.

## DIETARY-SUPPLEMENT ENZYMES

Aspergillus niger prolyl endoprotease (AN-PEP) is a supplemental gluten-digesting enzyme. This enzyme was evaluated in a placebo-controlled clinical trial in 2013. In this study, participants were given a dose of gluten high enough to ensure symptoms (roughly seven grams per day, equivalent to roughly five pieces of bread). The supplemental enzymes did not prevent intestinal damage or reduce symptoms when compared to those receiving the placebo.[6] This is important to note, because this is a commonly recommended gluten enzyme in health-food stores and on the Internet.

Another study was performed using a compound called Glutenon.[7] What exactly this compound is has been hard to determine. Some research into this elusive compound suggests it may be an animal enzyme—perhaps similar to the enzyme formula we discussed earlier that is used as part of our Great-in-8 plan. Other information suggests this might be a papaya-derived compound that requires a prescription. In any case, when study participants ingested roughly 3.5 grams of gluten per day, Glutenon did reduce symptoms and slightly protected from intestinal damage compared to the placebo. Unfortunately, this compound is no longer available, perhaps because of side effects.

Speaking of papaya, a study using papaya enzymes (40 mg Carica papaya) did show benefit in a placebo-controlled trial. Six grams of gluten per day were given to patients with skin sores, rashes, and pimples (known as dermatitis herpetiformis, which is known to be caused by gluten ingestion). The papaya enzymes reduced skin reactions associated with gluten, but there did not appear to be an effect on digestive or other symptoms.[8]

Overall, it does not appear that gluten enzymes offer substantial benefit, although they may aid slightly. But how do we account for people who swear that their "Gluten-Blaster 500" enzymes have really helped them? Here are a few thoughts: It's good to remain open but also important not to be gullible. Someone taking Gluten-Blaster 500 could have experienced an unusually strong improvement from the enzyme. It's also possible that there is a strong placebo effect. The placebo effect can account for up to 70% of symptom improvement in those being treated for IBS (abdominal pain, bloating, discomfort, constipation, and diarrhea). The average level of placebo effect in well-performed scientific studies is 40%, and you can assume it will be higher for self-experimentation (up to 70%).[9] One study even showed that people felt better when receiving a placebo pill even when they knew it was a placebo pill![10]

Having a healthy outlook on supplements will help keep you grounded. It's not a good idea to look at a supplement as if it's a magical substance that will change your life forever. The chances of "placeboing" yourself will be extremely high. Rather, if we look at these treatments like tools that can be used temporarily to support, heal, repair, and rebalance, we should be able to find the minimal dose and duration needed—because we're not afraid to discontinue using them. If the placebo effect helps someone feel better, I'm open to it, especially if it's safe. A vitamin C placebo, for example, is much easier to justify than a surgical placebo. However, be cautious: many of these safe or natural placebos come at a financial cost and might be a waste of money.

This brings us to another important principle:

*The placebo effect can be strong, so it's important to have a healthy view on supplements.*

Supplements can help with healing, but in the long term most aren't necessary for normal functioning.

Trying gluten enzymes could be worth a shot because there is a potential for improvement; however, if you don't notice a *clear* benefit, don't waste your money.

*Those with diagnosed celiac disease are likely to have a greater chance for improvement from gluten enzymes than those who are gluten sensitive.*

Anyone who has gone gluten-free and noticed minimal or no improvement should be screened for SIBO, which we address in step 3. Addressing bacterial overgrowth has a much higher likelihood of improving your symptoms than gluten enzymes. I have not included gluten enzymes in our Great-in-8 because I'm not convinced they're necessary. If you do try a gluten enzyme, remember that the placebo effect with digestive symptoms is significant, up to 70%, so it's a good idea to find the minimal needed dose and repeatedly reevaluate whether they're helpful.

So far, we've discussed steps 1 and 2 of our Great-in-8 plan. For some people, these two steps will be all that's needed to improve their health noticeably. However, some will need more work on their guts to fully improve, so the next step that comes in our action plan is the removal or reduction of unwanted bacteria using antibacterial treatments.

# CONCEPT SUMMARY

- Supplementing with enzymes can improve symptoms and aid in gut healing.

- Once your gut heals, you will likely need less supplemental digestive enzymes.

- Testing is not needed before using enzymes.

- Gluten-digesting enzymes do not appear to offer substantial benefit but may provide minor aid.

- Be cautious of the placebo effect when using a new supplement, as it can be as high as 70% for digestive symptoms.

1   Marcellus Simadibrata et al., "Examination of Small Bowel Enzymes in Chronic Diarrhea," *Journal of Gastroenterology and Hepatology (Australia)* 18, no. 1 (2003): 53–56, doi:10.1046/j.1440-1746.2003.02917.x; Christine Kapral et al., "Conjugated Bile Acid Replacement Therapy in Short Bowel Syndrome Patients with a Residual Colon," *Zeitschrift Fur Gastroenterologie* 42, no. 7 (2004): 583–89, doi:10.1055/s-2004-813059; Katherine H. Little et al., "Treatment of Severe Steatorrhea with Ox Bile in an Ileectomy Patient with Residual Colon," *Digestive Diseases and Sciences* 37, no. 6 (1992): 929–33, doi:10.1007/BF01300393; G. R. Corazza et al., "Beta-Galactosidase from Aspergillus-Niger in Adult Lactose-Malabsorption—a Double-Blind Crossover Study," *Alimentary Pharmacology & Therapeutics* 6, no. 1 (1992): 61–66; Jorge L. Rosado et al., "Enzyme Replacement Therapy for Primary Adult Lactase Deficiency: Effective Reduction of Lactose Malabsorption and Milk Intolerance by Direct Addition of ß-Galactosidase to Milk at Mealtime," *Gastroenterology* 87, no. 5 (1984): 1072–82, doi:10.1016/S0016-5085(84)80067-0; Giovanni Di Nardo et al., "Efficacy and Tolerability of ß-Galactosidase in Treating Gas-Related Symptoms in Children: A Randomized, Double-Blind, Placebo Controlled Trial," *BMC Gastroenterology* 13, no. 1 (2013): 142, doi:10.1186/1471-230X-13-142; Khaled Saad et al., "A Randomized, Placebo-Controlled Trial of Digestive Enzymes in Children with Autism Spectrum Disorders," *Clinical Psychopharmacology and Neuroscience : The Official Scientific Journal of the Korean College of Neuropsychopharmacology* 13, no. 2 (2015): 188–93, doi:10.9758/cpn.2015.13.2.188; Mario Roxas, "The Role of Enzyme Supplementation in Digestive Disorders," *Alternative Medicine Review*, 2008.

2   Joachim Mössner and Volker Keim, "Pancreatic Enzyme Therapy," *Deutsches Arzteblatt International*, 2010, doi:10.3238/arztebl.2011.0578.

3   Alan Barkun et al., "Bile Acid Malabsorption in Chronic Diarrhea: Pathophysiology and Treatment," *Canadian Journal of Gastroenterology*, 2013.

4   X. Fan and J. H. Sellin, "Review Article: Small Intestinal Bacterial Overgrowth, Bile Acid Malabsorption and Gluten Intolerance as Possible Causes of Chronic Watery Diarrhoea," *Alimentary Pharmacology and Therapeutics*, 2009, doi:10.1111/j.1365-2036.2009.03970.x.

5   Marja Leena Lähdeaho et al., "Glutenase ALV003 Attenuates Gluten-Induced Mucosal Injury in Patients with Celiac Disease," *Gastroenterology* 146, no. 7 (2014): 1649–58, doi:10.1053/j.gastro.2014.02.031.

6   Greetje J. Tack et al., "Consumption of Gluten with Gluten-Degrading Enzyme by Celiac Patients: A Pilot-Study," *World Journal of Gastroenterology* 19, no. 35 (2013): 5837–47, doi:10.3748/wjg.v19.i35.5837.

7   Hugh J. Cornell et al., "Enzyme Therapy for Management of Coeliac Disease," *Scandinavian Journal of Gastroenterology* 40, no. 11 (2005): 1304–12, doi:10.1080/00365520510023855.

8   Agnieszka Zebrowska et al., "The Effect of Enzyme Therapy on Skin Symptoms and Immune Responses in Patients with Dermatitis Herpetiformis," *International Journal of Celiac Disease* 2, no. 2 (May 5, 2016): 58–63, doi:10.12691/ijcd-2-2-7.

9   S. M. Patel et al., "The Placebo Effect in Irritable Bowel Syndrome Trials: A Meta-Analysis," in *Neurogastroenterology and Motility*, 17:332–40, 2005, doi:10.1111/j.1365-2982.2005.00650.x.

10  Ted J. Kaptchuk et al., "Placebos without Deception: A Randomized Controlled Trial in Irritable Bowel Syndrome," *PloS One* 5, no. 12 (2010): e15591, doi:10.1371/journal.pone.0015591.

# CHAPTER 17

# ANTIBACTERIAL TREATMENTS: REMOVING THE BAD BUGS

## ANTIBIOTICS AND ANTIMICROBIAL HERBS

Earlier, we discussed how low-carb and low-FODMAP diets may decrease bacteria overgrowth by depriving bacteria of their food (carbs, fiber, and prebiotics). We can take things a step further with either antibiotics or antimicrobial herbs, which will also decrease bacterial growth and kill bacteria. Collectively, antibacterial treatments are well studied and important clinical interventions that can be very helpful for those who do not adequately respond to dietary and lifestyle changes or probiotics and enzymes.

I know what many of you are probably thinking—aren't antibiotics part of the reason why our guts are messed up to begin with? A fair question. Antibiotics are not the only factor responsible. Clearly, administering antibiotics to infants and children is something to avoid as much as possible, but antibiotics can save lives if used when

really needed. Remember our discussion about the tribe in Papua New Guinea? Even though they use antibiotics, their gut microbiotas are still much more diverse than those of Westerners. This illustrates that other environmental factors are strongly affecting your gut and microbiota health, not solely antibiotics.

I believe if we use the right antibiotics in the right way—to clean out excessive bacterial or other overgrowths or infections—we can heal the gut and realize health benefits. Does this mean we should all run out and take antibiotics to fix our problems? No. But if you have a doctor you trust will only use antibiotics when absolutely necessary, and you get to a point where your doctor feels an antibiotic is the best choice, you should be open to this treatment.

*My* preference is to first use herbal antimicrobials, which can clean out unwanted bacteria but may be a bit milder than antibiotics. Herbal medicines are remarkable in the sense that they can have side benefits rather than side effects. For example, oregano has the ability to kill bacteria, but there is some preliminary evidence that it may also function as an antidepressant.[1]

# WHAT NEEDS REMOVING AND WHY

We will be using antimicrobial herbs to remove pathogens (bad guys) that should not be in the gut and to reduce the number of organisms that belong but are just overgrown (as in SIBO). Think of it like pulling weeds and trimming the shrubs. The weeds are removed because they shouldn't be there. The shrubs are trimmed (reduced) because they belong but have just overgrown. But shouldn't we test before using antimicrobials so we know exactly what we're removing or reducing? Testing can be helpful in personalizing the antimicrobial approach; however, we should be able to resolve most problems without testing as we work through our Great-in-8 plan.

What are some of the microorganisms that might be removed or reduced as we start the antimicrobial step of the Great-in-8? We've already discussed some of these, but here is a list in order of most common to least common, in my experience:

- SIBO—bacterial overgrowths must be reduced
- Fungus (candida and yeast)—overgrowths of fungus must be reduced
- H. pylori bacteria—this is a normal inhabitant for many but can also cause disease in others; while we used to think these bacteria needed to be eradicated, more contemporary thinking suggests it needs to be reduced while improving the health of the rest of the microbiota
- Protozoa—Toxoplasmosis gondii, Blastocystis hominis, giardia, cryptosporidium in particular should be removed

- Pathogenic bacteria—Yersinia enterocolitis and Clostridium difficile must both be removed
- Worms—roundworms and tapeworms must be removed

For someone who has been dealing with a health ailment for a while, it's easy and tempting to get pulled into a search for the one kind of bug that is the hidden source of all your problems. It's tempting to imagine that if you could just determine which bug you have, you could get rid of it and finally heal. But what happens if you remove this bug but still don't feel any better? This happens more often than you might think. I have come to realize your gut is more complicated than one bug. This is why we're taking a holistic approach to your gut health and addressing *the entire ecosystem*, not just one bug. I encourage you to think globally and not obsess over one particular source of your problems. Your gut is an ecosystem, and to restore optimum function and balance, we'll need to do more than just kill one bug.

There are some people who only have one minor bacterial imbalance, but it's enough to make them very ill. Others may have several major imbalances and feel fine. Some people feel better after treating an imbalance; some don't. The Great-in-8 takes into consideration the idea that no two people are the same so you have to treat the whole ecosystem—the whole person—not just kill stuff or treat lab findings. We have already taken massive strides to improve your gut-microbiota ecosystem with the steps we've covered so far. Now we will build upon that by working on antimicrobials.

The importance of the microbial approach brings us to another principle:

*removing pathogens and/ or overgrowths helps balance*

*the ecosystem that is your gut microbiota.*

Earlier, we used a community analogy. If crime became rampant, it could drive out small businesses and local residents. The small businesses and local residents in that community would like to live and work there, and they would move in and open up shop if there wasn't so much crime. This is exactly what happens with antimicrobials. They remove the stuff that shouldn't be there and give healthy bacteria a chance to thrive. The antimicrobials help to rebalance the ecosystem that is your gut microbiota and help tip the balance in favor of the good guys.

This rebalancing effect has been described in the scientific literature. In 2016, in the journal *Alimentary Pharmacology & Therapeutics*, the authors theorized that Rifaximin (an antibiotic that targets the small intestine and SIBO) may help *reset* the small-intestinal microbiota.[2] We discussed earlier how certain herbal antimicrobials have been shown equally effective in addressing SIBO as the antibiotic Rifaximin. So, reason would suggest we can reset the small-intestinal microbiota using herbal antimicrobials.

Herbal antimicrobials are powerful, and the effect of some of them has been fairly well documented.[3] Many of these herbs have been used by cultures around the world for those suffering from digestive distress.

We've already established, though, that in order for the ecosystem to rebalance, we need to do more than just kill the bad bugs. Inflammation is another factor that can thwart the rebalancing of your microbiota. An article in *Pharmacological Research* states: "Inflammation per se may also be a key driver of the failure to resolve dysbiosis."[4] ("Dysbiosis" means "imbalance.") Certain types of unhealthy bacteria are more prone to overgrow when in an inflammatory intestinal environment; they actually seem to thrive in inflammation.

These same bacteria can damage the lining of your gut and trick your immune system into attacking the good bacteria![5]

Inflammation is a key issue because it appears to create an environment where bad guys flourish and good guys struggle. We've already taken steps to greatly reduce intestinal inflammation by improving your diet and lifestyle and by using probiotics and enzymes. The antimicrobial herbs we use in step 3 will build upon this by removing certain microorganisms that can cause inflammation.

## CLEANING OUT HARD-TO-KILL BAD BUGS AND REDUCING INFLAMMATION

### INFLAMMATION, BIOFILMS, AND PROTOZOA

Sometimes, even after we have given the microbiota a nudge with antimicrobial herbs, we still haven't tipped the balance in favor of the good guys and reestablished a healthy equilibrium of your gut ecosystem. Perhaps you have been treated by your doctor for SIBO and haven't fully responded. Or perhaps you have tried a self-help herbal antifungal treatment and have seen only a slight improvement. Or perhaps when you went through step 3, you only felt slightly better. There are three factors that often cause this resistance to rebalancing:

- Inflammation
- Biofilms
- Protozoa

### INFLAMMATION

You already know that inflammation can feed unhealthy bacteria in the gut. You've learned about all the supports that can contribute to healing inflammation: diet, lifestyle, adrenal support, probiotics, and antimicrobials. Even with all these, you might need a little more anti-inflammatory support. What's nice about one herbal medicine we can add next is this agent can be used as a powerful anti-inflammatory but also has a side benefit of being an antiprotozoal agent.

Artemisia is a derivative of the herb wormwood. It has been used in clinical trials in those with IBD. A systematic review with meta-analysis found this herb to be an effective treatment for IBD due to its anti-inflammatory effects.[6] This has been supported by other systematic reviews.[7]

Similar herbs have been shown to be as effective as the anti-inflammatory drug mesalamine in inducing remission in IBD.[8]

## PROTOZOA

Artemisia has some nice anti-inflammatory effects, but it also has the ability to remove protozoa. Wondering what protozoa are? You can think of protozoa like a highly advanced bacteria. Many protozoa, such as Toxoplasmosis ghondii, Blastocystis hominis, giardia, cryptosporidium, are harmful. Fortunately, artemisia has been shown to be a powerful antiprotozoal agent.[9]

If you don't have protozoa, can you still use artemisia? Yes. As we mentioned, artemisia has been used to treat inflammation in the intestines. Adding this herb into another round of antimicrobial treatment makes sense, because it can lower inflammation and remove or reduce protozoa, should you have any—both of which can help your microbiota rebalance and achieve a healthy equilibrium. But a word of caution, herbal antimicrobials should not be used indiscriminately, because overuse might cause antimicrobial resistance,[10] just like overuse of antibiotics can cause antibiotic resistance. Be sure to follow our Great-in-8 plan.

If our initial herbal protocol in step 3 does not fully address symptoms, we add artemisia because it has both anti-inflammatory and antiprotozoal

effects. No testing is needed before using this herb. We will go through a self-assessment in step 3 to help you determine exactly what to do.

## BIOFILMS

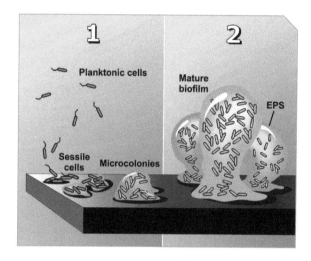

Biofilms are protective coatings that can form over bacteria and fungus and make them resistant to treatment. As shown in this illustration, bacteria and fungus can have two general forms in the body. When they first arrive, they are spread out in what's known as planktonic form (named after *plankton*, which are tiny vegetable fragments that float freely in the ocean). But after some time, bacteria and fungus start to aggregate and form a colony. The colony members all work together to build a protective fence-like barrier known as a biofilm. The biofilm protects the colony from eradication by antibiotics and antimicrobials, which makes it hard to treat.[11]

The good news is that we have already been working to address biofilms, because probiotics and antimicrobials have antibiofilm properties.[12]

However, when someone responds only partially to antimicrobials, it can mean that a biofilm is present and needs to be addressed directly. This is an area where the clinical science is fairly sparse and we have no choice but to try and make the best decisions we can based on lower-level science, because it's the only science we have available. There is a fair amount of bacterial-culture research (performed in vitro or a petri dish), but the clinical research is fairly sparse.[13]

There is one clinical biofilm study that is noteworthy, however. Two groups of patients were treated for an H. pylori bacterial infection. One group received an antibiotic, and the other group received an antibiotic plus an antibiofilm agent. Of those receiving the antibiotic alone, 20% cleared the infection, whereas 65% of those receiving the antibiotic plus the antibiofilm agent cleared the infection.[14] The antibiofilm agent used in this study was N-acetylcysteine (NAC). NAC is a very safe and natural compound that is also a powerful antioxidant. It has been well studied for its anti-biofilm properties.[15]

There are many natural treatments that are antibiofilm, in addition to NAC.[16] We will cover some options when we get into treatment details in part 5.

I am also very happy to announce that our office has shown, for the first time, certain anti-biofilm agents enhance the treatment effect of antimicrobial herbs in treating SIBO. At the time of writing this book, we are preparing our results to be published in a peer-reviewed medical journal. Essentially, we have shown that antibiofilm agents administered with herbal antimicrobials work better than antimicrobials alone, for hydrogen SIBO.

So, if you find you've gone through the initial herbal-antimicrobial protocol in step 3 and you haven't fully responded, adding in some specific biofilm treatment makes sense. Remember Jen from the introduction, who lost over fifty pounds after treating a fungal overgrowth in her intestines? Treating the biofilm that protected this fungus was a key component to her success. This will all be covered in the action plan we're working toward. Right now, let's continue our discussion regarding antibacterial treatments as they pertain to specific conditions.

# SUMMARY OF THE EVIDENCE— ANTIBACTERIAL TREATMENTS

## ANTIBACTERIAL TREATMENTS (DIETS, HERBAL ANTIMICROBIALS, AND ANTIBIOTICS)

- **IBS and SIBO**—Interventions that kill bacteria (herbal antimicrobials, antibiotics, and low-carb/prebiotic diets) have all been shown to be effective treatments for IBS in many RCTs. A short-term low-fiber diet may also be helpful. Intestinal parasites are an overlooked cause of IBS. Low-carb and low-prebiotic diets (such as the low-FODMAP diet) have impressive evidence for improving IBS.
- **Weight loss**—Preliminary evidence shows treating SIBO may lead to weight loss, improved blood sugar, and improved cholesterol. Low-carb diets have also been shown superior for weight loss, according to two systematic reviews.
- **Thyroid autoimmunity**—There is some exciting preliminary evidence that treating bacterial infections can help decrease thyroid autoimmunity. This reinforces a body of anecdotal clinical observations. One study has found a low-carb diet can decrease thyroid autoimmunity.
- **IBD (ulcerative colitis and Crohn's disease)**—Diets that are low in prebiotics, like the low-FODMAP diet and SCD, have shown impressive results in several RCTs. A short-term low-fiber diet may also be helpful. Systematic

reviews and clinical trials have shown antibiotics or herbal antimicrobials to induce remission in IBD, though the types of herbs and dosages used vary.

- **Celiac disease**—If you have celiac disease and have gone gluten-free but still have symptoms, you should be evaluated for gut infections and SIBO. Antibiotic treatment of these has been shown to eliminate symptoms; antimicrobial herbs appear to offer the same benefit. A low-FODMAP diet may improve symptoms in those with NCGS (nonceliac gluten sensitivity).
- **Insulin resistance**—Preliminary evidence shows treating SIBO may lead to weight loss, improved blood sugar, and improved cholesterol. The herb berberine is an effective antibacterial/antimicrobial and is also an effective treatment for lowering blood sugar/treating diabetes. Two systematic reviews have shown berberine works as well as the diabetes drug metformin. The dosages of berberine used ranged from 1 gram to 1.5 grams per day for diabetes and up to 5 grams per day for SIBO.
- **Depression and mood**—Preliminary evidence has shown treatments that kill bacteria, like antibiotics and antimicrobial herbs, may also help with depression.

# ANTIBACTERIAL TREATMENTS FOR SPECIFIC CONDITIONS

## IBS, SIBO, AND ANTIBACTERIAL TREATMENTS

What benefits are there to limiting dietary prebiotics and thus starving bacteria and having an antimicrobial effect? The low-FODMAP diet is low in prebiotics and has shown impressive results in the treatment of IBS. A systematic review with meta-analysis concluded that a low-FODMAP diet is effective for IBS. Once RCT showed 68% improvement in IBS in those using a low-FODMAP diet compared to only 23% improvement in the control subjects.[17] Numerous other studies have shown the low-FODMAP diet to help in IBS.[18]

The low-FODMAP diet does decrease bacteria in the intestines, even good bacteria like bifidobacteria.[19] However, remember that many with IBS have too much bacteria (even beneficial bacteria like bifidobacteria), so some bacterial loss is actually a good thing. But even more confusing is patients with IBS respond very well to Bifidobacterium probiotics. Maybe because supplemental Bifidobacterium probiotics are killing bifidobacteria overgrowth? So, what to do? Follow the results of clinical trials rather than speculating on what an effective treatment *might* be, based upon observations or mechanisms.

What about prebiotics and fungal or candida overgrowth? According to Elaine Gottschall, of the Specific Carbohydrate Diet, some prebiotics can also feed fungus (yeast or candida).[20] There is not much in the way of published medical science looking at prebiotic effect on candida; however, I feel caution is still warranted. If you follow our Great-in-8 recommendations, you will minimize risk of feeding overgrowths with prebiotics.

What about fiber? Even though fiber is generally considered good for you, in part because it feeds your microbiota, a clinical trial has shown reducing fiber intake aids with constipation and bloating.[21] It is possible that the patients in the study had SIBO and the low-fiber diet starved and killed these bacteria, thus improving their symptoms. The reduction in symptoms was quite dramatic, and the lower the fiber intake, the better the symptomatic improvement. A low-fiber diet is usually best used in the short term, to allow the gut a break from roughage and to have a chance to heal. Once symptoms have improved, slowly increasing fiber is advised.[22] This is exactly the process we will work through.

What about herbal antimicrobials or even antibiotic treatments? It appears that in many cases of IBS and, of course, with SIBO, an antibacterial approach is superior to a bacterial-feeding approach. Herbal antimicrobials or certain antibiotics have been shown to work very well, especially when followed by a low-FODMAP diet.[23] In fact, one systematic review with meta-analysis has shown that the antibiotic Rifaximin is an effective treatment for IBS.[24]

Herbal antimicrobials can have both antibacterial and antiparasitic effects. Parasites can be an overlooked cause of IBS.[25] Perhaps this is another reason why antimicrobials work well for IBS. Parasites are bugs that should not be there, like giardia, cryptosporidium, and amoebas, and you might also apply the term to Blastocystis hominis.[26] In my experience, a thorough evaluation for intestinal parasites is one of the most important steps toward optimizing your health. I learned this myself when I discovered an intestinal parasite in my twenties. Unfortunately, I have found some of the most popular functional-medicine tests for pathogens and parasites to be highly inaccurate, which is likely why, in the clinic, we routinely find infections that other doctors have missed.

Gut infections need to be addressed because they alter your microbiota. Gut infections cause inflammation, which changes the environment in your gut and makes it more favorable for the overgrowth of bad guys. It has been suggested that the microbiota can't normalize until infections have been addressed.[27]

This again hints at the concept that we can't "custom manipulate" our microbiota, but we can optimize the environment. This leads us to another principle:

> *you must remove the bad bugs before your gut and microbiota can rebalance and before you attempt to feed the good bacteria.*

This is why our removal step comes before our feeding step.

## WEIGHT LOSS AND ANTIBACTERIAL TREATMENTS

Two systematic reviews have shown low-carb diets are better for weight loss than higher-carb diets (and remember low-carb diets can also starve bacteria).[28] Other clinical trials using a low-carb diet have shown benefit for those who are overweight or diabetic.[29] However, this does not mean a low-carb diet is the best approach for everyone. If you follow the Great-in-8 steps, you will find your ideal level of carbohydrate intake.

There is some preliminary evidence that shows treating SIBO may help improve blood sugar, cholesterol, and even weight.[30] What might be happening here is the extra bacteria seen in SIBO increase calorie absorption from your diet, which leads to weight gain.[31]

There is some preliminary evidence that treating SIBO and improving someone's IBS can lead to weight loss. This is an area where there is not yet much published science. Here is what I see clinically regarding weight after treating SIBO and other gut infections with treatments that kill bacteria. Some patients lose a remarkable amount of weight, like Jen and Christine, whom we discussed in the intro. Most patients lose a moderate amount of weight—"moderate" meaning it's enough for the patient and his or her friends to notice. While some patients do not lose weight, almost every patient feels much better. So, this is exactly what I tell my patients when they ask me if treating a gut infection or overgrowth will cause weight loss: some lose a lot, most lose some, and some lose none—but they all feel better. Let's focus on getting you healthy first and hope for the best weight loss we can. I should also mention that those who are underweight will gain weight once their guts heal.

## THYROID AUTOIMMUNITY AND ANTIBACTERIAL TREATMENTS

Thyroid autoimmunity, like Hashimoto's disease, may also be helped by antibacterial treatments. One study, currently the only study looking at this issue, has found a low-carb diet decreases thyroid autoimmunity by over 40%.[32] Breath testing in these patients revealed that 80% of them might have difficulty digesting certain carbohydrates.

Additionally, thyroid antibodies have been shown to decrease after treating H. pylori, according to exciting preliminary findings (see diagram). A study was performed in Italy that illustrated how powerful treatment of infections can be in halting the autoimmune process. Ten patients who had Hashimoto's disease and also had an H. pylori infection were selected. Five underwent treatment for H. pylori, and five did not. Here is a breakdown of the findings (please note adequate data was only available for three patients from each group).

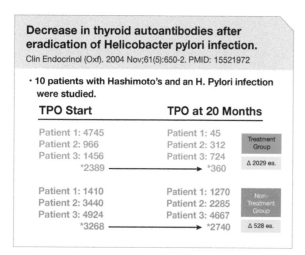

**Decrease in thyroid autoantibodies after eradication of Helicobacter pylori infection.**
Clin Endocrinol (Oxf). 2004 Nov;61(5):650-2. PMID: 15521972

· **10 patients with Hashimoto's and an H. Pylori infection were studied.**

| TPO Start | TPO at 20 Months | |
|---|---|---|
| Patient 1: 4745 | Patient 1: 45 | Treatment Group |
| Patient 2: 966 | Patient 2: 312 | |
| Patient 3: 1456 | Patient 3: 724 | |
| *2389 ——————→ | *360 | Δ 2029 ea. |
| Patient 1: 1410 | Patient 1: 1270 | Non-Treatment Group |
| Patient 2: 3440 | Patient 2: 2285 | |
| Patient 3: 4924 | Patient 3: 4667 | |
| *3268 ——————→ | *2740 | Δ 528 ea. |

The patients who were treated for the H. pylori bacterial infection (treatment group, in green) experienced a significant drop in their antibody levels (TPO), while those who did not undergo treatment (nontreatment, in red) did not. The treatment group experienced an average decrease of 2,029 points in their TPO antibodies, while the nontreatment group experienced an average of 528. The higher these TPO antibodies, the more thyroid damage and inflammation are occurring. Here you can clearly see a significant reduction in the TPO antibodies in the patients who were treated for the bacterial infection.[33]

One case study also showed a decrease in thyroid autoimmunity and an improvement in thyroid-hormone levels after treating a gut infection (Blastocystis hominis) with the antibiotic metronidazole.[34] These findings were preliminary but interesting nonetheless.

## IBD (ULCERATIVE COLITIS AND CROHN'S DISEASE) AND ANTIBACTERIAL TREATMENTS

Several RCT studies have shown diets that are low in prebiotics and discourage bacterial growth (specifically the low-FODMAP diet and the SCD) can help IBD.[35]

Both of these diets have shown impressive results. The positive impact of a low-prebiotic diet has been reinforced by systematic reviews with meta-analyses,[36] and other clinical trials have even shown this type of diet can help heal your intestinal lining.[37]

When IBD is active, or in a flare, low-fiber diets can aid in recovery. Again, a low-fiber diet is usually best used in the short term. Once symptoms have improved, slowly increasing fiber is advised.[38]

Antibiotics[39] or antimicrobial herbs[40] have been shown to induce remission in IBD, according to systematic reviews and clinical trials. The types of herbs and dosages used vary, so you will want to check in with a clinician on this one.

Another study also found that when patients with IBD who were in remission (meaning they were doing well) went on a high-prebiotic diet (a high-FODMAP diet, feeding gut bacteria), they experienced a doubling of their symptoms.[41]

## CELIAC DISEASE AND ANTIBACTERIAL TREATMENTS

What do you do if you have celiac disease, go gluten-free, but still have symptoms? You should have an evaluation for any gut infections, imbalances in fungus and bacteria, and for SIBO. A pivotal study illustrates this concept. Included in this study were fifteen celiac patients who all had gone gluten-free but still had some lingering symptoms.

These patients were then tested, and the following was found:

- Two patients could not digest dairy
- One patient had a Giardia lamblia infection, and one patient had a giant roundworm infection (Ascaris lumbricoides)
- **Ten patients showed SIBO!**

The two patients went off dairy. Giardia and roundworm were treated with antibiotics in the other two patients. And the ten SIBO patients were treated with a different antibiotic (Rifaximin). A month after treatment, all of these patients were symptom-free.[42] This study beautifully illustrates the point that

> *if diet doesn't work, the next step should be investigating a gut infection, overgrowth, or imbalance.*

This recommendation has been echoed by other researchers as well.[43]

Does this mean you *must* use an antibiotic? No. Herbal medicine works very well for treating infections and overgrowths, as we will expand upon in our removal step (step 3). If you follow the steps of our Great-in-8 plan in order, you'll navigate through this in the proper sequence—which will ensure your health improves as quickly and efficiently as possible.

What about antibacterial diets, like the low-FODMAP diet, for people who don't have celiac disease but suspect they have a problem with gluten (nonceliac gluten sensitivity, or NCGS)? One RCT suggests a low-FODMAP diet may help those with NCGS.[44]

## INSULIN RESISTANCE & ANTIBACTERIAL TREATMENTS

As discussed earlier, there is preliminary evidence that shows treating SIBO may help improve blood sugar, cholesterol, and even weight.[45] However, certain antibiotics, like vancomycin, have been shown to worsen insulin sensitivity.[46] Fortunately, there are other antibiotics available for treating gut infections that may help with insulin sensitivity. Rifaximin, Flagyl (metronidazole), and neomycin are common antibiotics used for treating SIBO, and they may help with insulin resistance. However, check in with your doctor on this also.

If, for whatever reason, you'd rather not use antibiotics, natural medicines are a fantastic option. The herb berberine has antimicrobial function, and it's often used to treat gut infections and SIBO. Berberine has been shown to be an effective treatment for IBS in a recent clinical trial.[47] It has also been demonstrated that berberine is effective in treating diabetes[48] and is even as effective as the diabetes drug metformin![49] Two systematic reviews have also found berberine to be a viable treatment for type 2 diabetes and cholesterol levels.[50] Dosages used ranged from 1 gram to 1.5 grams per day for diabetes but up to 5 grams per day when used to treat SIBO.

## DEPRESSION, MOOD, AND ANTIBACTERIAL TREATMENTS

My preference is to use herbal antimicrobials to kill bacteria rather than antibiotics. For certain conditions, we have more studies on antibiotics than herbal antimicrobials, but we can use these studies to support the concept of using something that kills bacteria to help improve that condition. With this in mind, there is some clinical-trial evidence that antibiotics decrease depression.

Preliminary data has shown antibiotics help with depression,[51] and this has been supported by other studies.[52] One study showed 70% of depression patients improved, and over 50% of them improved substantially, after treatment with an antibiotic. The improvement was sustained after ending the antibiotic. No patient worsened, and the antibiotics appeared to be well tolerated.[53] An RCT also showed antibiotics help with schizophrenia.[54]

The herb oregano can kill bacteria, but there is some preliminary evidence that it may also function as an antidepressant.[55] There will be more on oregano in step 3. Remember, antibacterial treatments may work so well because they reduce bacterial overgrowths and leaky gut, thus decreasing inflammation. This allows your healthy bacteria to grow, and once you've nudged the microbiota, it can rebalance.

There is one more antibacterial treatment, which we'll discuss next: liquid-elemental diets.

## CONCEPT SUMMARY

- We can use antimicrobial herbs to reduce overgrowths (trim the shrubs) or eradicate infection (weed).

- For more stubborn cases, we may need to add additional support in order to achieve balance in the microbiota. This support includes anti-inflammatory, antibiofilm, and antiprotozoal agents.

- Antimicrobial treatment can be helpful for IBS, IBD, thyroid autoimmunity, weight loss, insulin resistance, and mood.

1    Annis O. Mechan et al., "Monoamine Reuptake Inhibition and Mood-Enhancing Potential of a Specified Oregano Extract," *British Journal of Nutrition* 105, no. 8 (2011): 1150–63, doi:10.1017/S0007114510004940.

2    Mark Pimentel, "Review Article: Potential Mechanisms of Action of Rifaximin in the Management of Irritable Bowel Syndrome with Diarrhoea," *Alimentary Pharmacology & Therapeutics* 43 Suppl. 1 (2016): 37–49, doi:10.1111/apt.13437.

3    Fabien Juteau et al., "Composition and Antimicrobial Activity of the Essential Oil of Artemisia Absinthium from Croatia and France," *Planta Medica* 69, no. 2 (2003): 158–61, doi:10.1055/s-2003-37714; Kisaburo Nagamune et al., "Artemisinin-Resistant Mutants of Toxoplasma Gondii Have Altered Calcium Homeostasis," *Antimicrobial Agents and Chemotherapy* 51, no. 11 (2007): 3816–23, doi:10.1128/AAC.00582-07; Junling Han et al., "Modulating Gut Microbiota as an Anti-Diabetic Mechanism of Berberine," *Medical Science Monitor: International Medical Journal of Experimental and Clinical Research* 17, no. 7 (2011): RA164–A167, doi:881842 [pii]; Yang Yong et al., "Synthesis and Antimicrobial Activity of 8-Alkylberberine Derivatives with a Long Aliphatic Chain," *Planta Medica* 73, no. 6 (2007): 602–4, doi:10.1055/s-2007-967180; Padmaja V. Joshi et al., "Antidiarrheal Activity, Chemical and Toxicity Profile of Berberis Aristata," *Pharmaceutical Biology* 49, no. 1 (2011): 94–100, doi:10.3109/13880209.2010.500295; Suck Hee Chae et al., "Growth-Inhibiting Effects of Coptis Japonica Root-Derived Isoquinoline Alkaloids on Human Intestinal Bacteria," *Journal of Agricultural and Food Chemistry* 47, no. 3 (1999): 934–38, doi:10.1021/jf980991o; Niko Radulović et al., "Composition and Antimicrobial Activity of Equisetum Arvense L. Essential Oil," *Phytotherapy Research: PTR* 20, no. 1 (2006): 85–88, doi:10.1002/ptr.1815; Cynthia Cristina Arcila-Lozano et al., "Oregano: Properties, Composition and Biological Activity," [In Spanish.] *Archivos Latinoamericanos de Nutrición* 54, no. 1 (2004): 100–111, www.ncbi.nlm.nih.gov/pubmed/15332363; Sabahat Saeed and Perween Tariq, "Antibacterial Activity of Oregano (Origanum Vulgare Linn.) against Gram Positive Bacteria," *Pakistan Journal of*

*Pharmaceutical Sciences* 22, no. 4 (2009): 421–24; Isabella Savini et al., "Origanum Vulgare Induces Apoptosis in Human Colon Cancer Caco$_2$ Cells," *Nutrition and Cancer* 61, no. 3 (2009): 381–89, doi:10.1080/01635580802582769; Maryam Zarringhalam et al., "Inhibitory Effect of Black and Red Pepper and Thyme Extracts and Essential Oils on Enterohemorrhagic Escherichia Coli and DNase Activity of Staphylococcus Aureus," *Iranian Journal of Pharmaceutical Research* 12, no. 3 (2013): 363–69; D. Esmaeili et al., "Anti-Helicobacter Pylori Activities of Shoya Powder and Essential Oils of Thymus Vulgaris and Eucalyptus Globulus," *Open Microbiology Journal* 6, no. 1 (2012): 65–69, doi:10.2174/1874285801206010065.

4    Alan W. Walker and Trevor D. Lawley, "Therapeutic Modulation of Intestinal Dysbiosis," *Pharmacological Research*, 2013, doi:10.1016/j.phrs.2012.09.008.

5    Ibid.

6    Roja Rahimi et al., "Induction of Clinical Response and Remission of Inflammatory Bowel Disease by Use of Herbal Medicines: A Meta-Analysis," *World Journal of Gastroenterology* 19, no. 34 (2013): 5738–49, doi:10.3748/wjg.v19.i34.5738.

7    S. C. Ng et al., "Systematic Review: The Efficacy of Herbal Therapy in Inflammatory Bowel Disease," *Alimentary Pharmacology and Therapeutics*, 2013, doi:10.1111/apt.12464.

8    T. Tang et al., "Randomised Clinical Trial: Herbal Extract HMPL-004 in Active Ulcerative Colitis—A Double-Blind Comparison with Sustained Release Mesalazine," *Alimentary Pharmacology and Therapeutics* 33, no. 2 (2011): 194–202, doi:10.1111/j.1365-2036.2010.04515.x.

9    Christoph H. Blanke et al., "Herba Artemisiae Annuae Tea Preparation Compared to Sulfadoxine-Pyrimethamine in the Treatment of Uncomplicated Falciparum Malaria in Adults: A Randomized Double-Blind Clinical Trial," *Tropical Doctor* 38, no. 2 (2008): 113–16, doi:10.1258/td.2007.060184; Fabien Juteau et al., "Composition and Antimicrobial Activity of the Essential Oil of Artemisia Absinthium from Croatia and France," *Planta Medica* 69, no. 2 (2003): 158–61, doi:10.1055/s-2003-37714; Markus S. Mueller et al., "Randomized Controlled Trial of a Traditional Preparation of Artemisia Annua L. (Annual Wormwood) in the Treatment of Malaria," *Transactions of the Royal Society of Tropical Medicine and Hygiene* 98, no. 5 (2004): 318–21, doi:10.1016/j.trstmh.2003.09.001; Gerardo Priotto et al., "Artesunate and Sulfadoxine-Pyrimethamine Combinations for the Treatment of Uncomplicated Plasmodium Falciparum Malaria in Uganda: A Randomized, Double-Blind, Placebo-Controlled Trial," *Transactions of the Royal Society of Tropical Medicine and Hygiene* 97, no. 3 (2003): 325–30, doi:10.1016/S0035-9203(03)90161-1.

10   Kisaburo Nagamune et al., "Artemisinin-Resistant Mutants of Toxoplasma Gondii Have Altered Calcium Homeostasis," *Antimicrobial Agents and Chemotherapy* 51, no. 11 (2007): 3816–23, doi:10.1128/AAC.00582-07.

11   J. L. del Pozo and R. Patel, "The Challenge of Treating Biofilm-Associated Bacterial Infections," *Clinical Pharmacology & Therapeutics* 82, no. 2 (2007): 204–9, doi:10.1038/sj.clpt.6100247.

12   Anna Krasowska et al., "The Antagonistic Effect of Saccharomyces Boulardii on Candida Albicans Filamentation, Adhesion and Biofilm Formation," *FEMS Yeast Research* 9, no. 8 (2009): 1312–21, doi:10.1111/j.1567-1364.2009.00559.x; Samir Jawhara and Daniel Poulain, "Saccharomyces Boulardii Decreases Inflammation and Intestinal Colonization by Candida Albicans in a Mouse Model of Chemically-Induced Colitis," *Medical Mycology* 45, no. 8 (2007): 691–700, doi:10.1080/13693780701523013; E. B. Avalueva et al., "Use of Saccharomyces Boulardii in Treating Patients Inflammatory Bowel Diseases (Clinical Trial)," [In Russian.] *Eksperimental'naia I Klinicheskaia Gastroenterologiia*, no. 7 (2010): 103–11, http://europepmc.org/abstract/med/21033091.

13   S. Dinicola et al., "N-Acetylcysteine as Powerful Molecule to Destroy Bacterial Biofilms. A Systematic Review," *European Review for Medical and Pharmacological Sciences* 18, no. 19 (2014): 2942–48; Jie Feng et al., "Eradication of Biofilm-like Microcolony Structures of Borrelia Burgdorferi by Daunomycin and Daptomycin but Not Mitomycin C in Combination with Doxycycline and Cefuroxime," *Frontiers in Microbiology* 7, no. FEB (2016), doi:10.3389/fmicb.2016.00062; P. A. S. Theophilus et al., "Effectiveness of Stevia Rebaudiana Whole Leaf Extract against the Various Morphological Forms of Borrelia Burgdorferi in Vitro," *European Journal of Microbiology and Immunology* 5 (2015): 1–13, doi:10.1556/1886.2015.00031; A. Goc et al., "In Vitro Evaluation of Antibacterial Activity of Phytochemicals and Micronutrients against Borrelia Burgdorferi and Borrelia Garinii," *Journal of Applied Microbiology* 119, no. 6 (2015): 1561–72, doi:10.1111/jam.12970; Eva Sapi et al., "Evaluation of In-Vitro Antibiotic Susceptibility of Different Morphological Forms of Borrelia Burgdorferi," *Infection and Drug Resistance* 4, no. 1 (2011): 97–113, doi:10.2147/IDR.S19201; Alba A. Chavez-Dozal et al., "In Vitro Analysis of Flufenamic Acid Activity against Candida Albicans Biofilms," *International Journal of Antimicrobial Agents* 43, no. 1 (2014): 86–91, doi:10.1016/j.ijantimicag.2013.08.018.

14   Giovanni Cammarota et al., "Biofilm Demolition and Antibiotic Treatment to Eradicate Resistant Helicobacter Pylori: A Clinical Trial," *Clinical Gastroenterology and Hepatology* 8, no. 9 (2010), doi:10.1016/j.cgh.2010.05.006.

15    Alan W. Walker and Trevor D. Lawley, "Therapeutic Modulation of Intestinal Dysbiosis," *Pharmacological Research*, 2013, doi:10.1016/j.phrs.2012.09.008.

16    G. Cammarota et al., "Review Article: Biofilm Formation by Helicobacter Pylori as a Target for Eradication of Resistant Infection," *Alimentary Pharmacology and Therapeutics*, 2012, doi:10.1111/j.1365-2036.2012.05165.x.

17    H. M. Staudacher et al., "Fermentable Carbohydrate Restriction Reduces Luminal Bifidobacteria and Gastrointestinal Symptoms in Patients with Irritable Bowel Syndrome," *Journal of Nutrition* 142, no. 8 (2012): 1510–18, doi:10.3945/jn.112.159285.

18    Abigail Marsh et al., "Does a Diet Low in FODMAPs Reduce Symptoms Associated with Functional Gastrointestinal Disorders? A Comprehensive Systematic Review and Meta-Analysis," *European Journal of Nutrition* 55, no. 3 (2016): 897–906, doi:10.1007/s00394-015-0922-1; B. P. Chumpitazi et al., "Randomised Clinical Trial: Gut Microbiome Biomarkers Are Associated with Clinical Response to a Low FODMAP Diet in Children with the Irritable Bowel Syndrome," *Alimentary Pharmacology & Therapeutics* 42, no. 4 (2015): 418–27, doi:10.1111/apt.13286.

19    H. M. Staudacher et al., "Fermentable Carbohydrate Restriction Reduces Luminal Bifidobacteria and Gastrointestinal Symptoms in Patients with Irritable Bowel Syndrome," *Journal of Nutrition* 142, no. 8 (2012): 1510–18, doi:10.3945/jn.112.159285.

20    "Inulin—Breaking the Vicious Cycle," 2017, accessed October 11, 2017, www.breakingtheviciouscycle.info/knowledge_base/detail/inulin/.

21    Kok Sun Ho et al., "Stopping or Reducing Dietary-Fiber Intake Reduces Constipation and Its Associated Symptoms," *World Journal of Gastroenterology* 18, no. 33 (2012): 4593–96, doi:10.3748/wjg.v18.i33.4593.

22    Nancy Ling et al., "What Are High and Low Fiber Diets? | Cedars-Sinai Cancer Institute," 2017, accessed October 11, 2017, www.cedars-sinai.edu/Patients/Programs-and-Services/Colorectal-Cancer-Center/For-Patients/High-and-Low-Fiber-Diets.aspx.

23    Mark Pimentel, "An Evidence-Based Treatment Algorithm for IBS Based on a Bacterial/SIBO Hypothesis: Part 2," *American Journal of Gastroenterology* 105, no. 6 (2010): 1227–30, doi:10.1038/ajg.2010.125; Victor Chedid et al., "Herbal Therapy Is Equivalent to Rifaximin for the Treatment of Small Intestinal Bacterial Overgrowth," *Global Advances in Health and Medicine* 3, no. 3 (2014): 16–24, doi:10.7453/gahmj.2014.019.

24    Stacy B. Menees et al., "The Efficacy and Safety of Rifaximin for the Irritable Bowel Syndrome: A Systematic Review and Meta-Analysis," *American Journal of Gastroenterology* 107, no. 1 (2012): 28–35, doi:10.1038/ajg.2011.355.

25    D. Stark et al., "Irritable Bowel Syndrome: A Review on the Role of Intestinal Protozoa and the Importance of Their Detection and Diagnosis," *International Journal for Parasitology*, 2007, doi:10.1016/j.ijpara.2006.09.009.

26    Uday C. Ghoshal et al., "Bugs and Irritable Bowel Syndrome: The Good, the Bad and the Ugly," *Journal of Gastroenterology and Hepatology* 25, no. 2 (2010): 244–51, doi:10.1111/j.1440-1746.2009.06133.x.

27    Alan W. Walker and Trevor D. Lawley, "Therapeutic Modulation of Intestinal Dysbiosis," *Pharmacological Research*, 2013, doi:10.1016/j.phrs.2012.09.008.

28    M. Hession et al., "Systematic Review of Randomized Controlled Trials of Low-Carbohydrate vs. Low-Fat/Low-Calorie Diets in the Management of Obesity and Its Comorbidities," *Obesity Reviews*, 2009, doi:10.1111/j.1467-789X.2008.00518.x; Deirdre K. Tobias et al., "Effect of Low-Fat Diet Interventions versus Other Diet Interventions on Long-Term Weight Change in Adults: A Systematic Review and Meta-Analysis," *Lancet Diabetes and Endocrinology* 3, no. 12 (2015): 968–79, doi:10.1016/S2213-8587(15)00367-8.

29    Cara B. Ebbeling et al., "Effects of a Low-Glycemic Load vs Low-Fat Diet in Obese Young Adults," *JAMA* 297, no. 19 (2007): 2092, doi:10.1001/jama.297.19.2092; Christopher D. Gardner et al., "And LEARN Diets for Change in Weight and Related Risk Factors among Overweight," *Journal of the American Medical Association* 297, no. 9 (2007): 969–78, doi:10.1001/jama.297.9.969.

30    Ruchi Mathur et al., "Metabolic Effects of Eradicating Breath Methane Using Antibiotics in Prediabetic Subjects with Obesity," *Obesity* 24, no. 3 (2016): 576–82, doi:10.1002/oby.21385; Robert J. Basseri et al., "Intestinal Methane Production in Obese Individuals Is Associated with a Higher Body Mass Index," *Gastroenterology & Hepatology* 8, no. 1 (2012): 22–28, www.pubmedcentral.nih.gov/articlerender.fcgi?artid=3277195&tool=pmcentrez&rendertype=abstract; Ruchi Mathur et al., "Methane and Hydrogen Positivity on Breath Test Is Associated with Greater Body Mass Index and Body Fat," *Journal of Clinical Endocrinology and Metabolism* 98, no. 4 (2013): E698–702, doi:10.1210/jc.2012-3144; Andrew Curry, "Certain Bacteria Might Make Type 2 More Likely," *Diabetes Forecast*, November 2012, accessed October 9, 2017, www.diabetesforecast.org/2012/nov/certain-bacteria-might-make-type-2-more-likely.html.

31    Husen Zhang et al., "Human Gut Microbiota in Obesity and after Gastric Bypass," *Proceedings of the National Academy of Sciences of the United States of America* 106, no. 7 (2009): 2365–70, doi:10.1073/pnas.0812600106.

32  Teresa Esposito et al., "Effects of Low-Carbohydrate Diet Therapy in Overweight Subjects with Autoimmune Thyroiditis: Possible Synergism with ChREBP," *Drug Design, Development and Therapy* 10 (2016): 2939–46, doi:10.2147/DDDT.S106440.

33  Giovanni Bertalot et al., "Decrease in Thyroid Autoantibodies after Eradication of Helicobacter Pylori Infection [2]," *Clinical Endocrinology*, 2004, doi:10.1111/j.1365-2265.2004.02137.x.

34  Borko Rajik et al., "Eradication of Blastocystis Hominis Prevents the Development of Symptomatic Hashimoto's Thyroiditis: A Case Report," *Journal of Infection in Developing Countries* 9, no. 7 (2015): 788–91, doi:10.3855/jidc.4851.

35  Ashley Charlebois et al., "The Impact of Dietary Interventions on the Symptoms of Inflammatory Bowel Disease: A Systematic Review," *Critical Reviews in Food Science and Nutrition* 56, no. 8 (2016): 1370–78, doi:10.1080/10408398.2012.760515; Richard B. Gearry et al., "Reduction of Dietary Poorly Absorbed Short-Chain Carbohydrates (FODMAPs) Improves Abdominal Symptoms in Patients with Inflammatory Bowel Disease—A Pilot Study," *Journal of Crohn's and Colitis* 3, no. 1 (2009): 8–14, doi:10.1016/j.crohns.2008.09.004; Raquel Nieves and Roger T. Jackson, "Specific Carbohydrate Diet in Treatment of Inflammatory Bowel Disease," *Tennessee Medicine: Journal of the Tennessee Medical Association* 97, no. 9 (September 2004): 407, www.ncbi.nlm.nih.gov/pubmed/15497569; Stanley A. Cohen et al., "Clinical and Mucosal Improvement with Specific Carbohydrate Diet in Pediatric Crohn Disease," *Journal of Pediatric Gastroenterology and Nutrition* 59, no. 4 (2014): 516–21, doi:10.1097/MPG.0000000000000449.

36  Abigail Marsh et al., "Does a Diet Low in FODMAPs Reduce Symptoms Associated with Functional Gastrointestinal Disorders? A Comprehensive Systematic Review and Meta-Analysis," *European Journal of Nutrition* 55, no. 3 (2016): 897–906, doi:10.1007/s00394-015-0922-1.

37  David L. Suskind et al., "Nutritional Therapy in Pediatric Crohn Disease: The Specific Carbohydrate Diet," *Journal of Pediatric Gastroenterology and Nutrition* 58, no. 1 (2014): 87–91, doi:10.1097/MPG.0000000000000103.

38  Nancy Ling, "What Are High and Low Fiber Diets? | Cedars-Sinai Cancer Institute," 2017, accessed October 11, 2017, www.cedars-sinai.edu/Patients/Programs-and-Services/Colorectal-Cancer-Center/For-Patients/High-and-Low-Fiber-Diets.aspx.

39  Khurram J. Khan et al., "Antibiotic Therapy in Inflammatory Bowel Disease: A Systematic Review and Meta-Analysis," *American Journal of Gastroenterology* 106, no. 4 (2011): 661–73, doi:10.1038/ajg.2011.72.

40  Ahmed Salih Sahib, "Treatment of Irritable Bowel Syndrome Using a Selected Herbal Combination of Iraqi Folk Medicines," *Journal of Ethnopharmacology* 148, no. 3 (2013): 1008–12, doi:10.1016/j.jep.2013.05.034; S. C. Ng et al., "Systematic Review: The Efficacy of Herbal Therapy in Inflammatory Bowel Disease," *Alimentary Pharmacology and Therapeutics*, 2013, doi:10.1111/apt.12464.

41  Emma P. Halmos et al., "Consistent Prebiotic Effect on Gut Microbiota with Altered FODMAP Intake in Patients with Crohn's Disease: A Randomised, Controlled Crossover Trial of Well-Defined Diets," *Clinical and Translational Gastroenterology* 7, no. 4 (2016): e164, doi:10.1038/ctg.2016.22.

42  Antonio Tursi et al., "High Prevalence of Small Intestinal Bacterial Overgrowth in Celiac Patients with Persistence of Gastrointestinal Symptoms after Gluten Withdrawal," *American Journal of Gastroenterology* 98, no. 4 (2003): 839–43, doi:10.1111/j.1572-0241.2003.07379.x.

43  Ujjal Poddar, "Pediatric and Adult Celiac Disease: Similarities and Differences," *Indian Journal of Gastroenterology: Official Journal of the Indian Society of Gastroenterology* 32, no. 5 (2013): 283–88, doi:10.1007/s12664-013-0339-9; S. V. Rana et al., "Small Intestinal Bacterial Overgrowth in North Indian Patients with Celiac Disease," *Tropical Gastroenterology* 28, no. 4 (2007): 159–61, www.ncbi.nlm.nih.gov/pubmed/18416345; U. C. Ghoshal et al., "Partially Responsive Celiac Disease Resulting from Small Intestinal Bacterial Overgrowth and Lactose Intolerance," *BMC Gastroenterology* 4 (2004): 10, doi:10.1186/1471-230X-4-10.

44  Jessica R. Biesiekierski et al., "No Effects of Gluten in Patients with Self-Reported Nonceliac Gluten Sensitivity after Dietary Reduction of Fermentable, Poorly Absorbed, Short-Chain Carbohydrates," *Gastroenterology* 145, no. 2 (2013), doi:10.1053/j.gastro.2013.04.051.

45  Andrew Curry, "Certain Bacteria Might Make Type 2 More Likely," *Diabetes Forecast*, November 2012, accessed October 9, 2017, www.diabetesforecast.org/2012/nov/certain-bacteria-might-make-type-2-more-likely.html; Robert J. Basseri et al., "Intestinal Methane Production in Obese Individuals Is Associated with a Higher Body Mass Index," *Gastroenterology & Hepatology* 8, no. 1 (2012): 22–28, www.pubmedcentral.nih.gov/articlerender.fcgi?artid=3277195&tool=pmcentrez&rendertype=abstract; Ruchi Mathur et al., "Methane and Hydrogen Positivity on Breath Test Is Associated with Greater Body Mass Index and Body Fat," *Journal of Clinical Endocrinology and Metabolism* 98, no. 4 (2013): E698-702, doi:10.1210/jc.2012-3144.

46  Anne Vrieze et al., "Impact of Oral Vancomycin on Gut Microbiota, Bile Acid Metabolism, and Insulin Sensitivity," *Journal of Hepatology* 60, no. 4 (2014): 824–31, doi:10.1016/j.jhep.2013.11.034.

47 Chunqiu Chen et al., "A Randomized Clinical Trial of Berberine Hydrochloride in Patients with Diarrhea-Predominant Irritable Bowel Syndrome," *Phytotherapy Research* 29, no. 11 (2015): 1822–27, doi:10.1002/ptr.5475.

48 Yifei Zhang et al., "Treatment of Type 2 Diabetes and Dyslipidemia with the Natural Plant Alkaloid Berberine," *Journal of Clinical Endocrinology and Metabolism* 93, no. 7 (2008): 2559–65, doi:10.1210/jc.2007-2404.

49 Jun Yin et al., "Efficacy of Berberine in Patients with Type 2 Diabetes Mellitus," *Metabolism: Clinical and Experimental* 57, no. 5 (2008): 712–17, doi:10.1016/j.metabol.2008.01.013.

50 Jiarong Lan et al., "Meta-Analysis of the Effect and Safety of Berberine in the Treatment of Type 2 Diabetes Mellitus, Hyperlipemia and Hypertension," *Journal of Ethnopharmacology*, 2015, doi:10.1016/j.jep.2014.09.049; Hui Dong et al., "Berberine in the Treatment of Type 2 Diabetes Mellitus: A Systemic Review and Meta-Analysis," *Evidence-Based Complementary and Alternative Medicine: eCAM* 2012 (2012): 591654, doi:10.1155/2012/591654.

51 Uriel Heresco-Levy et al., "A Randomized Add-on Trial of High-Dose D-Cycloserine for Treatment-Resistant Depression," *International Journal of Neuropsychopharmacology / Official Scientific Journal of the Collegium Internationale Neuropsychopharmacologicum (CINP)* 16, no. 3 (2013): 501–6, doi:10.1017/S1461145712000910.

52 Joshua T. Kantrowitz et al., "Single-Dose Ketamine Followed by Daily D-Cycloserine in Treatment-Resistant Bipolar Depression," *Journal of Clinical Psychiatry*, 2015, doi:10.4088/JCP.14l09527.

53 V. G. Joshi, "Isoniazid (INH) in the Treatment of Depressive Syndrome: A Pilot Trial," *Diseases of the Nervous System* 73, no. 2 (1976): 106–11.

54 Ahmad Ghanizadeh et al., "Minocycline as Add-on Treatment Decreases the Negative Symptoms of Schizophrenia; a Randomized Placebo-Controlled Clinical Trial," *Recent Patents on Inflammation & Allergy Drug Discovery* 8, no. 3 (2014): 211–15.

55 Annis O. Mechan et al., "Monoamine Reuptake Inhibition and Mood-Enhancing Potential of a Specified Oregano Extract," *British Journal of Nutrition* 105, no. 8 (2011): 1150–63, doi:10.1017/S0007114510004940.

# CHAPTER 18

# THE LIQUID-ELEMENTAL AND SEMIELEMENTAL DIETS

## A LITTLE LESS TO CHEW ON

I hope the information in the last chapter on antibacterial treatments has made something clear: yes, much of the early research science on microbiota suggests we all need more bacteria (especially when compared to African hunter-gatherers), but when we examine the *clinical science*, we see a different picture emerge. We see that reducing bacterial overgrowths is very important for balancing the ecosystem of your gut—and, more importantly, for alleviating your symptoms. This is likely because once you remove what shouldn't be there, your gut-microbiota ecosystem can rebalance itself—as long as you are providing a healthy environment with proper diet and lifestyle. This reinforces our principle that we can't custom manipulate our microbiota, but we can optimize the environment. OK, on to the liquid-elemental diets.

## SUMMARY OF EVIDENCE— ELEMENTAL DIET

### SUMMARY

The elemental diet is not something that should be done as an initial therapy. However, for those who do not fully respond to the diets we have already discussed and who also do not respond well to things like probiotics or antimicrobial therapy, the elemental diet can be very helpful. Elemental diets have been shown to be highly effective for IBD. Preliminary data also shows elemental diets can improve IBS, SIBO, and rheumatoid arthritis. They may also be helpful for those with celiac disease.

# HYPOALLERGENIC LIQUID DIETS AS A POWERFUL HEALING TOOL

What is an elemental diet? An elemental diet is a liquid diet that can be both antibacterial and anti-inflammatory and is also reparative and hypoallergenic. It's similar to the modified fast we discussed earlier, but there are also some important differences. In elemental diets, the contents are fully digested or broken down into *elements*. For example, when protein is broken down (digested) into its most elemental form, you have amino acids. The carbohydrate contained in an elemental diet is also fully digested and contains essentially no fiber. The low-fiber content, as we have discussed, can be helpful for gut inflammation and SIBO.

The elemental diet is more well balanced than the modified fasts and provides a balance of essential proteins (amino acids), carbohydrates, fats, and vitamins. Because of this, the elemental diet can be used more frequently and for longer periods of time—it can be used exclusively for up to three weeks. As with the modified fast, the elemental diet can help give your intestines a break, and for many people, this break can provide valuable time to heal. For those who have not responded to other therapies, the elemental diet can often be the treatment that makes the difference.

There are a few different versions of the elemental diet available. There is a prescription version: Vivonex Plus. This works well and has been well studied, but the taste is hard for many to get past. There are some commercial versions available that are semielemental or polymeric, which makes them more filling and better tasting, and they still work well. What does "semielemental" or "polymeric" mean? Semielemental means the ingredients are not 100% digested as they are in the elemental version. This mainly has to do

with how digested or broken down the proteins are. Polymeric versions have the least broken down—thus largest—protein molecules, while the elemental version has the most broken down, smallest protein molecules (see illustration below). These differences do not seem to make much of a difference clinically,[1] but the larger molecules in the semielemental or polymeric version do make the formulas better tasting and more filling. If you are getting a little lost in the molecule-size details, don't worry. We will cover simple recommendations for how, when, and what to use as we work through our Great-in-8 plan. Going forward, I will refer to these diets as either elemental or semielemental, because this is what we will use in our Great-in-8.

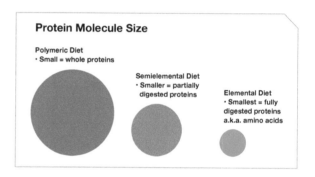

**Protein Molecule Size**

Polymeric Diet
· Small = whole proteins

Semielemental Diet
· Smaller = partially digested proteins

Elemental Diet
· Smallest = fully digested proteins a.k.a. amino acids

Here is a quick recap of key points of the elemental/semielemental diets:

- Both versions are antibacterial.
- Both are low in fiber and prebiotics.
- Both give the intestines a break.
- Both are anti-inflammatory.
- Their molecule size varies and influences taste but not clinical effect.
- Both are hypoallergenic.
- Both are easy to digest.

# THE ELEMENTAL DIET FOR SPECIFIC CONDITIONS

## SIBO, IBS, AND THE ELEMENTAL DIET

A 2004 study examined the effect of the elemental diet (using Vivonex Plus) on ninety-three patients who had SIBO and also had IBS symptoms. After two weeks on the elemental diet, 80% of subjects saw their SIBO breath test normalize, and 65% experienced an improvement in their IBS symptoms.[2]

There is also a large amount of observational data from clinicians using all types of the elemental or semielemental diet for SIBO and IBS. There seems to be general agreement that this is a highly effective treatment option. We do have to be careful here, because observational data is not high quality. However, it's my feeling that this is an area where the clinical science is ahead of the published science. Our office is taking steps to publish another clinical trial using a formula we are developing in the treatment of SIBO and IBS.

## IBD (ULCERATIVE COLITIS & CROHN'S) AND THE ELEMENTAL DIET

The elemental diet is probably the most well researched regarding its effect on intestinal inflammation and autoimmunity as seen in IBD. It has been shown to be an effective treatment in numerous clinical trials.[3] There are several studies showing that in the treatment of IBD, any type of elemental diet (elemental or semielemental) is as effective as anti-inflammatory corticosteroid drugs like prednisone or Cortef.[4] Because this is a nondrug treatment and because the corticosteroid drugs can carry substantial side effects, many researchers and clinicians feel an elemental diet should be used before steroids for IBD.

It has also been shown that using any type of elemental diet can help prevent relapse of IBD,

meaning it doesn't matter if the diet is technically elemental or semielemental.[5] This hints at a way in which we can incorporate elemental diets into your care plan. We can use periodic short courses of an elemental diet to help you maintain your improvements—for any gut condition. Again, we will cover guidelines as we work through our Great-in-8.

There are some studies showing an elemental diet is *not* as effective as steroids.[6] So then, what to do? Remember, this doesn't have to be an either/or situation. It seems reasonable to start with an elemental diet, and if this doesn't bring improvement, then consider steroids, if this is something your doctor has suggested. This brings us to another principle:

> *treatment is not either/or. You don't have to choose between natural medicine and conventional medicine.*

## WEIGHT AND THE ELEMENTAL DIET

To my knowledge, elemental diets have not been studied as a treatment for weight loss, but here is what I have observed clinically: People who are overweight and have gut problems tend to lose weight to the degree that the elemental or semielemental diet heals their gut. People who are underweight and need to gain weight tend to gain weight to the degree that the elemental diet heals their gut. In some underweight patients, there is a small amount of weight loss before weight gain. This can be minimized if you drink ample amounts of the solution. I have also noticed the semielemental versions tend to be better at preventing weight loss (or aiding in weight gain) in those who are underweight, and one clinical trial has shown the same.[7] Remember, if you are underweight, your weight might get a little worse before it gets better. I know this can be hard to hear for those who are underweight—it's a bit of a leap of faith, but you will get there.

### CELIAC DISEASE AND THE ELEMENTAL DIET

An elemental diet has been shown to help repair intestinal damage, reduce intestinal inflammation, and improve symptoms in those with celiac disease who did not respond fully to a gluten-free diet, according to one clinical trial.[8] Perhaps the improvements seen here were because of the anti-inflammatory and intestinally reparative nature of elemental diets. Or perhaps the improvements were due to treating underlying SIBO. One of the common reasons celiac patients do not respond fully to a gluten-free diet is SIBO.

### AUTOIMMUNITY AND THE ELEMENTAL DIET

Rheumatoid arthritis is an autoimmune condition resulting in joint inflammation and pain. A clinical trial has shown that an elemental diet was as effective as the anti-inflammatory steroid drug prednisone.[9] Elemental diets as a treatment for autoimmunity has not been well researched. However, I hope it's clear by this point that your gut has a very strong influence on your immune system, and thus anything you do to improve your gut health might help with an autoimmune condition. This is not a guarantee, but it's certainly worth a shot. My thinking is the degree to which an elemental diet improves your gut health, it may improve an autoimmune condition.

### MOOD, FATIGUE, SLEEP, MENTAL CLARITY, AND THE ELEMENTAL DIET

Again, there is little research looking directly at an elemental diet as a treatment for these problems. Fortunately, these symptoms often improve, sometimes quite dramatically, when you improve the health of your gut.

# HOW DOES THIS LIQUID DIET HELP?

A liquid-only diet can be incredibly reparative, antibacterial, and anti-inflammatory for your gut. In an earlier chapter, we used the analogy of a runner who sprains an ankle—and has to give it a chance to heal. This same concept applies to the gut. If you have a gut "injury" and are eating three times a day, it can be hard for the gut to heal. Using a liquid diet can give your gut a break and aid in healing the same way avoiding activity can help heal an ankle sprain.

I suspect that another reason an elemental diet works so well is because it has an especially favorable impact on the small intestine. Earlier, we discussed how the small intestine houses the majority of your immune system and is most prone to damage (leaky gut). The small intestine is a very important but underappreciated part of your digestive system. There is some published support for my small-intestinal theory.

It has been shown in numerous clinical trials that any type of elemental diet (elemental or semielemental) is highly beneficial for small-intestinal inflammation and autoimmunity, as seen in Crohn's disease. (Note, 80% of Crohn's disease affects the small intestine.) Preliminary research has shown that elemental/semielemental diets can decrease bacteria known to cause intestinal inflammation and can increase diversity of healthy bacteria in the small and large intestine.[10] So, how is it that we saw increased levels of healthy bacteria when using an elemental diet, which starves bacteria? Because the ecosystems of these people required an approach that reduced inflammation. Once the inflammation was reduced, the healthy bacteria could grow!

It has also been shown that fasting increases good bacteria in the gut, specifically Faecalibacterium prausnitzii and Akkermansia.[11]

Maybe this is an additional reason elemental and semielemental diets work so well, because they are liquid-only diets and similar to a fast. Regardless of *how* they are working, if you haven't reached the level of improvement you would like yet, now is the time to implement one of the elemental diets.

## VERSIONS OF THE ELEMENTAL DIET AND HELPFUL TIPS

There are a few versions of the elemental and semielemental diets available:

- Homemade elemental diet—see www.DrRuscio .com/GutBook for a handout on how to make your own at home
- Commercial elemental diet—Physicians Elemental, by Integrative Therapeutics
- Prescription elemental diet—Vivonex Plus, by Nestlé
- Commercial semielemental diet—Elemental Heal, by Functional Medicine Formulations (my preference)

There are also a few other commercial semielemental formulas available, listed below. These are not recommended unless someone has already tried the above versions and has not been able to tolerate them. The following formulas aren't preferred because they may contain undesired ingredients, such as corn, soy, or preservatives. Despite this, these formulas work well for some, so they are worth a try if you do not tolerate the other formulas. The formulas are

- EleCare, by Abbott (my favorite of these three);
- TwoCal HN, by Abbott;
- Peptamen, by Nestlé.

A question that naturally arises is, what version is the best—elemental or semielemental? The full elemental diet has the most digested and, therefore, smallest-sized protein molecules, which makes the molecules easier to absorb but also can make them taste bad. The semielemental proteins are not as fully digested and small, so they may be slightly harder to absorb, but they taste better. Many believe you have to do the full elemental diet to obtain good results. However, this is not what I have seen clinically. In my experience, semielemental diets seem to work just as well as the full elemental diets. My observation has been supported by an impressive number of clinical trials.

There have been two Cochrane systematic reviews that found a semielemental diet works just as well as the full elemental diet.[12] (The Cochrane Database does a good job of ensuring there is no bias in a body of research.) This has been reinforced by clinical trials that compared these diets.[13] It has also been shown that the semielemental diet may be more filling and better for those who are underweight and need to gain weight.[14] This does not mean you will gain weight if you are overweight, but this is good news for those with very impaired absorption who desperately need to gain weight. Remember what we discussed earlier—if you are overweight, the degree to which you heal your gut is the degree to which you can expect weight loss. This is not a guarantee but certainly seems to be true for many.

It has also been shown that the elemental and semielemental diets work equally as well as corticosteroids in treating intestinal inflammation and autoimmunity, as seen in Crohn's disease.[15]

So, if the diets are equally effective, how do you decide which version is right for you? I would recommend you try them in the order listed below. The order below starts with the easiest, cheapest, and best tasting. Once you find a version that is palatable and you react well to, use it. Most will do well with the first formula listed, the Elemental Heal formula, and won't need to try the others. But I will list all the options here just so you have them.

1. Commercial semielemental diet—Elemental Heal, by Functional Medicine Formulations (my preference)
2. Commercial elemental diet—Physicians Elemental (prescription not needed, but only available through a licensed health-care provider)
3. Commercial semielemental diet—EleCare by Abbott
4. Homemade elemental diet—see www.DrRuscio .com/GutBook for instructions; this includes a high-carb and a low-carb version
5. Commercial semielemental formula—TwoCal HN, by Abbott
6. Commercial semielemental formula—Peptamen, by Nestlé
7. Prescription elemental diet—Vivonex Plus, by Nestlé (doctor's prescription required; the taste is hard for many to get past)

## WHAT ABOUT TASTE?

Both the homemade and prescription elemental diets taste bad, really bad. However, there is good news: Elemental Heal is very palatable. This version is my preference because it's the perfect balance of being clean and tasting good. The other commercial semielemental diets (EleCare, Peptamen, and TwoCal HN) taste good but contain some undesirable ingredients. The commercial elemental diet (Physicians Elemental) also tastes good, but you will need a health-care provider to obtain it.

## HOW MUCH?

You can consume as much of the liquid as you desire. If you're feeling hungry, drink some more. It's best to sip on the solution throughout the day, instead of consuming large amounts in short periods. Sipping throughout the day will help keep a steady supply of nutrients and calories in your system, which will help prevent hunger and fatigue (it will also help prevent low blood sugar, if you have this tendency). While you're on the diet, you can engage in normal activity, but you might want to avoid highly rigorous exercise. Be sure to get plenty of rest and to drink water throughout the day.

## HOW LONG?

Elemental diets can be used in one of three general ways in terms of length.

### Short term, as a reset

The elemental or semielemental diet is used exclusively (your only source of calories) for two to four days. This can be very helpful to quell a flare.

### One to three weeks, as exclusive liquid nutrition

For one to three weeks, the liquid shakes you make are your only source of calories. This is done when using the elemental diet as a more formal treatment. As we saw in the research, this approach has been shown to be very helpful; however, this should be done under the supervision of a doctor.

It may sound daunting, but many patients tell me:

- they feel so good that they don't even miss food;
- they were not hungry and had no cravings;
- it was actually very convenient not to have to worry about food and to be able to simply sip on their shakes throughout the day.

### Longer term, with intermittent or hybrid use

Elemental diets can also be used intermittently as a gut-healing tool. The intermittent or hybrid use means that you get some of your calories from an elemental/semielemental formula and the rest of your calories from normal food; it's a combination of normal food plus the elemental diet. This could be a daily use, with half food and and half elemental, or it could be 70% food and 30% elemental or vice versa. If you use the hybrid approach, I recommend you experiment to find a method of incorporation that feels best to you—there is no set rule. For example, many patients like using one of these shakes as a meal replacement for breakfast, every day or most days. Some use the shakes as a meal replacement for breakfast *and* lunch and then eat a nice, big whole-foods dinner. Or some patients will do one full day of exclusive liquid nutrition per week. Others may only use elemental diets on and off, occasionally, when they feel like their guts are in need of a break. They may do anywhere from one to four days until symptoms have subsided—this is more like the reset approach.

## WHICH APPROACH IS BEST FOR YOU?

Again, it's best to use the elemental diet under a doctor's or health-care provider's supervision, but here are some guidelines to discuss with your doctor regarding an intermittent or hybrid use of the elemental diet.

A good way to start is with a two-to-four-day trial. Depending on how well you do with that, you may want to extend it for one to three weeks. How long you perform the diet really depends on the severity of your condition and how quickly you respond. As a general rule

> ## the greater the severity, the longer the duration.

Listen to your body, and when you feel like you have achieved the maximum benefit, then it's a good time to transition to the hybrid approach. The longer you are on the elemental diet, the more important it is to transition to a hybrid approach.

For example, if you performed the elemental diet for two days and felt 90% improved, you could simply transition back to whole foods using the "Transitioning Back to Whole Foods" tips we cover in step 1a of the Great-in-8 plan (part 5). However, if you were on the elemental diet for two weeks, you should transition to the hybrid approach. Again, the hybrid approach is when some of your daily nutrition is from whole foods and some is from the elemental-diet shakes. For example, you could have a shake for breakfast, a shake for lunch, and then have a whole-foods dinner. Over time, you'd gradually decrease the number of shakes while increasing the amount of whole foods you eat in a day.

Elemental/semielemental diets have been used like this in long-term studies. These studies have shown consuming as much as half your calories from a liquid solution can decrease inflammation and autoimmunity in the small intestine and that this is safe. We will cover this information when we discuss safety.

Bear in mind that over time, you should be continually working toward the minimum use of elemental diets. While these diets are designed to be a complete nutritional source and have been shown to be safe when used long-term, it's still best to get as much of your nutrition from whole foods as possible.

## HOW TO MAKE THEM

It's actually very simple. Just follow the instructions on the bottle. The elemental and semielemental formulas come in powder form, and you blend them with ice and water to make a shake. If the label instructs you to, you can add in a source of healthy fat. It's that simple. Mix and drink. There are only two exceptions: the homemade diet and some of the commercial semielemental diets. For the homemade elemental diet—just follow the instructions located at www.DrRuscio.com /GutBook. Some of the commercial semielemental diets come premixed, in a can, similar to other diet shakes. Simply open and drink. You may want to dilute these with some water or even blend with water and ice.

Elemental Heal calls for the addition of fat. If you are highly sensitive, you may want to try it for a day or two without fat and see how you do and then gradually add in fat. Udo's Oil 3·6·9 Blend is a good option that will work well for most. An MCT oil (medium-chain-triglyceride oil) can also work well, especially if you are constipated. MCT oil can have a laxative effect, so be careful with it if you are prone to diarrhea. You can also try coconut oil, olive oil, cod-liver oil, or fish oil. Follow the dosing instructions if listed on the Elemental Heal bottle.

## SAFETY

Whenever a fasting or liquid-fasting intervention hits the mainstream, there always appears to be some credentialed nutritionist who warns against it because of the risk for nutrient deficiencies. There are a few important pieces that are left out of this nutrient-centered way of thinking. Food, and the nutrients contained in it, are only good for you if you have a digestive tract that is working properly. Those with severe intestinal disorders can become very underweight even when eating a normal diet, because they can't absorb the nutrients in their food. An intervention, like liquid fasting, can aid in healing so that you can improve your ability to absorb nutrients from your diet. It's also important to mention that the elemental and semielemental formulas are designed to provide all essential nutrients. Yes, a man-made liquid diet probably won't have the same depth of nutrients that a healthy and diverse whole-foods diet will. But if you can't tolerate a healthy, diverse whole-foods diet, an elemental diet is your best option because it provides nutrients and aids with healing.

What does the science say about safety? The bulk of the research has been done for those with inflammation and autoimmunity of the small intestine, as seen in Crohn's disease. A Cochrane systematic review examined long-term use of elemental diets and found them to improve these patients' health. The patients examined used the elemental/semielemental diet interchangeably with whole foods and obtained anywhere from 30% to 50% of their calories from an elemental diet over a period as long as *three years*.[16] We certainly have support showing elemental diets are safe and can be used long-term when people need to heal their guts.

Until I began the research for this book, I was unaware of the studies showing long-term use of elemental diets were safe, but I had been doing them with some patients for well over a year. It clearly helped patients and appeared very safe. The question I pondered was, if a patient feels sick from eating two to three meals a day but feels fine when eating one liquid meal and two regular meals, do you force the patient to eat three meals because it's what we are told we should do? It was nice to see I was not the only one who came to the conclusion that longer-term hybrid use was justifiable and that the conclusion had been supported by science.

Another RCT looked at this hybrid approach of mixing food with the elemental diet in the long term. Patients with Crohn's disease were divided into two groups. Over a three-year period, one group ate a normal diet. The other group followed a hybrid diet and got half their calories from an elemental diet and half from normal foods. Those on the hybrid diet cut their risk for digestive flares in half! The food-only group had a 64% relapse rate, compared to a 34% relapse rate in the hybrid group. There were no adverse events reported, which illustrates the safety of this approach.[17]

Similar studies have reinforced the finding that this hybrid approach is helpful and safe. One study showed those doing the half-and-half approach had an improved quality of life.[18]

Other studies have even shown that those who consumed more of the elemental-liquid-diet solution did better than those who consumed less, when being tracked over two to four years.[19]

But, again, please remember that to be on the safe side, it's best to have your doctor monitor you when using an elemental diet. I should mention that none of the long-term studies found any lab markers were consistently negatively affected, so lab monitoring may not be needed.[20] Here are the markers your doctor may want to monitor if you are using an elemental diet long-term:

- Your vital signs
  » weight, blood pressure, and pulse rate

- Two simple and cheap blood tests
  » comprehensive metabolic panel
  » complete blood count, with differential

There are a few other tests that are not essential but your doctor might want to consider:

- Iron panel
- Lipids
- Vitamins A, D, E, $B_{12}$
- Serum magnesium, zinc, selenium, copper, manganese

This takes us to the end of our antimicrobial options that remove and reduce infections or overgrowths. In recap, they are

- herbal antimicrobials;
- herbal antimicrobials plus anti-inflammatory, antiprotozoal, and antibiofilm agents;
- liquid-elemental diets.

Later, when we start step 3 of the Great-in-8, we will check in along the way and guide you through exactly what to do and what to use during this step. By step 3 of our action plan, you will have taken enormous steps toward improving your gut health. The process will become easier from there on out. The next step involves ensuring unwanted imbalances do not return after ridding ourselves of them.

## CONCEPT SUMMARY

- A liquid-elemental or semielemental diet can work very well to improve gut health for those who have not responded to other interventions.

- Liquid-elemental and semielemental diets have shown impressive results for IBS, SIBO, and IBD.

- They are very safe but should be used under a doctor's supervision.

1   F. González-Huix et al., "Polymeric Enteral Diets as Primary Treatment of Active Crohn's Disease: A Prospective Steroid Controlled Trial," *Gut* 34, no. 6 (1993): 778–82, doi:10.1136/gut.34.6.778; S. Verma et al., "Polymeric versus Elemental Diet as Primary Treatment in Active Crohn's Disease: A Randomized, Double-Blind Trial," *American Journal of Gastroenterology* 95, no. 3 (2000): 735–39, doi:10.1111/j.1572-0241.2000.01527.x; Osvaldo Borrelli et al., "Polymeric Diet Alone Versus Corticosteroids in the Treatment of Active Pediatric Crohn's Disease: A Randomized Controlled Open-Label Trial," *Clinical Gastroenterology and Hepatology* 4, no. 6 (2006): 744–53, doi:10.1016/j.cgh.2006.03.010.

2   Mark Pimentel et al., "A Fourteen-Day Elemental Diet Is Highly Effective in Normalizing the Lactulose Breath Test," *Digestive Diseases and Sciences* 49, no. 1 (2004): 73–77, doi:10.1023/B:DDAS.0000011605.43979.e1.

3   Alexander Tsertsvadze et al., "Clinical Effectiveness and Cost-Effectiveness of Elemental Nutrition for the Maintenance of Remission in Crohn's Disease: A Systematic Review and Meta-Analysis," *Health Technology Assessment* 19, no. 26 (2015): 1–138, doi:10.3310/hta19260; A. S. Day et al., "Systematic Review: Nutritional Therapy in Paediatric Crohn's Disease," *Alimentary Pharmacology and Therapeutics*, 2008, doi:10.1111/j.1365-2036.2007.03578.x; Robert Heuschkel, "Enteral Nutrition Should Be Used to Induce Remission in Childhood Crohn's Disease," *Digestive Diseases*, 27: 297–305, 2009, doi:10.1159/000228564; S. Verma et al., "Polymeric versus Elemental Diet as Primary Treatment in Active Crohn's Disease: A Randomized, Double-Blind Trial," *American Journal of Gastroenterology* 95, no. 3 (2000): 735–39, doi:10.1111/j.1572-0241.2000.01527.x; N. Hiwatashi, "Enteral Nutrition for Crohn's Disease in Japan," *Diseases of the Colon and Rectum* 40, no. 10 Suppl. (1997): S48–53, www.ncbi.nlm.nih.gov/pubmed/9378012.

4   Nirooshun Rajendran and Devinder Kumar, "Role of Diet in the Management of Inflammatory Bowel Disease," *World Journal of Gastroenterology*, 2010, doi:10.3748/wjg.v16.i12.1442; R. B. Heuschkel et al., "Enteral Nutrition and Corticosteroids in the Treatment of Acute Crohn's Disease in Children," *Journal of Pediatric Gastroenterology and Nutrition* 31, no. 1 (2000): 8–15, www.ncbi.nlm.nih.gov/pubmed/10896064; Osvaldo Borrelli et al., "Polymeric Diet Alone Versus Corticosteroids in the Treatment of Active Pediatric Crohn's Disease: A Randomized Controlled Open-Label Trial," *Clinical Gastroenterology and Hepatology* 4, no. 6 (2006): 744–53, doi:10.1016/j.cgh.2006.03.010; R. Canani Berni et al., "Short- and Long-Term Therapeutic Efficacy of Nutritional Therapy and Corticosteroids in Paediatric Crohn's Disease," *Digestive and Liver Disease* 38, no. 6 (2006): 381–87, doi:10.1016/j.dld.2005.10.005; C. Knight et al., "Long-Term Outcome of Nutritional Therapy in Paediatric Crohn's Disease," *Clinical Nutrition* 24, no. 5 (2005): 775–79, doi:10.1016/j.clnu.2005.03.005.

5   Alexander Tsertsvadze et al., "Clinical Effectiveness and Cost-Effectiveness of Elemental Nutrition for the Maintenance of Remission in Crohn's Disease: A Systematic Review and Meta-Analysis," *Health Technology Assessment* 19, no. 26 (2015): 1–138, doi:10.3310/hta19260; Maki Nakahigashi et al., "Enteral Nutrition for Maintaining Remission in Patients with Quiescent Crohn's Disease: Current Status and Future Perspectives," *International Journal of Colorectal Disease*, 2016, doi:10.1007/s00384-015-2348-x.

6   M. Zachos et al., "Enteral Nutritional Therapy for Induction of Remission in Crohn's Disease," *Cochrane Database of Systematic Reviews*, no. 1 (2007): CD000542, doi:10.1002/14651858.CD000542.pub2; F. Fernández-Banares et al., "How Effective Is Enteral Nutrition in Inducing Clinical Remission in Active Crohn's Disease? A Meta-Analysis of the Randomized Clinical Trials," *Journal of Parenteral and Enteral Nutrition* 19, no. January 1984 (1994): 356–64; M. Zachos et al., "Enteral Nutritional Therapy for Inducing Remission of Crohn's Disease," *Cochrane Database of Systematic Reviews*, no. 3 (2001): CD000542, doi:10.1002/14651858.CD000542.

7   J. F. Ludvigsson et al., "Elemental versus Polymeric Enteral Nutrition in Paediatric Crohn's Disease: A Multicentre Randomized Controlled Trial," *Acta Paediatrica, International Journal of Paediatrics* 93, no. 3 (2004): 327–35, doi:10.1080/08035250310008050.

8   Richard Willfred Olaussen et al., "Effect of Elemental Diet on Mucosal Immunopathology and Clinical Symptoms in Type 1 Refractory Celiac Disease," *Clinical Gastroenterology and Hepatology* 3, no. 9 (2005): 875–85, doi:10.1016/S1542-3565(05)00295-8.

9   T. Podas et al., "Is Rheumatoid Arthritis a Disease That Starts in the Intestine? A Pilot Study Comparing an Elemental Diet with Oral Prednisolone," *Postgraduate Medical Journal* 83, no. 976 (2007): 128–31, doi:10.1136/pgmj.2006.050245.

10  Valeria D'Argenio et al., "An Altered Gut Microbiome Profile in a Child Affected by Crohn's Disease Normalized after Nutritional Therapy," *American Journal of Gastroenterology* 108, no. 5 (May 1, 2013): 851–52, doi:10.1038/ajg.2013.46; Hisashi Shiga et al., "Changes of Faecal Microbiota in Patients with Crohn's Disease Treated with an Elemental Diet and Total Parenteral Nutrition," *Digestive and Liver Disease : Official Journal of the Italian Society of Gastroenterology and the Italian Association for the Study of the Liver* 44, no. 9 (2012): 736–42, doi:10.1016/j.dld.2012.04.014.

11  Marlene Remely et al., "Increased Gut Microbiota Diversity and Abundance of Faecalibacterium Prausnitzii and Akkermansia after Fasting: A Pilot Study," *Wiener Klinische Wochenschrift* 127, no. 9–10 (2015): 394–98, doi:10.1007/s00508-015-0755-1.

12  M. Zachos et al., "Enteral Nutritional Therapy for Induction of Remission in Crohn's Disease," *Cochrane Database of Systematic Reviews*, no. 1 (2007): CD000542, doi:10.1002/14651858.CD000542.pub2.

13  D. Rigaud et al., "Controlled Trial Comparing Two Types of Enteral Nutrition in Treatment of Active Crohn's Disease: Elemental versus Polymeric Diet," *Gut* 32, no. 12 (1991): 1492–97, doi:10.1136/gut.32.12.1492l; S. Verma et al., "Polymeric versus Elemental Diet as Primary Treatment in Active Crohn's Disease: A Randomized, Double-Blind Trial," *American Journal of Gastroenterology* 95, no. 3 (2000): 735–39, doi:10.1111/j.1572-0241.2000.01527.x; M. Okada et al., "Controlled Trial Comparing an Elemental Diet with Prednisolone in the Treatment of Active Crohn's Disease," *Hepato-Gastroenterology* 37, no. 1 (1990): 72–80.

14  J. F. Ludvigsson et al., "Elemental versus Polymeric Enteral Nutrition in Paediatric Crohn's Disease: A Multicentre Randomized Controlled Trial," *Acta Paediatrica, International Journal of Paediatrics* 93, no. 3 (2004): 327–35, doi:10.1080/08035250310008050.

15   Osvaldo Borrelli et al., "Polymeric Diet Alone Versus Corticosteroids in the Treatment of Active Pediatric Crohn's Disease: A Randomized Controlled Open-Label Trial," *Clinical Gastroenterology and Hepatology* 4, no. 6 (2006): 744–53, doi:10.1016/j.cgh.2006.03.010; R. B. Heuschkel et al., "Enteral Nutrition and Corticosteroids in the Treatment of Acute Crohn's Disease in Children," *Journal of Pediatric Gastroenterology and Nutrition* 31, no. 1 (2000): 8–15, www.ncbi.nlm.nih.gov/pubmed/10896064; F. González-Huix et al., "Polymeric Enteral Diets as Primary Treatment of Active Crohn's Disease: A Prospective Steroid Controlled Trial," *Gut* 34, no. 6 (1993): 778–82, doi:10.1136/gut.34.6.778.

16   A. K. Akobeng and A. G. Thomas, "Enteral Nutrition for Maintenance of Remission in Crohn's Disease," *Cochrane Database of Systematic Reviews (Online)*, 2007, doi:10.1002/14651858.CD005984.pub2.

17   S. Takagi et al., "Effectiveness of an 'Half Elemental Diet' as Maintenance Therapy for Crohn's Disease: A Randomized-Controlled Trial," *Alimentary Pharmacology and Therapeutics* 24, no. 9 (2006): 1333–40, doi:10.1111/j.1365-2036.2006.03120.x.

18   S. Takagi et al., "Quality of Life of Patients and Medical Cost of 'Half Elemental Diet' as Maintenance Therapy for Crohn's Disease: Secondary Outcomes of a Randomised Controlled Trial," *Digestive and Liver Disease: Official Journal of the Italian Society of Gastroenterology and the Italian Association for the Study of the Liver* 41, no. 6 (2009): 390–94, doi:10.1016/j.dld.2008.09.007.

19   H. Koga et al., "[Long-Term Efficacy of Low Residue Diet for the Maintenance of Remission in Patients with Crohn's Disease]," *Nihon Shokakibyo Gakkai Zasshi* 90, no. 11 (1993): 2882–88; H. Hirakawa et al., "Home Elemental Enteral Hyperalimentation (HEEH) for the Maintenance of Remission in Patients with Crohn's Disease," *Gastroenterologia Japonica* 28, no. 3 (1993): 379–84.

20   S. Verma et al., "Does Adjuvant Nutritional Support Diminish Steroid Dependency in Crohn Disease?," *Scandinavian Journal of Gastroenterology* 36, no. 4 (2001): 383–88; Akira Andoh et al., "Serum Selenoprotein-P Levels in Patients with Inflammatory Bowel Disease," *Nutrition* 21, no. 5 (2005): 574–79, doi:10.1016/j.nut.2004.08.025; Anthony Goode et al., "Use of an Elemental Diet for Long-Term Nutritional Support in Crohn's Disease," *Lancet* 307, no. 7951 (1976): 122–24, doi:10.1016/S0140-6736(76)93159-7; Cassie Jo Davis et al., "The Use of Prealbumin and C-Reactive Protein for Monitoring Nutrition Support in Adult Patients Receiving Enteral Nutrition in an Urban Medical Center," *Journal of Parenteral and Enteral Nutrition* 36, no. 2 (2012): 197–204, doi:10.1177/0148607111413896; K. Nikaki and G. L. Gupte, "Assessment of Intestinal Malabsorption," *Best Practice and Research: Clinical Gastroenterology* 30, no. 2 (2016): 225–35, doi:10.1016/j.bpg.2016.03.003.

# CHAPTER 19

# PROKINETICS AND INTESTINAL MOTILITY— PREVENTING IMBALANCES FROM RETURNING

## KEEPING THINGS MOVING

To help ensure your gut ecosystem returns to and maintains an optimum balance after the nudge we provide in the antimicrobial phase, we next add a prokinetic. What is a prokinetic? Prokinetics are agents that support healthy motility in your stomach and intestines. Motility just means that food moves through your intestinal tract at the right pace. When food moves through at the appropriate pace, it keeps your intestinal ecosystem (mostly fungi and bacteria) in balance. However, if food is moving too slowly, it can cause bacteria and fungi to overgrow. The flowing water of a river or stream doesn't foster bacterial growth. Stagnant pond water does. We want to prevent small-intestinal bacterial (or fungal) overgrowth by ensuring things are flowing through your intestinal tract and are not stagnant.

If you have a history of diarrhea, doesn't that mean things are moving too fast and you don't need a prokinetic? No. If you have diarrhea, you may still benefit from a prokinetic. Certain types of bacterial overgrowth can cause diarrhea, and a prokinetic will prevent this type of bacterial overgrowth from coming back after we've cleaned it out with the antimicrobials in step 3. Prokinetics are not the same as laxatives (magnesium and vitamin C, for example).

Is there any scientific documentation that prokinetics prevent bacterial overgrowths from returning after they've been cleaned out with antimicrobials? Yes. One study found two different prokinetic medications slowed or prevented the return of bacterial overgrowth.[1] The medications are low-dose erythromycin and tegaserod. Erythromycin is an antibiotic, but when used in very low doses, it appears not to function as an antibiotic but rather as a prokinetic. The other prokinetic medication, tegaserod, is no longer available in the United States due to potential cardiovascular side effects. The graph from this study shows the length of time participants were in remission from SIBO after receiving antimicrobial therapy. As you can see, the low-dose erythromycin led to roughly 140 days SIBO-free, while tegaserod led to roughly 220 days SIBO-free. Those who did nothing were SIBO-free for roughly 60 days.

There are a few natural prokinetics. Iberogast is a compound that has been well studied. Iberogast

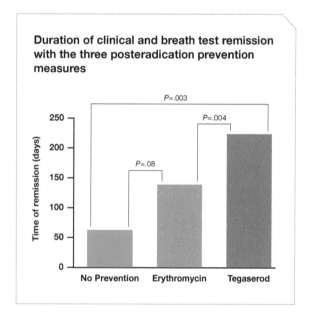

**Duration of clinical and breath test remission with the three posteradication prevention measures**

has been shown to be equivalent to the medication cisapride in treating certain types of motility impairment.[2] One meta-analysis,[3] one systematic review,[4] and numerous other clinical trials have shown Iberogast to be helpful for motility-related conditions.[5] So, there is some great research on Iberogast and its prokinetic function that strongly suggests it can help prevent bacterial overgrowths from returning. However, we don't know this for sure. A study *specifically* examining if Iberogast prevents bacterial overgrowth from returning has not yet been performed. Unfortunately, at the time

of writing, Iberogast is no longer available in the United States. I hope this will change soon.

MotilPro is another natural compound that functions as a prokinetic. This compound doesn't have the same wealth of clinical research that Iberogast has, but there is data supporting the theory that its ingredients function as a prokinetic.[6]

Diet might even be a prokinetic. Many prokinetics work by boosting serotonin levels in the gut. It has been shown that a low-FODMAP diet can actually increase the number of serotonin cells in your gut. In these studies, those with IBS experienced an increase in the number of serotonin cells in their guts, thus making them more similar to healthy controls.[7]

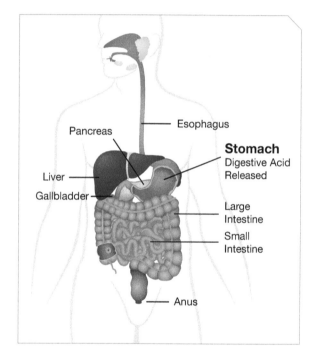

## HOW YOU CAN RESTORE HEALTHY INTESTINAL MOTILITY

You may have heard that impaired motility can be an autoimmune process. If you haven't heard this before, the short story is that some people may form autoimmunity in their intestines against the intestinal cells that regulate motility.[8] When this happens, their intestinal motility becomes damaged, and bacterial overgrowth can occur. This autoimmunity can form after a bout of food poisoning, stomach flu, or traveler's diarrhea. In other words, if someone has food poisoning, stomach flu, or traveler's diarrhea, this can start an autoimmune attack against the cells in the intestines that regulate motility. This altered (slowed) motility can then allow bacterial overgrowth to occur.

What is often left out in the telling of this scenario is that this damage can be repaired! I have seen several patients who went on the Internet and read that "SIBO is caused by autoimmunity and is extremely difficult to recover from." When patients who've read this receive the SIBO diagnosis, they think their lives are ruined. This could not be further from the truth. Yes, there are challenging and severe cases of any condition, but be cautious about what you read on the Internet. Every day, the Great-in-8 allows people to beat SIBO and never look back. But here is the thing—these people are not hanging out in online chat groups venting about their SIBO—they're out there enjoying their lives.

I think that many of the horror stories you read on the Internet are from the small percentage of people who have severe SIBO or, more likely, from people who are not working with a well-trained doctor but rather self-diagnosing and -treating or from those who are just starting with their treatment and have not yet seen improvements but need someplace to vent. In any case, you often get a very negative view from the Internet that is not representative of the experience most people will have. So, be very cautious about information you get from Internet sources. Take the useful information; leave the fear mongering and pessimism.

We covered how motility problems can be caused by autoimmune damage. Specifically, the autoimmune damage occurs to cells in your intestines known as the ICC or interstitial cells of Cajal. Why am I torturing you with these details? Because when we understand these ICC, we see that there is much hope for the ability to recover healthy intestinal motility.

Experiments in animals have shown that

> ## the ICC can regenerate—the cells that regulate intestinal motility can repair themselves!

This regeneration has been observed to occur after surgical damage[9] and, in another study, after drug/chemical damage.[10] Why are we citing animal data? Isn't this low-level science? Yes, you are correct! However, it would be unethical for us to intentionally inflict damage on these cells in humans and then study their response. We have already covered the clinical data regarding the use of prokinetics to restore motility in humans, which shows clinical benefit, so we have our bases covered here. This animal data just helps us better understand how and why prokinetics work and how your motility can be repaired.

In addition to being able to repair/regenerate, the ICC can also restore motility through what's known as plasticity. This means the electrical system in your gut can rewire itself to avoid damaged wires and focus on healthy wires in order to maintain normal function.[11] This frequently observed reparative ability of your ICC has led some researchers to conclude "ICC display a rather robust degree of plasticity or ability to regenerate."[12]

But what does this look like in the real world? Are people who have developed this autoimmunity able to recover normal function? Yes! Clinical studies have shown that if you have an autoimmune attack that damages your motility, it's likely you will recover motility with time, usually within six months to two years.[13] That's why *most* people who get food poisoning, stomach flu, or traveler's diarrhea return to normal with a little time. This is probably because the ICC are continuously recycled, which means that even if these cells are damaged, in a number of months they will be replaced with fresh, new cells. Think of them like your skin cells, which are constantly replacing themselves.[14]

We previously discussed the concept of creating a healthy internal environment. It has been shown that environment can either aid in or hinder the ability of your ICC to repair. If you can reduce inflammation and balance blood sugar, you can create an environment that helps these cells repair optimally.[15]

ICC are located throughout your entire gastrointestinal tract, from esophagus to rectum. If you have trouble swallowing or gallbladder problems or constipation, there is a chance that by going through our steps, which help repair the ICC, you will see these issues improve as well.[16]

We covered how reducing inflammation and controlling blood sugar, both of which we address in our Great-in-8, can help repair ICC. What else can we do to help repair our ICC? Use prokinetics. Prokinetics create an environment that encourages ICC regeneration. This happens because prokinetics essentially help boost serotonin in the gut and serotonin stimulates ICC regeneration.[17] Serotonin is a neurotransmitter—a molecule that helps nerve cells communicate with one another. Prokinetics help prevent the return of bacterial overgrowth by helping to repair the ICC.

The highest density of these ICC is found in the ileocecal valve region.[18] The ileocecal valve separates the small intestine from the large intestine. In this diagram, you can see the last section of the small intestine, the ileum, flows into the colon (large intestine). This is where the ileocecal valve is located. This valve helps prevent bacteria from the colon from sneaking backward into the small intestine, which can cause bacterial overgrowth. Because of this, it's thought the ileocecal valve must be functioning properly to prevent bacterial

overgrowths, like SIBO, from coming back after treatment.[19] If you can repair the ICC and restore your motility, you should restore function to this valve.

Is motility all about bacteria and preventing bacterial overgrowth? No, bacteria are just what we understand the best. These same motility problems may cause fungal overgrowths, even SIFO.[20]

Once we have gotten rid of overgrowths and unwanted bacteria, it can sometimes be helpful to support the growth of good bacteria. We want to first rebalance your microbiota, and *then* support growth so that we're supporting balanced growth. We don't support growth first because if imbalances are present, we might be supporting *imbalanced* growth. This is also why in our Great-in-8, we *remove* in step 3 before we *feed* in step 6.

## THE GREAT-IN-8 ACTION PLAN

1. Reset—reset your diet and lifestyle
2. Support—support your gut with probiotics and digestive enzymes/acid
3. Remove—remove/reduce unwanted gut bacteria with antimicrobial herbs
4. Rebalance—rebalance gut bacteria after treatment with antimicrobial herbs
5. Reintroduce—reintroduce foods you removed in step 3
6. Feed—feed the good bacteria
7. Wean—wean yourself off the supplements in your plan
8. Maintenance and fun—maintain your improvements, and enjoy your newfound health

# CONCEPT SUMMARY

- Prokinetics are agents that help ensure you have optimal intestinal motility, meaning the ability to move food through your intestinal tract.

- After using antimicrobials, it is helpful to use prokinetics to prevent imbalances from returning.

- It is possible to regain and improve motility. In time, your body can repair itself.

1   Mark Pimentel et al., "Low-Dose Nocturnal Tegaserod or Erythromycin Delays Symptom Recurrence after Treatment of Irritable Bowel Syndrome Based on Presumed Bacterial Overgrowth," *Gastroenterology and Hepatology* 5, no. 6 (2009): 435–42.

2   W. Rösch et al., "A Randomised Clinical Trial Comparing the Efficacy of a Herbal Preparation STW 5 with the Prokinetic Drug Cisapride in Patients with Dysmotility Type of Functional Dyspepsia," *Zeitschrift Fur Gastroenterologie* 40, no. 6 (2002): 401–8, doi:10.1055/s-2002-32130.

3   J. Melzer et al., "Meta-Analysis: Phytotherapy of Functional Dyspepsia with the Herbal Drug Preparation STW 5 (Iberogast)," *Alimentary Pharmacology and Therapeutics* 20, no. 11–12 (2004): 1279–87, doi:10.1111/j.1365-2036.2004.02275.x.

4   J. Melzer et al., "Iberis Amara L. and Iberogast—Results of a Systematic Review Concerning Functional Dyspepsia," *Journal of Herbal Pharmacotherapy* 4, no. 4 (2004): 51–59, doi:10.1300/J157v04n04_05.

5   Ulrike von Arnim et al., "STW 5, a Phytopharmacon for Patients with Functional Dyspepsia: Results of a Multicenter, Placebo-Controlled Double-Blind Study," *American Journal of Gastroenterology* 102, no. 6 (2007): 1268–75, doi:10.1111/j.1572-0241.2006 .01183.x; A. Madisch et al., "A Plant Extract and Its Modified Preparation in Functional Dyspepsia. Results of a Double-Blind Placebo Controlled Comparative Study," [In German.] *Zeitschrift Fur Gastroenterologie* 39, no. 7 (2001): 511–17, doi:10.1055/s-2001-16142; R. Saller et al., "Iberogast(r): Eine Moderne Phytotherapeutische Arzneimittelkombination Zur Behandlung Funktioneller Erkrankungen Des Magen-Darm-Trakts (Dyspepsie, Colon Irritabile)—von Der Pflanzenheilkunde Zur «Evidence Based Phytotherapy».Eine Systematische Übersicht," *Forschende Komplementärmedizin / Research in Complementary Medicine* 9, no. 1 (November 17, 2004): 1–20, doi:10.1159/000068645; B. Braden et al., "Clinical Effects of STW 5 (Iberogast) Are Not Based on Acceleration of Gastric Emptying in Patients with Functional Dyspepsia and Gastroparesis," *Neurogastroenterology and Motility* 21, no. 6 (2009), doi:10.1111/j.1365-2982.2008.01249.x; Amelia N. Pilichiewicz et al., "Effects of Iberogast® on Proximal Gastric Volume, Antropyloroduodenal Motility and Gastric Emptying in Healthy Men," *American Journal of Gastroenterology* 102, no. 6 (2007): 1276–83, doi:10.1111/j.1572-0241.2007.01142.x.

6   Keng-Liang Wu et al., "Effects of Ginger on Gastric Emptying and Motility in Healthy Humans," *European Journal of Gastroenterology & Hepatology* 20, no. 5 (2008): 436–40, doi:10.1097/MEG.0b013e3282f4b224; Ming Luen Hu et al., "Effect of Ginger on Gastric Motility and Symptoms of Functional Dyspepsia," *World Journal of Gastroenterology* 17, no. 1 (2011): 105–10, doi:10.3748/wjg.v17 .i1.105; Edith Bülbring and A. Crema, "The Action of 5-Hydroxytryptamine, 5-Hydroxytryptophan and Reserpine on Intestinal Peristalsis in Anaesthetized Guinea-Pigs," *Journal of Physiology* 146, no. 1 (April 23, 1959): 29–53, doi:10.1113/jphysiol.1959.sp006176; Edith Bülbring and R .C. Lin, "The Effect of Intraluminal Application of 5-Hydroxytryptamine and 5-Hydroxytryptophan on Peristalsis; the Local Production of 5-HT and Its Release in Relation to Intraluminal Pressure and Propulsive Activity," *Journal of Physiology* 140, no. 3 (1958): 381–407, doi:10.1113/jphysiol.1958.sp005940; Edith Bülbring and A. Crema, "Observations Concerning the Action of 5-Hydroxytryptamine on the Peristaltic Reflex," *British Journal of Pharmacology and Chemotherapy* 13, no. 4 (1958): 444–57, www.pubmedcentral.nih.gov/articlerender.fcgi?artid=1481872&tool=pmcentrez&rendertype=abstract; Edith Bülbring et al., "An Investigation of the Peristaltic Reflex in Relation to Anatomical Observations," *Quarterly Journal of Experimental Physiology and Cognate Medical Sciences* 43, no. 1 (January 22, 1958): 26–37, doi:10.1113/expphysiol.1958.sp001305; Edith Bülbring and A. Crema, "The Release of 5-Hydroxytryptamine in Relation to Pressure Exerted on the Intestinal Mucosa," *Journal of Physiology* 146, no. 1 (April 23, 1959): 18–28, doi:10.1113/jphysiol.1959.sp006175.

7   T. Mazzawi et al., "Dietary Guidance Normalizes Large Intestinal Endocrine Cell Densities in Patients with Irritable Bowel Syndrome," *European Journal of Clinical Nutrition* 70, no. 2 (2016): 175–81, doi:10.1038/ejcn.2015.191; Benedikt Weber et al., "25-Hydroxyvitamin-D3 Serum Modulation after Use of Sunbeds Compliant with European Union Standards: A Randomized Open Observational Controlled Trial," *Journal of the American Academy of Dermatology* 77, no. 1 (2017): 48–54, doi:10.1016 /j.jaad.2017.02.029.

8   Mark Pimentel et al., "Development and Validation of a Biomarker for Diarrhea-Predominant Irritable Bowel Syndrome in Human Subjects," *PLoS ONE* 10, no. 5 (2015), doi:10.1371/journal.pone.0126438.

9   Feng Mei et al., "Interstitial Cells of Cajal Could Regenerate and Restore Their Normal Distribution after Disrupted by Intestinal Transection and Anastomosis in the Adult Guinea Pigs," *Virchows Archiv* 449, no. 3 (2006): 348–57, doi:10.1007/s00428-006-0258-6.

10  Feng Mei et al., "Plasticity of Interstitial Cells of Cajal: A Study in the Small Intestine of Adult Guinea Pigs," *Anatomical Record (Hoboken, N.J. : 2007)* 292, no. 7 (2009): 985–93, doi:10.1002/ar.20928.

11  Sabine Klein et al., "Interstitial Cells of Cajal Plasticity rather than Regeneration Restores Slow-Wave Activity and Enteric Neurotransmission upon Acute Damage," *BMC Pharmacology & Toxicology* 14, no. Suppl. 1 (2013): P34, doi:10.1186/2050-6511-14-S1-P34.

12  K. M. Sanders, "Interstitial Cells of Cajal at the Clinical and Scientific Interface," *Journal of Physiology* 576, no. Pt. 3 (2006): 683–87, doi:10.1113/jphysiol.2006.116814.

13  Luther Sigurdsson et al., "Postviral Gastroparesis: Presentation, Treatment, and Outcome," *Journal of Pediatrics* 131, no. 5 (1997): 751–54, doi:10.1016/S0022-3476(97)70106-9.

14  Jan D. Huizinga et al., "Physiology, Injury, and Recovery of Interstitial Cells of Cajal: Basic and Clinical Science," *Gastroenterology* 137, no. 5 (2009): 1548–56, doi:10.1053/j.gastro.2009.09.023.

15  Satya Vati Rana et al., "Relationship of Cytokines, Oxidative Stress and GI Motility with Bacterial Overgrowth in Ulcerative Colitis Patients," *Journal of Crohn's and Colitis* 8, no. 8 (2014): 859–65, doi:10.1016/j.crohns.2014.01.007; Feng Mei et al., "Interstitial Cells of Cajal Could Regenerate and Restore Their Normal Distribution after Disrupted by Intestinal Transection and Anastomosis in the Adult Guinea Pigs," *Virchows Archiv* 449, no. 3 (2006): 348–57, doi:10.1007/s00428-006-0258-6.

16  Othman A. Al-Shboul, "The Importance of Interstitial Cells of Cajal in the Gastrointestinal Tract," *Saudi Journal of Gastroenterology: Official Journal of the Saudi Gastroenterology Association* 19, no. 1 (2013): 3–15, doi:10.4103/1319-3767.105909.

17  Jan D. Huizinga et al., "Physiology, Injury, and Recovery of Interstitial Cells of Cajal: Basic and Clinical Science," *Gastroenterology* 137, no. 5 (2009): 1548–56, doi:10.1053/j.gastro.2009.09.023.

18  Othman A. Al-Shboul, "The Importance of Interstitial Cells of Cajal in the Gastrointestinal Tract," *Saudi Journal of Gastroenterology: Official Journal of the Saudi Gastroenterology Association* 19, no. 1 (2013): 3–15, doi:10.4103/1319-3767.105909.

19  Bani Chander Roland et al., "Low Ileocecal Valve Pressure Is Significantly Associated with Small Intestinal Bacterial Overgrowth (SIBO)," *Digestive Diseases and Sciences* 59, no. 6 (2014): 1269–77, doi:10.1007/s10620-014-3166-7.

20  Askin Erdogan and Satish S. C. Rao, "Small Intestinal Fungal Overgrowth," *Current Gastroenterology Reports*, 2015, doi:10.1007/s11894-015-0436-2.

# CHAPTER 20

# FIBER SUPPLEMENTS

## PROS AND CONS OF FIBER SUPPLEMENTS

We already discussed *dietary* fiber, but let's specifically cover fiber *supplements*. This is an important discussion for a few reasons:

- Fiber can help some but make others feel worse, so we want to make sure we use fiber correctly.
- Because fiber feeds gut bacteria and there is much interest in gut bacteria at the moment, you're sure to hear exaggerated claims regarding fiber. We want to make sure you have an accurate and factual understanding of the benefits of fiber supplements so you don't fall victim to marketing hype.

See step 6 of the Great-in-8 for ideal timing and approach for using supplemental fiber.

- **Digestive-tract cancers**—Unfortunately, the overall impact of supplemental fiber, including resistant starch, on colorectal-cancer risk appears to be minimal at best. Most of the data show no positive impact.
- **IBD**—RCTs have shown fiber to be helpful for IBD, but fiber is likely best used when IBD is in remission. Low-fiber diets have been shown to be helpful for active IBD. For dosing and types, see step 6 of the Great-in-8.
- **IBS**—Fiber has been shown to help IBS symptoms, including stool frequency and consistency, and quality of life. However high-fiber intake can be problematic for some IBS and correspondingly low-fiber diets have also been shown to be helpful in IBS. If IBS is being caused by SIBO, you should avoid fiber until the SIBO is under control. Fiber has the most benefit for those with constipation. For dosing and types see Step 6.
- **Celiac disease**—There is no quality data available for supplemental fiber's impact on celiac disease.

- **Diabetes**—High-level science shows supplemental fiber can help lower fasting blood glucose by about thirty-five points and hemoglobin A1c by about 1% in patients with type 2 diabetes. The healthier your blood sugar already is, the less effect supplemental fiber has.
- **Heart health**—Supplemental fiber may cause a small decrease in blood pressure and cholesterol levels. However, there does not appear to be a clear benefit on heart disease from fiber supplementation.
- **Obesity and weight loss**—A review paper has shown the average weight loss from fiber supplementation to be 4.2 pounds. Viscous fibers (gel forming) might be best for weight loss but also may carry the highest risk of digestive side effects.

As we've done before, we will again take a dive into the pool of research on fiber, this time on *supplemental* fiber. We'll discuss the research that actually matters to you, the research that asks questions like

- what happens when someone like you supplements with fiber;
- if you supplement with fiber, can you affect your chances of getting certain diseases like colon cancer or heart disease?

We will cover supplemental fiber's impact on

- digestive-tract cancer;
- IBD;
- IBS;
- celiac disease;
- diabetes;
- heart disease;
- obesity and weight loss.

We'll work through each condition that might be affected by supplemental fiber. I will summarize the data that shows supplemental fiber is helpful for a condition, summarize the data showing supplemental fiber is *not* helpful for that condition, and provide a summary of supplemental fiber's impact on that condition.

There are a few conditions where there is so little data that only a conclusion is needed. If you don't care to cover the details, you could skim this section, reading only the conclusion paragraph for each topic.

## DIGESTIVE-TRACT CANCERS

*Digestive-tract cancers—supplemental fiber helpful*
A clinical trial examined if supplementing the diet with different forms of resistant starch (resistant starch is a type of fiber/prebiotic contained in many foods that has been of interest in both the research community and on certain nutritional websites) influenced risk factors for colorectal cancer. Although some positive effects were shown, the researchers concluded the overall effect was "limited."[1] Another study supplementing with resistant starch found similar results: a minor positive impact but most of the markers that were tracked remained unchanged.[2]

*Digestive-tract cancers—supplemental fiber no effect*
One systematic review of clinical trials on fiber supplements to prevent colorectal-cancer recurrence found

- no effect from folic acid supplementation (based upon four clinical trials);
- not enough data to conclude if there is an effect from antioxidants, green tea extract, prebiotic fiber, or insoluble fiber.[3]

One clinical trial showed no benefit from supplemental fiber, and one showed potential benefit.[4]

In a systematic review of nine clinical trials, eight of the studies did not find supplementation with prebiotics reduced colorectal-cancer risk.[5] Interestingly, six of these studies were with resistant starch, and none of these six were found to reduce cancer risk. This is likely because the effect of resistant starch on colorectal-cancer risk markers was found to be limited, as we discussed earlier.

### Digestive-tract cancers and supplemental fiber conclusion

Unfortunately, the overall impact of supplemental fiber, including resistant starch, on colorectal-cancer risk appears to be minimal at best. Most of the data show no positive impact.

## IBD

### IBD and supplemental fiber conclusion

A systematic review of twenty-three randomized control trials examined if supplemental fiber improves ulcerative colitis or Crohn's disease. Of the twenty-three studies, only four showed supplemental fiber was beneficial.[6] What this means is supplemental fiber might be helpful, but it's not very likely. The best time to experiment to determine whether it's helpful for you is when you're in remission, which is why we have waited to add in fiber until step 6.

## IBS

### IBS—supplemental fiber helpful

Fiber has been shown to help IBS symptoms, including stool frequency and consistency, and quality of life.[7]

Fiber supplementation has been shown most helpful for constipation. Fiber supplementation may also help general IBS symptoms, but the symptoms of pain and bloating appear to benefit the least. Soluble fiber works better and causes fewer reactions than insoluble fiber. (Soluble fiber dissolves in water; insoluble does not. Don't fret over this detail right now; we'll help you find the best fiber type in our protocol recommendations.) But the studies have also found there is a chance that fiber supplementation could make IBS worse.[8]

One study of 275 IBS patients compared 10 g soluble fiber (psyllium) to 10 g insoluble fiber (bran) for twelve weeks.[9] The soluble psyllium was more effective. If patients were able to stay on the fiber for three months, symptoms could be reduced by 50% by the bran and up to 90% by the psyllium. However, the chance of a negative reaction causing patients to stop was about 40%. Fiber supplementation appears to be a double-edged sword.

### IBS—supplemental fiber no effect

A systematic review by the Cochrane Database found no benefit of fiber supplementation for IBS.[10] This was regardless of fiber type—soluble or insoluble. These results were reinforced by another review paper that examined the results of 121 trials.[11] Another systematic review of twelve studies found fiber supplementation, specifically psyllium, may or may not be helpful for IBS.[12]

So, some studies show supplemental fiber helps, while others do not. Part of this inconsistency may be due to the quality of the studies. When a meta-analysis of double-blinded clinical trials was performed and poor-quality studies were thrown out, fiber did not show any benefit for IBS over placebos.[13]

A higher-fiber intake can be problematic for some with IBS and may need to be avoided. Low-fiber diets have also been shown to be helpful in IBS.[14]

### IBS and supplemental fiber conclusion

In conclusion, fiber supplementation is worth trying. You may experience benefit from it, and if you do, great, continue with it. However, you may also have a negative reaction; if you do, discontinue. If you notice no change, you may want to use fiber for some of its other potential health benefits, but it's not required.

If your IBS is being caused by SIBO, then you may want to avoid fiber until the SIBO is under control. We will address how and when to incorporate fiber in more detail in step 6. For now, just know it's best to start with a healthy diet, as we have discussed already, and not worry about the fiber content. Do not use any supplemental fiber until step 6.

## CELIAC DISEASE AND FIBER

To my knowledge, there are no clinical trials on fiber supplementation in celiac disease.

## DIABETES

### Diabetes and supplemental fiber conclusion

High-level science shows supplemental fiber can help lower fasting blood glucose by about thirty-five points and hemoglobin A1c by about 1% in patients with type 2 diabetes. The healthier your blood sugar already is, the less effect supplemental fiber has.[15] I consider these results to be clinically meaningful.

## HEART HEALTH

### Heart health—supplemental fiber helpful

A meta-analysis of clinical trials showed flaxseed may cause a small reduction in blood pressure, roughly a 1.5- to 2-point reduction.[16] Soluble fiber (oat beta-glucan at three grams or more per day) may yield an eleven-point reduction in total cholesterol and a nine-point reduction in LDL cholesterol—which I do not consider meaningful. The effect appears to be stronger in those with diabetes.[17]

One systematic review summarized the data from four clinical trials using the highly viscous

fiber glucomannan (konjac).[18] There was a significant reduction in cholesterol levels; however, adverse reactions of bloating and diarrhea were reported.

### Heart health—supplemental fiber no effect

Many other studies have shown supplemental fiber to have no impact on cholesterol levels or heart-disease risk.[19]

### Heart health and supplemental fiber conclusion

Supplemental fiber may cause a small decrease in blood pressure and cholesterol levels. However, there does not appear to be a clear benefit on heart disease from fiber supplementation.

## WEIGHT LOSS AND OBESITY

### Weight loss and obesity—supplemental fiber helpful

As we mentioned earlier, one review showed supplemental fiber's average weight-loss effect was 4.2 lb.,[20] and this is a reasonable expectation. When selecting a fiber for weight loss, it appears viscous fibers may be more effective, according to a review of clinical trials.[21]

### Weight loss and obesity—supplemental fiber not helpful

A systematic review of six clinical trials examined the effect of supplemental glucomannan fiber on weight loss.[22] Unfortunately, no effect from the fiber was seen, and the placebo may have actually been more effective.

A meta-analysis of nine trials using glucomannan-fiber supplementation in overweight and obese subjects did not find any benefit of glucomannan supplementation for weight loss.[23] Subjects did report adverse events of abdominal discomfort, diarrhea, and constipation. We discussed earlier that the best weight-loss results using fiber for weight loss occurred with glucomannan fiber. This is true. However, as we have been discussing throughout this book, one study can show unusually good or bad results. One study did show promise for using fiber supplementation for weight loss, but the majority of the research has shown no weight loss and even adverse abdominal side effects.[24]

You may have heard that fiber fills you up and makes you less hungry, and you, therefore, eat less. A systematic review of forty-four studies found that most fibers do not lead to a feeling of fullness that causes a decreased intake of calories.[25]

Supplemental fiber has shown varying levels of benefit with metabolic syndrome, blood sugar levels, and body weight. At worst, no results are seen; at best, marginal results are seen.[26]

### *Weight loss and obesity and supplemental fiber conclusion*

Overall, supplemental fiber does not appear effective for weight loss. There is a small probability that you may lose a small amount of weight (a few pounds) from supplemental fiber. There is a higher likelihood that you will not lose any weight but may experience negative digestive side effects from weight-loss fibers like glucomannan.

# SUPPLEMENTAL FIBER CONCLUSION

As with dietary fiber, when we take a look at both sides of the evidence, it's clear to see supplemental fiber can be a double-edged sword. It may help some, and it may harm others.

Unfortunately for digestive-tract cancers, the overall impact of supplemental fiber, including resistant starch, appear to be minimal at best. Most of the data show no positive impact. Supplemental fiber may help or harm IBS and IBD. It is best used when in remission. It may have a slight benefit for diabetes.

Supplemental fiber may cause a *small* decrease in blood pressure and cholesterol levels. However, there does not appear to be a clear benefit for heart disease from fiber supplementation. Overall, supplemental fiber does not appear effective for weight loss. There is a minor probability that you may lose a small amount of weight (a few pounds) from supplemental fiber. There is a higher likelihood that you will not lose any weight but will experience negative digestive side effects from weight-loss fibers like glucomannan.

Bear in mind the evidence we've looked at when you hear people proclaiming that feeding our gut bugs supplemental fiber is the next miracle cure for a given disease or condition. This doesn't mean fiber will not help—we just want to have a reasonable understanding and expectation. We will try fiber at the right time during our Great-in-8 plan.

## CONCEPT SUMMARY

- Most of the data show no positive impact of supplemental fiber on digestive-tract cancers.

- Supplemental fiber is likely best used when IBD is in remission.

- Fiber has the most benefit for constipation-type IBS but can also be problematic for some with IBS, so it should be used cautiously.

- Supplemental fiber can be helpful for lowering blood sugar and hemoglobin A1c.

- There does not appear to be a clear benefit on heart disease from fiber supplementation.

- Fiber appears to have a minimal impact on obesity and weight.

1　Marie Louise A. Heijnen et al., "Limited Effect of Consumption of Uncooked (RS2) or Retrograded (RS3) Resistant Starch on Putative Risk Factors for Colon Cancer in Healthy Men," *American Journal of Clinical Nutrition* 67, no. 2 (1998): 322–31.

2　M. J. Grubben et al., "Effect of Resistant Starch on Potential Biomarkers for Colonic Cancer Risk Patients with Colonic Adenomas: A Controlled Trial," *Digestive Diseases and Sciences* 46, no. 4 (2001): 750–56, doi:10.1023/A:1010787931002.

3　M. van Dijk and G. K. Pot, "The Effects of Nutritional Interventions on Recurrence in Survivors of Colorectal Adenomas and Cancer: A Systematic Review of Randomised Controlled Trials," *European Journal of Clinical Nutrition* 70, no. 5 (2016): 566–73, doi:10.1038/ejcn.2015.210.

4　Paul J. Limburg et al., "Randomized Phase II Trial of Sulindac, Atorvastatin, and Prebiotic Dietary Fiber for Colorectal Cancer Chemoprevention," *Cancer Prevention Research (Philadelphia, Pa.)* 4, no. 2 (2011): 259–69, doi:10.1158/1940-6207.CAPR-10-0215; Mariabeatrice Principi et al., "Phytoestrogens/Insoluble Fibers and Colonic Estrogen Receptor: Randomized, Double-Blind, Placebo-Controlled Study," *World Journal of Gastroenterology* 19, no. 27 (2013): 4325, doi:10.3748/wjg.v19.i27.4325.

5　Michelle J. Clark et al., "Effect of Prebiotics on Biomarkers of Colorectal Cancer in Humans: A Systematic Review," *Nutrition Reviews* 70, no. 8 (2012): 436–43, doi:10.1111/j.1753-4887.2012.00495.x.

6　Linda Wedlake et al., "Fiber in the Treatment and Maintenance of Inflammatory Bowel Disease: A Systematic Review of Randomized Controlled Trials," *Inflammatory Bowel Diseases* 20, no. 3 (2014): 576–86, doi:10.1097/01.MIB.0000437984.92565.31.

7　G. Parisi et al., "High-Fiber Diet Supplementation in Patients with Irritable Bowel Syndrome (IBS): A Multicenter, Randomized, Open Trial Comparison between Wheat Bran Diet and Partially Hydrolyzed Guar Gum (PHGG)," *Digestive Diseases and Sciences* 47, no. 8 (2002): 1697–1704, doi:10.1023/A:1016419906546; Lin Xu et al., "Efficacy of Pectin in the Treatment of Diarrhea Predominant Irritable Bowel Syndrome," *Chinese Journal of Gastrointestinal Surgery* 18, no. 3 (2015): 267–71; Luigi Russo et al., "Partially Hydrolyzed Guar Gum in the Treatment of Irritable Bowel Syndrome with Constipation: Effects of Gender, Age, and Body Mass Index," *Saudi Journal of Gastroenterology: Official Journal of the Saudi Gastroenterology Association* 21, no. 2 (2015): 104–10, doi:10.4103/1319-3767.153835.

8　C. J. Bijkerk et al., "Systematic Review: The Role of Different Types of Fibre in the Treatment of Irritable Bowel Syndrome," *Alimentary Pharmacology and Therapeutics*, 2004, doi:10.1111/j.0269-2813.2004.01862.x; Neeraja Nagarajan et al., "The Role of Fiber Supplementation in the Treatment of Irritable Bowel Syndrome: A Systematic Review and Meta-Analysis," *European Journal of Gastroenterology & Hepatology* 27, no. 9 (2015): 1002–10, doi:10.1097/MEG.0000000000000425; N. C. Suares and A. C. Ford, "Systematic Review: The Effects of Fibre in the Management of Chronic Idiopathic Constipation," *Alimentary Pharmacology & Therapeutics* 33, no. 8 (2011): 895–901, doi:10.1111/j.1365-2036.2011.04602.x; Jing Yang et al., "Effect of Dietary Fiber on Constipation: A Meta Analysis," *World Journal of Gastroenterology* 18, no. 48 (2012): 7378–83, doi:10.3748/wjg.v18.i48.7378.

9　C. J. Bijkerk et al., "Soluble or Insoluble Fibre in Irritable Bowel Syndrome in Primary Care? Randomised Placebo Controlled Trial," *BMJ* 339, no. aug27_2 (2009): b3154+, doi:10.1136/bmj.b3154.

10　Lisa Ruepert et al., "Bulking Agents, Antispasmodics and Antidepressants for the Treatment of Irritable Bowel Syndrome," *Cochrane Database of Systematic Reviews (Online)*, no. 8 (2011): CD003460, doi:10.1002/14651858.CD003460.pub3.

11　Paul Enck et al., "Therapy Options in Irritable Bowel Syndrome," *European Journal of Gastroenterology & Hepatology* 22, no. 12 (2010): 1402–11, doi:10.1097/MEG.0b013e3283405a17.

12　Laura E. Chouinard, "The Role of Psyllium Fibre Supplementation: In Treating Irritable Bowel Syndrome," *Canadian Journal of Dietetic Practice and Research*, 2011, doi:10.3148/72.1.2011.48.

13　D. Lesbros-Pantoflickova et al., "Meta-Analysis: The Treatment of Irritable Bowel Syndrome," *Alimentary Pharmacology & Therapeutics* 20, no. 11–12 (2004): 1253–69, doi:10.1111/j.1365-2036.2004.02267.x.

14　Kok Sun Ho et al., "Stopping or Reducing Dietary-Fiber Intake Reduces Constipation and Its Associated Symptoms," *World Journal of Gastroenterology* 18, no. 33 (2012): 4593–96, doi:10.3748/wjg.v18.i33.4593.

15　Roger D. Gibb et al., "Psyllium Fiber Improves Glycemic Control Proportional to Loss of Glycemic Control: A Meta-Analysis of Data in Euglycemic Subjects, Patients at Risk of Type 2 Diabetes Mellitus, and Patients Being Treated for Type 2 Diabetes Mellitus," *American Journal of Clinical Nutrition* 102, no. 6 (December 1, 2015): 1604–14, doi:10.3945/ajcn.115.106989.

16　Saman Khalesi et al., "Flaxseed Consumption May Reduce Blood Pressure: A Systematic Review and Meta-Analysis of Controlled Trials," *Journal of Nutrition* 145, no. 4 (2015): 758–65, doi:10.3945/jn.114.205302.

17  Anne Whitehead et al., "Cholesterol-Lowering Effects of Oat B-Glucan: A Meta-Analysis of Randomized Controlled Trials 1–4," *American Journal of Clinical Nutrition* 100, no. 6 (2014): 1413–21, doi:10.3945/ajcn.114.086108.1.

18  Igho J. Onakpoya and Carl J. Heneghan, "Effect of the Novel Functional Fibre, Polyglycoplex (PGX), on Body Weight and Metabolic Parameters: A Systematic Review of Randomized Clinical Trials," *Clinical Nutrition* 34, no. 6 (2015): 1109–14, doi:10.1016/j.clnu.2015.01.004.

19  J. F. Swain et al., "Comparison of the Effects of Oat Bran and Low-Fiber Wheat on Serum Lipoprotein Levels and Blood Pressure," *New England Journal of Medicine* 322, no. 3 (1990): 147–152, doi:10.1056/nejm199001183220302; B. M. Burton-Freeman et al., "Red Raspberries and Their Bioactive Polyphenols: Cardiometabolic and Neuronal Health Links," *Advances in Nutrition: An International Review Journal* 7, no. 1 (2016): 44–65, doi:10.3945/an.115.009639; J. Leadbetter et al., "Effects of Increasing Quantities of Oat Bran in Hypercholesterolemic People," *American Journal of Clinical Nutrition* 54, no. 5 (1991): 841–45; L. V. van Horn et al., "Serum Lipid Response to Oat Product Intake with a Fat-Modified Diet," *Journal of the American Dietetic Association* 86, no. 6 (1986): 759–64, www.ncbi.nlm.nih.gov/pubmed/3011876.

20  N. C. Howarth et al., "Dietary Fiber and Weight Regulation," *Nutrition Reviews* 59, no. 5 (2001): 129–39, doi:10.1111/j.1753-4887.2001.tb07001.x.

21  A. J. Wanders et al., "Effects of Dietary Fibre on Subjective Appetite, Energy Intake and Body Weight: A Systematic Review of Randomized Controlled Trials," *Obesity Reviews* 12, no. 9 (2011): 724–39, doi:10.1111/j.1467-789X.2011.00895.x.

22  Bartlomieij M. Zalewski et al., "The Effect of Glucomannan on Body Weight in Overweight or Obese Children and Adults: A Systematic Review of Randomized Controlled Trials," *Nutrition*, 2015, doi:10.1016/j.nut.2014.09.004.

23  Igho J. Onakpoya et al., "The Efficacy of Glucomannan Supplementation in Overweight and Obesity: A Systematic Review and Meta-Analysis of Randomized Clinical Trials," *Journal of the American College of Nutrition* 33, no. 1 (2014): 70–78, doi:10.1080/07315724.2014.870013.

24  Max H. Pittler and Edzard Ernst, "Guar Gum for Body Weight Reduction: Meta-Analysis of Randomized Trials," *American Journal of Medicine* 110, no. 9 (2001): 724–30, doi:10.1016/S0002-9343(01)00702-1.

25  Michelle J. Clark and Joanne L. Slavin, "The Effect of Fiber on Satiety and Food Intake: A Systematic Review," *Journal of the American College of Nutrition* 32, no. 3 (2013): 200–211, doi:10.1080/07315724.2013.791194.

26  Blanca R. Balcazar-Munoz et al., "Effect of Oral Inulin Administration on Lipid Profile and Insulin Sensitivity in Subjects with Obesity and Dyslipidemia," [In Spanish.] *Revista Medica de Chile* 131, no. 6 (2003): 597–604; D. A. Luis et al., "Randomized Clinical Trial with a Inulin Enriched Cookie on Risk Cardiovascular Factor in Obese Patients," [In Spanish.] *Nutrición Hospitalaria*, 2010, doi:10.3305/nh.2010.25.1.4535; Akira Kobayakawa et al., "Improvement of Fasting Plasma Glucose Level after Ingesting Moderate Amount of Dietary Fiber in Japanese Men with Mild Hyperglycemia and Visceral Fat Obesity," *Journal of Dietary Supplements* 10 no. 2 (2013): 129–41, doi:10.3109/19390211.2013.790335; Jorge L. Ble-Castillo et al., "Effects of Native Banana Starch Supplementation on Body Weight and Insulin Sensitivity in Obese Type 2 Diabetics," *International Journal of Environmental Research and Public Health* 7, no. 5 (2010): 1953–62, doi:10.3390/ijerph7051953; Valesca Dall'Alba et al., "Improvement of the Metabolic Syndrome Profile by Soluble Fibre—Guar Gum—in Patients with Type 2 Diabetes: A Randomised Clinical Trial," *British Journal of Nutrition* 110, no. 9 (2013): 1601–10, doi:10.1017/S0007114513001025.

# CHAPTER 21

# *PREBIOTICS*

## PROS AND CONS OF PREBIOTICS

Prebiotics are compounds in foods, usually carbohydrates, that feed bacteria in your gut. To provide you a more detailed definition, we can paraphrase the UpToDate medical database: "Prebiotics" generally refers to nondigestible food ingredients that affect the host by selectively stimulating the growth and/or activity of one or a limited number of beneficial bacteria in the large intestine. The most widely accepted prebiotics are the fermentable oligosaccharides inulin, fructooligosaccharides (FOS or fructans), galactooligosaccharides (GOS), and lactulose.

In case that definition is confusing, here is a simple way you can determine how many prebiotics you are getting in your diet. The more carbohydrates—fruits, vegetables, and starches—you are consuming and the greater the variety of them, the more and different types of prebiotics you are getting.

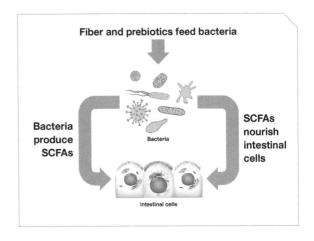

There is a bit of a prebiotic craze occurring, with many suggesting that everyone should ingest lots of prebiotics. However, my clinical observations and the medical research suggest that this is simply not the case. Aggressively feeding bacteria can be problematic for the many people who have bacterial overgrowths—which can be worsened by bacterial feeding. Do you remember how we discussed that some people do better on fewer carbs, fiber, and prebiotics while some do better on more? Our Great-in-8 plan will help guide you to a decision about what role prebiotics should play in your gut and microbiotal health.

Several studies have shown prebiotics have positive effects, like an increase in the health of the intestinal mucous membrane and a decrease in blood sugar levels, inflammation, insulin, and cholesterol. Prebiotics may help prevent traveler's diarrhea and aid in digestion of lactose in those who are lactose intolerant.[1]

This all sounds pretty good, right? To help give you an accurate understanding regarding the benefits of prebiotics, let's now cover what the research shows.

---

**SUMMARY OF THE EVIDENCE—PREBIOTICS**

See step 6 of the Great-in-8 for the ideal timing and approach for using prebiotics.

- **IBS and SIBO**—The best evidence suggests you should avoid prebiotics and use a low-prebiotic diet like the low-FODMAP diet. Some may benefit from a moderate dose of prebiotic supplementation; a moderate dose is about 3.5–5 grams of fructooligosaccharide (FOS) per day.
- **IBD (Crohn's disease and ulcerative colitis)**—The best evidence suggests you should avoid prebiotics and use a low-prebiotic diet like the low-FODMAP diet or the SCD. Some clinical trials have shown harm from using prebiotic supplementation in IBD. One clinical trial has shown harm from using a high-FODMAP (prebiotic) diet in IBD.
- **Weight loss**—Many studies show no effect; some studies show small effect. In the studies showing weight loss, the most weight lost was roughly 2.3 lb. using twenty-one grams per day of oligofructose—this is a high dose, and digestive side effects were reported.
- **Diabetes**—A systematic review of twenty-six clinical trials concluded that prebiotics are effective in lowering blood sugar. More importantly, the effect is meaningful—the best results have ranged from a twenty-point reduction to a more than sixty-point reduction in fasting blood sugar.

---

Prebiotics appear to be more effective than probiotics in lowering blood sugar. However, the doses of prebiotics have been high (ten to twenty-one grams/day) and might cause significant digestive distress in those with underlying digestive issues like SIBO, IBS, or IBD. These studies typically use oligofructose or inulin-enriched oligofructose.

- **Celiac disease**—There are no studies available; however, indirect evidence suggests avoiding prebiotics may be advised in celiac disease, especially in those who do not fully respond to a gluten-free diet. This is because bacterial overgrowths are common in those who don't fully respond to a gluten-free diet, and prebiotics may make bacterial overgrowths worse.

# PREBIOTICS FOR SPECIFIC CONDITIONS

## IBS, SIBO, AND PREBIOTICS

One review paper examining four clinical trials found two of these trials showed no effect of prebiotics on IBS. The other two trials showed benefit. In patients who may benefit from prebiotics, 3.5–5 grams per day of the prebiotic fructooligosaccharide (FOS) might be best.[2] Some other studies have shown low doses of prebiotics can reduce digestive symptoms, including diarrhea.[3]

Prebiotics can be helpful for those who tend to be deficient in bacteria. However, remember that there are many with IBS who have an excess of bacteria (SIBO), which makes prebiotics a bad idea for these people. The dose is important, because using the right dose can minimize side effects. Side effects when using prebiotics can be common and include gas, bloating, cramps, and pain—also the symptoms of SIBO.[4] This is likely why studies have concluded caution should be exercised when using prebiotics in IBS (because those with IBS often have SIBO as the underlying cause).[5] Again, the ideal dose may be around 3.5–5 g per day.[6]

What about limiting prebiotics? As we detailed in the antibacterial-treatments section, the best treatment evidence for IBS/SIBO appears to be an antibacterial approach. Prebiotics can help or harm, so using them at the right time is important. Let's now discuss IBD, another condition where similar rules apply.

## IBD (ULCERATIVE COLITIS AND CROHN'S DISEASE) AND PREBIOTICS

The low-FODMAP diet and the SCD both call for limiting prebiotic-rich foods. Both of these diets have good evidence supporting their use as a treatment for IBD.[7] Elimination diets, where you remove common food allergens, have outperformed steroids in maintaining remission in IBD.[8] So, IBD responds well to diets lower in prebiotics and allergens. Clinical trials using prebiotic supplements in Crohn's disease show a worsening of the disease.[9]

There was some initial excitement as one early trial showed prebiotic supplementation might help IBD,[10] but when a follow-up study was performed, no improvement was found, and, as we just discussed,[11] prebiotic supplementation may even cause harm.

What happens if we put people with IBD on a high-FODMAP diet that feeds gut bacteria? One study showed that after going on a high-FODMAP diet, the subjects experienced a near doubling of their symptoms—they became much worse![12] What else is noteworthy here is that, according to microbiota testing, the subjects saw an increase in bacteria that we think are healthy. This reflects our earlier points of not thinking small and that microbiota tests do not offer any clinical value.

## WEIGHT LOSS AND PREBIOTICS

A systematic review of clinical trials has found there is limited data showing prebiotics help with weight loss.[13] This means some studies show benefit, and some do not.

For example, some studies show no change in weight, even though more healthy bacteria appeared in the gut[14] or other metabolic markers improved.[15]

What about trials that *do* show weight loss? The best results achieved using a prebiotic for weight loss showed 2.3 pounds of weight loss using twenty-one grams per day of oligofructose.[16] It's important to mention these studies are studies that isolated for the effect of prebiotics on weight loss. I have seen misleading claims citing studies where subjects changed their diets, started exercising, *and* started using prebiotics but the author attributes the weight loss to prebiotics alone.

## INSULIN RESISTANCE AND PREBIOTICS

A systematic review of twenty-six clinical trials has shown that prebiotics decrease blood sugar and insulin levels.[17] Now the question is how *much* of an effect do prebiotics have? The greatest improvement in blood sugar was a sixty-three-point (mg/dL) drop in fasting glucose,[18] which is quite dramatic. This occurred in healthy but overweight or obese subjects, over the course of twelve weeks, while using twenty-one grams of oligofructose per day. Prebiotics were the only intervention. Other studies have also found meaningful improvements in blood glucose from prebiotics, showing a twenty-point drop and 34% decrease in fasting blood sugar. These two studies used roughly 10 g of either inulin or oligofructose-enriched inulin per day.[19]

However, no consistent relationship between altered microbiota species and diabetes has been shown.[20] This means it's impossible to treat diabetes by testing your microbiota. Skip the test, and try the treatment!

It's clear from the evidence that prebiotics are better for lowering blood sugar than probiotics. However, the doses used are high enough to cause gastrointestinal side effects. The higher doses will not be an issue for everyone, but those with IBS, SIBO, IBD, or a possible gluten allergy may not tolerate these high doses.

## CELIAC DISEASE AND PREBIOTICS

No studies are available on prebiotic supplementation in celiac disease. However, some studies have shown increased microbiotal *diversity* in those with celiac disease versus healthy study participants,[21] which may mean prebiotics will be problematic for those with celiac disease. We've already discussed the increased chance for SIBO in those with celiac disease,[22] and we know prebiotics should not be used in those with SIBO. Also, remember that SIBO has been shown to prevent people from responding to a gluten-free diet, and treating the SIBO then ameliorates these patients' symptoms.[23] So, it appears (at least initially) that prebiotics are not a good idea for celiac disease.

We've now reviewed all the components included in the Great-in-8 plan. The next step is to take what we've covered and apply it using the personalized step-by-step Great-in-8 plan. Before we do, however, there is one more therapy we should cover. For the very small number of people who do not fully heal with the Great-in-8 plan, this next therapy is worth considering.

## CONCEPT SUMMARY

- Prebiotics are compounds that feed bacteria.

- Supplemental prebiotics can be helpful but can also cause negative reactions, so they should be used with care.

- Prebiotics have been shown to have the most benefit for those with diabetes; however, the high dosages used increase the likelihood of negative digestive reactions, like bloating.

1    Jelena Vulevic et al., "A Mixture of Trans-Galactooligosaccharides Reduces Markers of Metabolic Syndrome and Modulates the Fecal Microbiota and Immune Function of Overweight Adults," *Journal of Nutrition* 143, no. 3 (March 1, 2013): 324–31, doi:10.3945/jn.112.166132; Parvin Dehghan et al., "Oligofructose-Enriched Inulin Improves Some Inflammatory Markers and Metabolic Endotoxemia in Women with Type 2 Diabetes Mellitus: A Randomized Controlled Clinical Trial," *Nutrition* 30, no. 4 (2014): 418–23, doi:10.1016/j.nut.2013.09.005; Nicole J. Kellow et al., "Metabolic Benefits of Dietary Prebiotics in Human Subjects: A Systematic Review of Randomised Controlled Trials," *British Journal of Nutrition* 111, no. 7 (2014): 1147–61, doi:10.1017/S0007114513003607; Sailendra N. Nichenametla et al., "Resistant Starch Type 4-Enriched Diet Lowered Blood Cholesterols and Improved Body Composition in a Double Blind Controlled Crossover Intervention," *Molecular Nutrition and Food Research* 58, no. 6 (2014): 1365–69, doi:10.1002/mnfr.201300829; Parvin Dehghan et al., "Inulin Controls Inflammation and Metabolic Endotoxemia in Women with Type 2 Diabetes Mellitus: A Randomized-Controlled Clinical Trial," *International Journal of Food Sciences and Nutrition* 65, no. 1 (2014): 117–23, doi:10.3109/09637486.2013.836738; Zatollah Asemi et al., "Effects of Synbiotic Food Consumption on Metabolic Status of Diabetic Patients: A Double-Blind Randomized Crossover Controlled Clinical Trial," *Clinical Nutrition (Edinburgh, Scotland)* 33, no. 2 (2014): 198–203, doi:10.1016/j.clnu.2013.05.015.

2    Kevin Whelan, "Mechanisms and Effectiveness of Prebiotics in Modifying the Gastrointestinal Microbiota for the Management of Digestive Disorders," *Proceedings of the Nutrition Society* 72, no. 3 (2013): 288–98, doi:10.1017/S0029665113001262.

3   A. Drakoularakou et al., "A Double-Blind, Placebo-Controlled, Randomized Human Study Assessing the Capacity of a Novel Galacto-Oligosaccharide Mixture in Reducing Travellers' Diarrhoea," *European Journal of Clinical Nutrition* 64, no. 2 (2010): 146–52, doi:10.1038/ejcn.2009.120; Christine Hughes et al., "Galactooligosaccharide Supplementation Reduces Stress-Induced Gastrointestinal Dysfunction and Days of Cold or Flu: A Randomized, Double-Blind, Controlled Trial in Healthy University Students," *American Journal of Clinical Nutrition* 93, no. 6 (2011): 1305–11, doi:10.3945/ajcn.111.014126.

4   Anna Liber and Hania Szajewska, "Effects of Inulin-Type Fructans on Appetite, Energy Intake, and Body Weight in Children and Adults: Systematic Review of Randomized Controlled Trials," *Annals of Nutrition & Metabolism* 63, no. 1–2 (2013): 42–54, doi:10.1159/000350312.

5   R. Spiller, "Review Article: Probiotics and Prebiotics in Irritable Bowel Syndrome," *Alimentary Pharmacology and Therapeutics*, 2008, doi:10.1111/j.1365-2036.2008.03750.x.

6   Kevin Whelan, "Probiotics and Prebiotics in the Management of Irritable Bowel Syndrome: A Review of Recent Clinical Trials and Systematic Reviews," *Current Opinion in Clinical Nutrition and Metabolic Care* 14, no. 6 (2011): 581–87, doi:10.1097/MCO .0b013e32834b8082.

7   Richard B. Gearry et al., "Reduction of Dietary Poorly Absorbed Short-Chain Carbohydrates (FODMAPs) Improves Abdominal Symptoms in Patients with Inflammatory Bowel Disease—A Pilot Study," *Journal of Crohn's and Colitis* 3, no. 1 (2009): 8–14, doi:10.1016/j.crohns.2008.09.004; Ashley Charlebois et al., "The Impact of Dietary Interventions on the Symptoms of Inflammatory Bowel Disease: A Systematic Review," *Critical Reviews in Food Science and Nutrition* 56, no. 8 (2016): 1370–78, doi:10.108 0/10408398.2012.760515; Raquel Nieves and Roger T. Jackson, "Specific Carbohydrate Diet in Treatment of Inflammatory Bowel Disease," *Tennessee Medicine: Journal of the Tennessee Medical Association* 97, no. 9 (September 2004): 407, www.ncbi.nlm .nih.gov/pubmed/15497569; David L. Suskind et al., "Nutritional Therapy in Pediatric Crohn Disease: The Specific Carbohydrate Diet," *Journal of Pediatric Gastroenterology and Nutrition* 58, no. 1 (2014): 87–91, doi:10.1097/MPG.0000000000000103; Stanley A. Cohen et al., "Clinical and Mucosal Improvement with Specific Carbohydrate Diet in Pediatric Crohn Disease," *Journal of Pediatric Gastroenterology and Nutrition* 59, no. 4 (2014): 516–21, doi:10.1097/MPG.0000000000000449.

8   A. M. Riordan et al., "Treatment of Active Crohn's Disease by Exclusion Diet: East Anglian Multicentre Controlled Trial," *Lancet* 342, no. 8880 (1993): 1131–34, doi:10.1016/0140-6736(93)92121-9.

9   Kevin Whelan, "Mechanisms and Effectiveness of Prebiotics in Modifying the Gastrointestinal Microbiota for the Management of Digestive Disorders," *Proceedings of the Nutrition Society* 72, no. 3 (2013): 288–98, doi:10.1017/S0029665113001262; Jane L. Benjamin et al., "Randomised, Double-Blind, Placebo-Controlled Trial of Fructo-Oligosaccharides in Active Crohn's Disease," *Gut* 60, no. 7 (2011): 923–29, doi:10.1136/gut.2010.232025; Marie Joossens et al., "Effect of Oligofructose-Enriched Inulin (OF-IN) on Bacterial Composition and Disease Activity of Patients with Crohn's Disease: Results from a Double-Blinded Randomised Controlled Trial," *Gut* 61, no. 6 (June 1, 2012): 958, doi:10.1136/gutjnl-2011-300413.

10  J. O. Lindsay et al., "Clinical, Microbiological, and Immunological Effects of Fructo-Oligosaccharide in Patients with Crohn's Disease," *Gut* 55, no. 3 (2006): 348–55, doi:10.1136/gut.2005.074971.

11  Jane L. Benjamin et al., "Randomised, Double-Blind, Placebo-Controlled Trial of Fructo-Oligosaccharides in Active Crohn's Disease," *Gut* 60, no. 7 (2011): 923–29, doi:10.1136/gut.2010.232025.

12  Emma P. Halmos et al., "Consistent Prebiotic Effect on Gut Microbiota with Altered FODMAP Intake in Patients with Crohn's Disease: A Randomised, Controlled Crossover Trial of Well-Defined Diets," *Clinical and Translational Gastroenterology* 7, no. 4 (2016): e164, doi:10.1038/ctg.2016.22.

13  Anna Liber and Hania Szajewska, "Effects of Inulin-Type Fructans on Appetite, Energy Intake, and Body Weight in Children and Adults: Systematic Review of Randomized Controlled Trials," *Annals of Nutrition & Metabolism* 63, no. 1–2 (2013): 42–54, doi:10.1159/000350312.

14  Evelyne M. Dewulf et al., "Insight into the Prebiotic Concept: Lessons from an Exploratory, Double Blind Intervention Study with Inulin-Type Fructans in Obese Women," *Gut* 62, no. 8 (2013): 1112–21, doi:10.1136/gutjnl-2012-303304.

15  Jelena Vulevic et al., "A Mixture of Trans-Galactooligosaccharides Reduces Markers of Metabolic Syndrome and Modulates the Fecal Microbiota and Immune Function of Overweight Adults," *Journal of Nutrition* 143, no. 3 (March 1, 2013): 324–31, doi:10.3945 /jn.112.166132.

16  Jill A. Parnell and Raylene A. Reimer, "Weight Loss during Oligofructose Supplementation Is Associated with Decreased Ghrelin and Increased Peptide YY in Overweight and Obese Adults," *American Journal of Clinical Nutrition* 89, no. 6 (2009): 1751–59, doi:10.3945/ajcn.2009.27465.

17    Nicole J. Kellow et al., "Metabolic Benefits of Dietary Prebiotics in Human Subjects: A Systematic Review of Randomised Controlled Trials," *British Journal of Nutrition* 111, no. 7 (2014): 1147–61, doi:10.1017/S0007114513003607.

18    Jill A. Parnell and Raylene A. Reimer, "Weight Loss during Oligofructose Supplementation Is Associated with Decreased Ghrelin and Increased Peptide YY in Overweight and Obese Adults," *American Journal of Clinical Nutrition* 89, no. 6 (2009): 1751–59, doi:10.3945/ajcn.2009.27465.

19    Parvin Dehghan et al., "Oligofructose-Enriched Inulin Improves Some Inflammatory Markers and Metabolic Endotoxemia in Women with Type 2 Diabetes Mellitus: A Randomized Controlled Clinical Trial," *Nutrition* 30, no. 4 (2014): 418–23, doi:10.1016/j.nut.2013.09.005.

20    Canxia He et al., "Targeting Gut Microbiota as a Possible Therapy for Diabetes," *Nutrition Research*, 2015, doi:10.1016/j.nutres.2015.03.002.

21    Yolanda Sanz et al., "Differences in Faecal Bacterial Communities in Coeliac and Healthy Children as Detected by PCR and Denaturing Gradient Gel Electrophoresis," *FEMS Immunology and Medical Microbiology* 51, no. 3 (2007): 562–68, doi:10.1111/j.1574-695X.2007.00337.x.

22    Antonio Tursi et al., "High Prevalence of Small Intestinal Bacterial Overgrowth in Celiac Patients with Persistence of Gastrointestinal Symptoms after Gluten Withdrawal," *American Journal of Gastroenterology* 98, no. 4 (2003): 839–43, doi:10.1111/j.1572-0241.2003.07379.x.

23    Ibid.

# CHAPTER 22

# FECAL MICROBIOTAL TRANSPLANT (FMT)

## WHAT IS FMT, AND WHO SHOULD CONSIDER IT?

We discussed how probiotics do not appear to colonize you but rather have a transient benefit. Remember, the reason probiotics do not colonize you is because your microbiota is resistant to colonization, which is a good thing, because this prevents colonization by bad guys. However, fecal microbiotal transplant (FMT) is an exception to this. In FMT, we take the microbiota of one person and implant it into someone else. How? With poop, often via enema. In FMT, we essentially use healthy stool as a probiotic. Stool contains an immense number of bacteria, enough bacteria to recolonize the recipient's microbiota. Under the guidance of a doctor, a healthy donor's stool is administered to the ill patient and creates an extremely powerful probiotic.

FMT has received much attention, so it's important to understand for whom and what conditions this treatment might make sense. A 2014 review paper provides a nice overview of FMT.[1] FMT is a highly effective treatment option for those with a recurring Clostridium difficile infection that is not responding to standard treatment. This is a situation where there is little question that FMT should be used, because it can save someone from the potentially life-threatening consequences of this chronic infection.[2]

Going into specifics about reoccurring Clostridium difficile infections is beyond the scope of this book. However, if you have this condition, you may want to look into FMT.

---

**SUMMARY OF THE EVIDENCE—FMT**

- **Chronic infection**—FMT is a highly effective treatment for *resistant* Clostridium difficile infections, according to numerous RCTs and a systematic review.
- **Obesity and insulin resistance**—In the one RCT that has been published, no meaningful effect was found.
- **IBS**—Only preliminary data are available, but they suggest FMT may help with IBS. However, since there are other effective therapies that have been well studied, I do not recommend FMT for

---

251

IBS until all other treatment options have been exhausted.

- **IBD**—Clinical trials have found FMT to be safe for IBD and variably effective. Results ranged from 20% to 60% effective in inducing remission, with an overall average of 45%. FMT may work better for Crohn's disease. Again, since there are other effective therapies that have been well studied, I do not recommend FMT for IBD until all other treatment options have been exhausted.
- **Chronic fatigue, MS, thyroid disease, celiac disease**—One study has shown FMT might benefit chronic fatigue, and one study has shown FMT might benefit MS. However, these studies have not been replicated, so they should be interpreted with caution. To my knowledge, there is no data available for FMT in thyroid disease or celiac disease.

# FMT FOR SPECIFIC CONDITIONS

## OBESITY, INSULIN RESISTANCE, AND FMT

Can FMT help obesity? An RCT study was performed where the feces of lean men were transplanted into recipients who were overweight and had high blood sugar levels.[3] Unfortunately, there was no change in weight or body fat.

## IBS AND FMT

FMT for IBS appears to be helpful;[4] however, these results are preliminary, and there is a high chance the improvement could be the placebo effect, which can be very high in IBS treatment.[5] I would recommend you start with the more well-established treatments for IBS, as we've discussed, and only use FMT once all other options have been exhausted.

## IBD (ULCERATIVE COLITIS AND CROHN'S DISEASE) AND FMT

In the clinical trials, there are mixed data on FMT in IBD (Crohn's disease, ulcerative colitis). FMT *may* induce remission in up to 63% of cases;[6] however, a recent double-blind study showed no effect.[7] A systematic review with meta-analysis showed FMT is safe but variably effective in IBD. The effectiveness ranged from 20% to 60%, with an overall effectiveness of 45% for inducing remission. This study also showed that FMT might work better for Crohn's disease than ulcerative colitis.[8] A second study showed clinical improvement in 86% and remission in 76% for Crohn's disease.[9] This has been reinforced by another study.[10]

Another study showed FMT induces remission in a significantly greater percentage of patients with active ulcerative colitis than treatment with placebo, with no difference in adverse events,[11] which has been reinforced by other studies.[12]

FMT is worth considering for those with IBD that has not responded to other therapies. However, I would like to emphasize that you should try preliminary therapies first, because we still lack long-term studies. If there is long-term harm from FMT (which I think unlikely), we may not know for several years.

## CHRONIC FATIGUE, MS, THYROID DISEASE, CELIAC DISEASE, AND FMT

One study showed improvement in 50% of subjects with chronic fatigue syndrome receiving FMT.[13] Another study showed FMT may yield a 70% success rate in MS. MS patients experienced improved sleep and less fatigue after one to three days of FMT, with the results lasting two to fifteen years. This paper was cited in a 2013 review;[14] however, when I attempted to check this reference, I was unable to find the original paper. The results with chronic fatigue and MS are preliminary and have not yet been replicated, so caution is certainly warranted.

To my knowledge, there are no studies on FMT for thyroid disease or celiac disease.

## CLOSING THOUGHTS ON FMT

Are you thinking, *if I might benefit from FMT, why not just try it?* Because there is still much we don't know, and there is a potential risk of negative reactions and long-term consequences. FMT might be worth considering for conditions that have not responded to other therapies or to our Great-in-8 plan. However, I would like to emphasize again that you should try preliminary therapies first, because negative side effects have been documented with FMT, and because we still lack long-term studies. If there is long-term harm from FMT, we may not know for several years. I would only recommend pursuing FMT under the guidance of a doctor or clinician skilled in the treatment. It is very important to have the donor screened for diseases, infections, and metabolic problems like diabetes. It is also very important to follow the appropriate protocol when preparing and administering the FMT solution. Only do FMT when working with a professional.

You now have the most up-to-date summary on what conditions the available gut and microbiota treatments can and cannot help. But what treatments do you use and when? This brings us to our action plan, which organizes everything into an efficient sequence of steps. Let's now pull all this information together into our personalized action plan—the Great-in-8.

## CONCEPT SUMMARY

- FMT is a process where stool from a healthy donor is used like a probiotic to transplant healthy microbiota into someone who is ill.

- It can be very helpful for resistant Clostridium difficile infections.

- It shows promise for IBD and potential promise for IBS.

- FMT should only be used under a doctor's supervision or guidance and only if your condition has not responded to other treatments.

1    Gianluca Ianiro et al., "Therapeutic Modulation of Gut Microbiota: Current Clinical Applications and Future Perspectives," *Current Drug Targets* 15 (2014): 762–70, doi:10.2174/1389450115666140606111402.

2    Kathryn A. Bowman et al., "Fecal Microbiota Transplantation: Current Clinical Efficacy and Future Prospects," *Clinical and Experimental Gastroenterology* 8 (2015): 285–91, doi:10.2147/CEG.S61305; Dimitri Drekonja et al., "Fecal Microbiota Transplantation for Clostridium Difficile Infection: A Systematic Review," *Annals of Internal Medicine*, 2015, doi:10.7326/M14-2693; Krishna Rao and Vincent B. Young, "Fecal Microbiota Transplantation for the Management of Clostridium Difficile Infection," *Infectious Disease Clinics of North America*, 2015, doi:10.1016/j.idc.2014.11.009.

3    Anne Vrieze et al., "Transfer of Intestinal Microbiota from Lean Donors Increases Insulin Sensitivity in Individuals with Metabolic Syndrome," *Gastroenterology* 143, no. 4 (2012), doi:10.1053/j.gastro.2012.06.031.

4    Ning Li et al., "Efficacy Analysis of Fecal Microbiota Transplantation in the Treatment of 406 Cases with Gastrointestinal Disorders," [In Chinese.] *Zhonghua Wei Chang Wai Ke Za Zhi = Chinese Journal of Gastrointestinal Surgery* 20, no. 1 (2017): 40–46, http://europepmc.org/abstract/med/28105618.

5    Gianluca Ianiro et al., "Therapeutic Modulation of Gut Microbiota: Current Clinical Applications and Future Perspectives," *Current Drug Targets* 15 (2014): 762–70, doi:10.2174/1389450115666140606111402.

6    Ibid.

7    Noortie G. Rossen et al., "Findings from a Randomized Controlled Trial of Fecal Transplantation for Patients with Ulcerative Colitis," *Gastroenterology* 149, no. 1 (2015): 110–18, doi:10.1053/j.gastro.2015.03.045.

8    Ruben J. Colman and David T. Rubin, "Fecal Microbiota Transplantation as Therapy for Inflammatory Bowel Disease: A Systematic Review and Meta-Analysis," *Journal of Crohn's and Colitis*, 2014, doi:10.1016/j.crohns.2014.08.006.

9    Bota Cui et al., "Fecal Microbiota Transplantation through Mid-Gut for Refractory Crohn's Disease: Safety, Feasibility, and Efficacy Trial Results," *Journal of Gastroenterology and Hepatology* 30, no. 1 (2015): 51–58, doi:10.1111/jgh.12727.

10   David L. Suskind et al., "Fecal Microbial Transplant Effect on Clinical Outcomes and Fecal Microbiome in Active Crohn's Disease," *Inflammatory Bowel Diseases* 21, no. 3 (2015): 556–63, doi:10.1097/MIB.0000000000000307.

11   Paul Moayyedi et al., "Fecal Microbiota Transplantation Induces Remission in Patients with Active Ulcerative Colitis in a Randomized Controlled Trial," *Gastroenterology* 149, no. 1 (2015): 102–9, doi:10.1053/j.gastro.2015.04.001.

12   Rongrong Ren et al., "A Pilot Study of Treating Ulcerative Colitis with Fecal Microbiota Transplantation," [In Chinese.] *Zhonghua Nei Ke Za Zhi* 54, no. 5 (2015): 411–15.

13   Tom Borody, "Bacteriotherapy for Chronic Fatigue Syndrome: A Long Term Follow-Up Study," Complementary Medicine in CFS National Consensus Conference. Sydney, 1995, www.cdd.com.au/pdf/publications/All Publications/1995-Bacteriotherapy for chronic fatigue syndrome a long term follow-up study.pdf.

14   A. Vrieze et al., "Fecal Transplant: A Safe and Sustainable Clinical Therapy for Restoring Intestinal Microbial Balance in Human Disease?," *Best Practice and Research: Clinical Gastroenterology* 27, no. 1 (2013): 127–37, doi:10.1016/j.bpg.2013.03.003.

# PART 5

## THE GREAT-IN-8 ACTION PLAN

# CHAPTER 23

# THE GREAT-IN-8—SIMPLE STEPS TO HEAL YOUR GUT AND REGAIN YOUR HEALTH

## GREAT-IN-8 OVERVIEW

*As to the methods there may be a million and then some, but principles are few. The man who grasps principles can successfully select his own methods. The man who tries methods, ignoring principles, is sure to have trouble.*

Harrington Emerson

We will now focus on the steps you need to take in order to improve your health. Just like the patients we discussed at the beginning of this book, you can expect to see improvement in a broad array of symptoms, because we will be addressing a major root cause of illness, the health of your gut. As a refresher, here are some common symptoms or conditions that can improve from going through our plan:

- Fatigue
- Brain fog, depression, anxiety, poor memory

- Insomnia
- Weight loss or weight gain
- Gas, bloating, constipation, diarrhea, heartburn, reflux, IBS
- Joint pain
- Food reactions
- Thyroid health
- Autoimmune conditions
- Cravings
- Hot flashes, mood swings, PMS
- Inflammatory bowel disease
- Skin health, including acne, breakouts, psoriasis, eczema

Let's start with a big-picture overview and then work through the steps in more detail.

The reason to have a sequence is to help you minimize unneeded interventions and get healthy as quickly as possible. This particular sequence organizes actions in such a way that the most commonly needed interventions are performed first. Then, if after going through these initial steps you're still not better (or are only partially improved), you move on to the less commonly needed interventions. I can't overemphasize how important this is. The main drawback I see from the wealth of information available to patients on the Internet is that patients end up trying treatments or performing tests completely at random. As a result—and unfortunately—there are people who know a lot about health but are still sick. It's like someone who has read a lot about playing soccer but never actually played trying to jump into a serious game. Or think of it this way: If you studied up on law, would you be willing to act as your own lawyer? Probably not, right? You can only get so good at doing something when you read about it from the sidelines.

Here is a quick example. A patient named Jon recently came into my office. After going through his initial history and exam, we established that Jon has chronic bloating, constipation, and brain fog. He eats a healthy, Paleo-like diet—he's not perfect, but he is doing rather well with his diet. He also gets an appropriate amount of exercise, has a life he enjoys, and gets adequate sleep. Jon has been to one doctor already and had a stool test and a blood test, both of which were normal. Jon is convinced he should be screened for heavy-metal toxicity, have his adrenals tested, and do FMT (fecal microbiotal transplant therapy). This would cost thousands of dollars and might require him to fly to a special clinic for the FMT therapy.

What Jon doesn't understand is that he has not yet been tested for small-intestinal bacterial overgrowth (SIBO), which can cause all of his symptoms, and that the stool test he did was a very poor-quality test. When we performed another stool test (which was covered by his insurance) and an inexpensive SIBO test, we found SIBO and candida (a type of fungus), both of which can be treated cheaply and often easily. Once we treated the conditions, all Jon's symptoms went away. Did Jon need the metal detox, adrenal testing,

and FMT? No. Are heavy-metal detox, adrenal testing, and FMT needed for some patients? Yes. But these were clearly not the first steps to take in Jon's case—or in most cases. The sequencing helps prevent us from making this kind of mistake.

Unfortunately, most of what you get from the media (including the alternative-health media) are just sound bites meant to pique your interest. A health writer doesn't spend every day in a clinical practice, figuring out how information can best be *applied*.

## The difference between knowledge and wisdom is experience.

You can get knowledge in seconds on the Internet; what is much harder to come by is wisdom.

Here are the steps in our sequence.

- The Great-in-8 Action Plan
    1. Reset—reset your diet and lifestyle
    2. Support—support your gut with probiotics and digestive enzymes/acid
    3. Remove—remove/reduce unwanted gut bacteria with antimicrobial herbs
    4. Rebalance—rebalance gut bacteria after treatment with antimicrobial herbs
    5. Reintroduce—reintroduce foods you removed in step 3
    6. Feed—feed the good bacteria
    7. Wean—wean yourself off the supplements in your plan
    8. Maintenance and fun—maintain your improvements, and enjoy your newfound health

How does the sequencing of the eight steps work? Does everyone have to do all eight? No. Here are a few important notes:

- If, after step 1 or step 2, your symptoms have improved to a point where you feel satisfied, move directly to step 5.
  » For example, if you feel better after step 1, proceed directly to step 5. If you feel better after, step 2, proceed directly to step 5.
- If you don't feel fully improved after steps 1 and 2, move on to step 3.
- If you perform step 3, you must also perform step 4. Steps 3 and 4 must always go together.
- Whether you've completed step 1, steps 1 and 2, or steps 1 through 4, you should complete steps 5 through 8.

If you have questions about the steps, don't worry: we'll work through them together, step by step.

Let's elaborate a little on these steps now and then go into detail on each step in the next several chapters.

### Step 1: Reset—reset diet and lifestyle

In this step, we start with a brief liquid-nutrition fast that can work wonders to calm down symptoms and allow your gut to heal quickly. After the brief fast, we transition to a healthy and gut-healing diet. There are a couple of diets that can be very helpful in improving gut health. The diets all have similarities, but there are a few nuances that distinguish one diet from another. In step 1, we will work through a process to guide you to the best diet for you and your gut ecosystem. After step 1, most people will experience at least a 30% improvement in how they feel, and some will experience a dramatic improvement.

### Step 2: Support—support your gut with probiotics and digestive enzymes/acid

Step 2 involves supporting your gut with probiotics, digestive support, and adrenal support. For many people who don't feel 100% improved after

step 1, step 2 is the extra push they need to get there.

### Step 3: Remove—remove/reduce unwanted gut bacteria with antimicrobial herbs, and Step 4: Rebalance—rebalance gut bacteria after treatment with antimicrobial herbs

If you are **not** feeling better after working through step 2, then it's time to move on to steps 3 and 4, which are a bit more clinical. In step 3, we will use target agents that can correct things like SIBO (small-intestinal bacterial overgrowth) or SIFO (small-intestinal fungal overgrowth). In step 4, we will make sure we *rebalance* your gut ecosystem and prevent any of the imbalances from returning. *Steps 3 and 4 should always be performed back to back.*

### Step 5: Reintroduce—reintroduce foods you removed in step 3

Once your gut is significantly healthier, we will work to broaden your diet so you have the fewest food restrictions possible. At this point, you should be feeling much better, even when you're not eating strictly according to plan all the time. Some people will end up able to eat a broader diet than others, but working through this process will enable *you* to determine what *your* dietary boundaries are. For example, can you have dairy or not? Can you eat a higher-carb diet, or do you have to be careful with your carbs? Step 5 is where we find out.

> *Step 5 is where you stop being a victim of dietary dogma and discover your own answers.*

### Step 6: Feed—feed the good bacteria, and Step 7: Wean—wean yourself off the supplements in your plan

Steps 6 and 7 are fairly straightforward. Now that we've balanced your gut ecosystem, in step 6 we give your gut bacteria some food. Just as different ecosystems do better or worse with more or less rain, different gut ecosystems do better or worse with more or less feeding of their bacteria. We will determine how much feeding your gut bacteria need. And then, maybe most important of all, in step 7 we work to wean your gut in order to find the minimum number and dose of supplements and supports needed to maintain your newfound level of health. Step 7 helps establish the minimum amount of stuff you need to take to maintain the maximum benefit. For many, this step is very liberating, because it frees them from dependence on supplements.

### Step 8: Maintenance and Fun—maintain your improvements, and enjoy your newfound health

Step 8 involves two things. First, a simple reminder to *have fun*. Now that you're healthier, enjoy your life. Don't live in a bubble, afraid to eat out or overly dependent on your trusted supplements. This may seem unimportant, but we want to ensure you don't fall into a health-obsession syndrome. Second, have a yearly checkup. We'll cover some tips on finding a good functional-medicine doctor for a yearly check-in. In step 8, we will also cover some simple tips for what to do if you have a setback or a flare. We will also cover tests to ask your doctor about, should you need some professional help.

One final point before we get started—***healing can take time***. We are trying to improve your internal ecosystem, and this will not happen overnight. Just like a garden requires time for soil health to improve and yield healthy plants, your gut will require time to heal and time for you to experience far-reaching health improvements. We will, of course, work to get you healthy as fast as we can, but if these improvements don't occur as quickly as you would like, stick with it, and be patient.

Let's get started.

# CHAPTER 24

# STEP 1: RESET

## STEP 1A: MODIFIED FAST (HITTING THE RESET BUTTON FOR QUICK SYMPTOM RELIEF)

Step 1 consists of a quick modified fast, which is then followed by diet and lifestyle changes. The modified fast is a liquid-only fast that can be incredibly reparative and anti-inflammatory for your gut.

There are two options available; choose whichever appeals most to you. One option is a cleansing lemonade, and the other is a homemade broth. See the *Modified Fast* handout at www.DrRuscio.com /GutBook for specific instructions on how to make both fast solutions.

Let's review the main action items regarding fasting that we covered earlier. You should perform the fast for two to four days. The first day is a transition day. Not everyone feels better on day one. It's usually by the second day that improvements are noticeable. Often, patients report improved energy, mental clarity, digestive symptoms, weight, sleep, and mood. For most people, modified fasting seems to work well and

can be used again in the future if they experience a flare-up of their symptoms. However, occasionally someone feels tired or hungry or has some other negative reaction that lasts the entire fast. For these people, it's generally best to avoid fasting or to try the other version, in case they're merely having a negative reaction to something in the first version they tried. If you try both and don't feel well on either version, simply move along to the next part of step 1. How long you perform the modified fast depends on how you're responding. If you're responding well, go for the full four days. If you're having a reaction that doesn't abate after the second day, stop at day two.

Before I tried a liquid fast, I was sure I wouldn't be able to. I was very wrong. My energy, sleep, and mental clarity were incredible. This can be a powerful healing tool for you to keep in your toolbox. It's not a guarantee, but giving the fast a trial is well worth it.

During the fast, it's best to stop taking any supplements, but continue to take any medications. You can engage in activity but might want to avoid highly rigorous exercise. Also, make sure to get plenty of rest and drink lots of water. A big glass of water can help quell hunger, if you're feeling it.

## TRANSITIONING BACK TO WHOLE FOODS

When you start eating solid foods again, go slow. Start with smaller meals rather than large ones. Opt for softer foods, like steamed veggies and soups, rather than hard foods, like raw veggies and charred meats. When transitioning back to solid foods, listen to how your body reacts to certain foods. After performing a fast, people will often notice they can pick out certain foods that don't agree with them. To help make this easier, it's best to limit the number of new foods you eat at once. The basic principle here is to eat simple meals that contain a minimal number of ingredients so it's easier to tell if a food doesn't sit well with you. For example, baked chicken seasoned with oregano and olive oil, accompanied by a side of steamed broccoli, is better than chicken tikka masala (with its multiple-ingredient sauce) and a side of a heavily seasoned vegetable medley. We will detail what diet you should transition to in a moment. The good news is as you start on a diet plan, you'll eat simpler and cleaner foods.

## YOUR RESPONSE TO MODIFIED FASTING HELPS DETERMINE WHAT YOUR MEAL FREQUENCY SHOULD BE

When we talk about meal frequency, we're referring to whether you eat small frequent meals or larger less frequent ones. The better you feel on the modified liquid fast, the more it suggests you will do better on infrequent meals (perhaps two meals per day). Of course, if in the past you noticed you feel better when you skip a meal, breakfast, for example, you too might do better on two meals a day compared to three or four.

Here are the basic points that will help you determine if you should eat small frequent meals (every three to four hours) or larger infrequent meals (skipping one or more meals per day). (Note, sometimes the practice of skipping a meal is described as "intermittent fasting.")

You'll probably do better skipping meals if

- you've noticed in the past that you feel better when you skip meals;
- you find you're not hungry at certain mealtimes;
- you felt good on the modified fast.

You'll probably do better with frequent meals if

- you've noticed you feel worse when you miss a meal (fatigued, irritable, hungry, foggy-headed);
- you're hungry at or before mealtimes;
- you didn't feel well on the modified fast.

## SUMMARY

We perform a short liquid fast and then transition back to whole foods. Do the best you can with the fast; if it's not perfect, that's OK. Perfect execution or not, you're taking a huge step to feeling better! See the handouts section at www.DrRuscio.com/GutBook for exact instructions for making the liquid for the fast. Next, we want to find the ideal diet for you and your unique gut ecosystem. Let's detail that now.

# STEP 1B: FINDING OUR OPTIMUM DIET FOR GUT HEALING

## MEAL FREQUENCY AND FASTING

If you felt a lot better when you performed the modified fast, you may do better when skipping a meal per day. If you feel better when skipping breakfast but are a little hungry, you can make a cup of the modified-fast solution (broth or the lemonade solution) and sip on that during the morning to help get you through. You can also have some tea or coffee, but make sure that whatever you add to it (cream and sugar, for example) is compliant with the diet plan you are on.

If you did *not* feel well on the modified fast or you're someone who gets tired, irritable, and jittery when you miss a meal, you should eat regularly. Let's discuss the diet plans now.

## THE PALEO DIET AND THE LOW-FODMAP DIET

In my opinion, diet is unquestionably the most impactful intervention for improving your gut and overall health. It's because of the importance of diet that this will be our longest and most important step. We will work through a process to help you determine the exact diet for *your* gut ecosystem. These steps address the most important principles of a healthy diet.

The principles of a healthy diet are listed here in order of importance:

1. A diet low in allergens/intolerances
2. A diet that contains the appropriate amount of bacterial feedings (prebiotics and FODMAPs)
3. A diet that regulates blood sugar and contains the appropriate amount of carbohydrate
4. A diet that focuses on fresh, whole, and unprocessed foods
5. A diet that focuses on organic and local foods

Fortunately, we have a few dietary plans that cover these points. Here is how to determine which diet is best for you:

- Start with the Paleo diet, and after two to three weeks, reevaluate. If you're happy with your results, stick with this diet.
- If you're not happy with your results on the Paleo diet, try the other diets one by one *in the order listed* for two to three weeks each until you find one that provides a satisfactory level of improvement.
- If none of the diets provides satisfactory improvement, stick with whichever one felt best, and then move on to step 2.

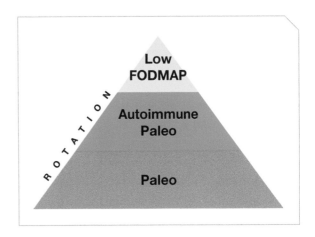

## OTHER DIETS

Other diet options include

- autoimmune Paleo (AIP);
- low FODMAP (either standard low FODMAP or Paleo low FODMAP ).

The Paleo diets remove allergens and inflammatory foods. The low-FODMAP diet helps to starve bacterial overgrowths. There are two versions of the low-FODMAP diet. It's pretty easy to determine which one is best for you (remember—if a diet is working for you, you should notice a difference within the first couple of weeks).

### *Which low-FODMAP is right for you?*

The following suggest the Paleo low-FODMAP diet is best for you:
- You felt better on the Paleo diet.
- You notice you feel better when avoiding grains or dairy.

The following suggest the standard low-FODMAP diet is best for you:
- You didn't notice any changes from the Paleo diet.
- You are underweight—you may need the potatoes, rice, and grains allowed on the standard low-FODMAP diet.

See www.DrRuscio.com/GutBook for a simple food guide for each one of these diets. Here is a *very* important concept to understand: you should view each one of these diets as a mini experiment. Each experiment is to identify if you are in the right dietary ballpark. If you're not, you'll move on. At first, keep the diet simple and basic. Once we find a diet you like, we can worry about finding delicious recipes. When you're first running the experiment, don't worry about making each meal super tasty but rather focus on testing the basic aspects of the diet and evaluating how it makes you feel. Once you find the diet you feel best on, you can find a cookbook that will provide ideas for how to put together tasty meals when you're on the diet long-term.

What I am trying to prevent you from doing is trying each diet at the expert level, meaning you eat a painstakingly compliant version and you work exhaustingly hard to make delicious meals in accordance with each dietary plan. Doing this will make the dietary-experiment phase feel daunting. Rather, what I recommend is to keep it simple. Do your best to be compliant with each diet, but don't fret over the small details—focus on the big picture. Also, don't worry about finding delicious meal plans at first; worry about that later, once you know what your long-term diet will be. There is no need to perform a two-week diet trial at an expert level if you might be moving on to a different diet after fourteen days. Remember, if a diet is working for you, you should notice a difference within the first couple of weeks.

We discussed this earlier, but it is so important it is worth visiting again. Trying to adhere to an increasing number of dietary rules and restrictions can make some people feel like there is nothing they can eat, which can create diet neurosis. This is not necessary and is something you should avoid. Sometimes people feel they must comply perfectly with a diet, which can be maddening and nearly impossible.

While the diets we have discussed have much overlap, there are some subtle differences as well. Please know there is no magic diet, so don't drive yourself crazy with trying to perfectly adhere to one diet's rules if it violates another diet's rules. The point of these diets is to help you uncover foods that are causing problems. They are tools to guide awareness, not a list of rigid mandates that cannot be broken. Many patients end up combining rules from the different diets as they observe the need. For example, they might avoid a few FODMAPs they notice don't agree with them but eat others. They may generally eat Paleo but also notice they feel OK with rice. The way to determine this is to work through these diets gradually, over several weeks, rather than trying to do this all at once. By doing it gradually, you will develop a sense for what rules from a given diet you should follow and what rules you don't need to follow. Take what you need, and leave the rest.

## CARB INTAKE

Do you have to hit a certain carb intake number when you start on one of these diets? No—you will naturally start to limit your carb intake as you work through each diet. However, in order to ensure you are at least in the right ballpark, check your total daily carb intake a few times. In chapter 8 we discussed some of the available carb-counting tools, such as the ones offered by the Atkins Center, MyFitnessPal, and even a general Internet search. Whatever tool you use to count carbs, shoot to be in the moderate or low range:

- *Moderate-carb intake is 100–175 grams per day*
- *Low-carb intake is fewer than 100 grams per day*

Here is the big picture: we start with a more restrictive diet of low-allergen and lower-carb foods. Then, as the gut heals, we slowly work to bring both types of restricted foods back into your diet during the reintroduction phase in step 5. Some will tolerate greater or lesser amounts of allergens and carbs upon reintroduction. This is how you determine your ideal long-term diet. For example, your ideal diet might be a Paleo diet that has you eating up to three hundred grams of carbs a day, or it might be one on which you eat fifty grams of carbs per day—this is what we will work to determine.

You may do better on a lower-carb diet (100 grams/day or less) if

- you have tried a lower-carb diet and felt good;
- you have family history of diabetes;
- you have diabetes or prediabetes (type 2);
- you are overweight;
- you crave carbs or can't stop eating carbs/sugar once you start eating them;
- you are of a more northern descent than equatorial descent (Irish versus Venezuelan, for example).

You may do better on a moderate-carb diet (100–175 grams/day or more) if

- you have tried a higher-carb diet and felt good;
- if you are an athlete or highly active;
- if you need to gain weight;
- if you are of a more equatorial descent than northern descent (Venezuelan versus Irish, for example).

**How to know if your carb intake is too low**
If you have been eating a lower-carb diet for a while and feel like your health is regressing, you may want to try increasing your carbs. Common symptoms of being too low carb include fatigue, insomnia, irritability, carb cravings, brain fog, feeling cold, and digestive upset. If you increase your carbs and feel better, you have confirmation that your diet was too low carb. If you increase your carbs but don't notice any change, carbs are probably not the issue.

**DIET—WHAT YOU SHOULD DO**

- First, spend a few weeks determining which diet you feel best on: Paleo, autoimmune Paleo, or low FODMAP.
- As you're doing this, periodically check to ensure you're eating a lower-carb diet (most people feel best on a lower-carb diet when they're eating roughly 100–175 grams of carbs per day or less. Don't get overly concerned about exact numbers, but do check to see roughly how many grams of carbs you are eating per day, and adjust accordingly if you are significantly over this range.
- When we get to step 5, you will increase your carb intake and determine at what level you feel best. We follow this sequencing because many do better with a lower-carb diet initially but then may need some additional carbs once their guts heal.
- Eat regular meals, every three to five hours, unless you notice you do better when skipping a meal.
- Remember to focus on fresh, whole, unprocessed foods. Buy organic and local when you can.

**FIBER TIP**

In step 5 of our Great-in-8 Action Plan, you will work to broaden your diet, and, as you do this, your fiber intake will increase. This will happen naturally as you start to eat more vegetables, fruits, and grains (if you tolerate them upon reintroduction). However, if you have IBS, SIBO, IBD, or just general digestive-tract inflammation, too much fiber might aggravate your gut. If you start eating lots of vegetables and dietary fiber and notice your gut is bothered by this, try eating a little less until your gut heals, and then slowly increase dietary fiber to see how much you can

tolerate. If your gut is sensitive, try focusing on softer fibers. Avoid lots of raw veggies and opt for veggies that are softened via steaming or sautéing. It might also be helpful to avoid the skins and seeds of fruits and vegetables, because they're rougher and can be irritating. Focus on things that are soft.

OK, that takes us through the main aspects of diet. In case you are feeling a little overwhelmed by the fact that you are in the driver's seat with the decisions about diet, it's extremely important for us to establish the fact that

> *the most powerful thing you can do to improve your health is learn to listen to your own body and stop listening to everyone else.*

**WHAT IF DIET HASN'T HELPED?**

What if you've worked through these diets and still don't feel like you've gotten your health back? The answer is probably to be stricter with the diet and work harder to make all these rules fit together. Right? No, no, no, no. Please do not go there—you will drive yourself crazy. If you have taken these dietary steps and have been, say, 80% perfect, and you don't feel much better, it means you need to do more than change your diet. So, relax with the diet, or you will drive yourself insane. To paraphrase the adage, which says it well, insanity is doing the same thing over and over again and expecting different results.

If you have done the diets—even imperfectly—and not seen results, it's time to refocus and move to nondietary interventions. Don't try to force a dietary answer on a nondietary problem. This concept can be the hardest for many patients to accept. Often, they come into my office quite neurotic about diet and expect me to have these magical dietary guidelines for them. We then have the conversation I'm having with you now, and for most patients, it's incredibly freeing—they can finally stop beating themselves up over diet.

## LIFESTYLE

In addition to dietary changes, changes to lifestyle can significantly impact your health. The most important lifestyle concepts for your health are

- avoid toxins to the best of your ability;
- obtain appropriate sun exposure;
- spend time in nature;
- exercise, enough but not too much;
- walk as much as you can;
- get enough sleep; if you notice you need more or less sleep than the normal range (seven to nine hours), you should see this improve as we work through our steps;
- mitigate stress, and/or practice stress management;
- nurture healthy relationships and social connections.

A key principle of mine is that food comes before exercise. If you can only focus on one, it should be food. Healthy food will have a larger impact on your health (weight, body composition, energy) than exercise will. They are both important, but focus on food first.

There is something I should share that many clinicians observe. Regardless of diagnosis or disease, the patients that have the most balanced lives tend to improve the most. As doctors, we can treat a disease, but we can't control what you do each day, every day. Those who let their illness become their life and identity have the hardest time healing, because there is no life to get back to without

the illness. This can be further compounded by the fact that these same people often get sucked into a black hole of health research and diet obsession that perpetuates their depression and anxiety while impeding important social relationships.

If this is where you are, don't be too hard on yourself. Simply start the process of gradually working to rebalance your life. Will it happen overnight? Probably not. However, if you work at it slowly and continuously, you will gradually achieve results. It is like starting an exercise program. If you're new to exercise, you probably won't be super fit right away, but with steady and repetitive exercise, you'll get there. The same principle applies to rebalancing your life. I know it can be tough if you're not feeling well, but do your best to get started, even if only in a small way.

## REASSESSING

Step 1 is the most important step you can take toward your health—it's the foundation. It also requires the most work on your part. So, if you've gone through step 1, give yourself some praise. Nice job. At this point you are most likely feeling better. For many, step 1 is all they'll need to do to feel great. But if you have a deeper imbalance in your gut or microbiota, you likely won't feel 100% improved after the dietary changes of step 1 and will need to move on to step 2.

*If you are feeling fully improved* after completing step 1, great! There is no need to move through the next three steps—move directly to the reintroduction phase, step 5. If you are feeling fully improved but still want to experiment (which is *not* necessary), you can continue to the support phase, step 2.

*If you feel partially improved (70% improved or less)*, or just not as well as you would like, move to step 2.

*What symptoms should be improving?*
Well, what have we covered so far? That the gut can affect a wide array of symptoms, correct? So, with that in mind, you should be looking for *any* symptomatic improvement that occurs during this time. It might be digestive, but it also might be sleep or mood or skin or mental clarity or joint pain.

Step 2 transitions us from the world of diet and lifestyle into the realm of gut and microbiota treatments. Step 2 involves helping to heal your gut with probiotics, digestive acid, enzymes, and adrenal support. Other gut and microbiota treatments like antimicrobial herbs and prebiotics are discussed in later steps. The Great-in-8 program organizes all the available treatments into the most logical and efficient sequence of action steps. Let's continue.

## STEP 1 ACTION-PLAN SUMMARY

- Reset things with a modified fast.

- Eat every three to five hours, unless you feel better when skipping a meal.

- Eliminate allergens via the Paleo (or possibly autoimmune Paleo) diet.

- Potentially reduce bacterial-feeding foods with the low-FODMAP diet.

- Reduce carb intake to around 100–150 grams per day.

- Focus on whole, fresh, minimally processed foods. Eat organic and local when possible.

- Keep your life balanced by adhering to good lifestyle principles: sleep, fun, friends, and nature.

- Do your best with diets, and do not look at them as needing to be followed 100%. You are human— allow yourself some room for error.

- If or when you feel greatly improved from the diet (anywhere from a few weeks to a few months into step 1), you can start the reintroduction process, covered in step 5.

- If you don't feel fully improved, keep working through our process by continuing to step 2.

# CHAPTER 25

# STEP 2: SUPPORT

## STEP 2: SUPPORT YOUR GUT WITH PROBIOTICS AND DIGESTIVE ENZYMES/ACID

As we move into gut-support protocols, it's important to establish that knowing when and how to use these tools (the process) is more important than merely knowing what to use (the protocol). The "magic protocol," which so many search for, simply does not exist. However, I can share with you some clinical wisdom I've accrued after using these tools with literally thousands of patients over several years. This is where the magic can occur—not merely knowing what to use but how to use it and in what order—the magic is in the *process* and not the *protocol*.

This process is codified into our Great-in-8 plan. We have already laid the groundwork with healthy lifestyle changes and by working our way through some dietary personalization in step 1. This usually helps people improve anywhere from 15% to 100%. Of course, if you're feeling 100% improved after step 1, you can move directly to step 5. If you're not yet where you would like to be after step 1, you'll now take step 2. With step 1, we've laid the important foundation. Step 2, our

support step, involves the addition of probiotics, digestive enzymes, and adrenal support.

### WHERE TO GET THESE SUPPLEMENTS

Everything you need for the steps of our Great-in-8 can be obtained through our clinic store at www.DrRuscio.com/GutBook. These are the same products I use in the clinic with my patients. Is there anything special about the products I recommend? Well, yes and no. I could tell you these are the "purest ingredients" or the "most bioavailable forms," but this is more supplement-company sales jargon than truth. Here's what *is* important regarding the specific product recommendations in our Great-in-8:

- The dosages and forms used approximate those that have been used in the clinical studies.
- The products are the ideal balance between quality and cost. Using a car as an analogy, we don't want you driving a lemon, but you probably don't need a Ferrari either. We don't want you using junk supplements, but this doesn't mean you need the most expensive supplements either—let's make this economical.

- The products are free of common allergens (hypo-allergenic) and irritants like gluten and emulsifiers, and are, therefore, gut friendly and good for sensitive patients.
- Proceeds from our clinic store help fund further research, which will improve health care in this area. For example, behind the scenes of the writing of this book, there was a team of people helping me sift through the research so I could generate the recommendations you see here. Another team helped perform the clinical research in my office. All of this benefits you as the consumer but is also dependent upon financial support from you.

# PROBIOTICS PROTOCOL

The Lactobacillus/Bifidobacterium blend is the probiotic mixture most studied and has been shown to help a wide variety of conditions. It's also very safe. We will use Lacto-Bifido Probiotic Blend at a dose of two hundred to three hundred billion per day (equal to ¼ teaspoon), one to two times per day, preferably on an empty stomach. It's often easiest to take with water first thing in the morning on an empty stomach and again before bed. Refer to chapter 14 for more information about probiotics.

We will also use Saccharomyces Boulardii Probiotic at a dose of 500 mg to 1,000 mg per day (two to four capsules per day). This isn't actually bacteria; it's a healthy probiotic fungus. Take this along with your Lacto-Bifido Probiotic Blend (preferably on an empty stomach).

Finally, there is also a Soil-Based Probiotic dosed at one to two capsules per day. This is best taken with food.

If you've tried probiotics like these before and not noticed much difference, you should still try them again. Remember, we are working through a multifaceted process, and many of these interventions will work together synergistically. Also, if you're concerned about a negative reaction (some people are more sensitive than others), you can start the probiotics one at a time, adding a new one every few days. This will help you pinpoint a negative reaction, should you have one.

## DOSE RANGES

Anytime you see a dose range ("one to two capsules," for example), it's best to start at the minimal dose. After a few days at this dose, see how you feel. If you're feeling great, stay at that dose. If you still need further improvement, increase to the full dose. This will help you find the minimal dose required, which is always our goal. More is not always better.

## WHAT TO EXPECT

After a couple of days or weeks on these probiotics, you will likely experience an improvement in how you're feeling. What *exactly* will you notice? Well, as we have covered in chapter 14, probiotics can help a wide array of conditions, so there is not a specific answer. Here is another way to approach this: if you notice anything improve around the time of taking the probiotics, it's likely this improvement is attributable to the probiotic. Listen to your body, and see what you notice. Maybe you have less bloating, clearer thinking, improved stool consistency, improved mood, better sleep, clearer skin, or less joint pain. Again, there are several things that might improve (not limited to this list), and if the improvement occurs after starting the probiotics, the probiotics are likely the reason for the improvement.

Are these probiotics safe for kids and infants? Yes, as we discussed in chapter 5 "How Early Life and Environment Impact Your Gut and Immune System," taking probiotics early in life can be helpful, so be sure to revisit this if you need clarification.

## REACTIONS

Reactions from probiotics are also possible. Probiotics can have antibacterial effects. When bad bacteria die inside your body, they can cause what's known as a die-off reaction. This often looks like a few days to a week of not feeling well, which can include feeling tired, headaches, irritability, digestive upset, and flu-like symptoms, among others. If you're experiencing a die-off reaction, it should last no more than a few days to a week and then disappear. This reaction isn't harmful, so don't be alarmed. You may also want to decrease your probiotic dose to help dissipate the die-off reaction. If, however, your reaction doesn't go away, it might not be a die-off reaction. A reaction like this is rare, but it can happen. If you do have this experience, experiment with trying one probiotic at a time to see if you can pinpoint which one is causing the reaction, and then discontinue that particular probiotic. The most common negative reaction people experience with probiotics is bloating. If bloating lasts longer than a few days to a week, you might do better with a lower dose or no probiotic at all.

## PERSONALIZATION AND MORE ISN'T ALWAYS BETTER

Should you take probiotics with or without food? In my opinion, it doesn't really matter. I have provided what might be the ideal recommendation for each probiotic, but I often instruct patients to disregard these instructions and simply take the probiotics with or without food, depending on what is easier for them—the best dose is the one you will take consistently.

What about optional add-ons to the protocol? This is actually a very important concept to understand. There is a lot of gray area in functional medicine, and the way I approach gray areas is to involve you—the patient—in the decision-making process.

I understand that in many cases it is easier to just have one single recommendation that everyone follows and that too many options can be overwhelming. However, I have noticed that most people really appreciate this approach of being involved in the decision-making process and having flexibility in the protocols used.

A final point here is doing **more** isn't always **better**. This is another point I feel is important for both doctors and patients to understand. In my observation, when we leave the conventional treatment model, we have the ability to do more. Whether you are a doctor or a patient, when you enter into the realm of functional and integrative medicine, there is a chance to do more. I think all doctors and patients like this idea. However, this sometimes causes what I think of as the freedom effect. It's similar to when teenagers who have been sheltered their entire lives finally get freedom in college. Because they haven't learned how to handle their freedom, they go crazy—they stay out late and drink too much, and their grades start to slip because of it. Although crude, I think this analogy speaks to what can happen in functional medicine. We, as doctors and practitioners, finally have the freedom to do more when we leave the constraints of a standard model that is highly restrictive. With this freedom sometimes comes excessive testing and treatment, just like the teenagers' excessive drinking and partying. Even though it's well intentioned, it can be too much.

I say this not to criticize but rather as someone who is doing much less testing and treatment today than I was several years ago *and* getting better results. I share this in the hope that we will all start to realize that more is not necessarily better. *Better* is better. Think, as an example, of two different doctors who both fix the same problem, but one does it in four months, spending $2,800, while the other does it in nine months, after spending $8,000. Which would you rather have? With the higher price-tag care comes more testing, which sometimes paints the illusion of more comprehensive care. Sometimes, less is better, because it allows us to focus on a small number of things rather than struggling to manage what an excessive array of test results mean and how to gauge effectiveness of several co-occurring treatments. Less information can prevent the crippling effect of information overload. More testing or treatment does not mean better results.

## DIGESTIVE-ENZYMES PROTOCOL

The digestive-enzymes protocol includes a formula that combines pancreatic enzymes, bile, and digestive acid. So, in addition to probiotics, we will use Digestive Enzyme with HCl as part of step 2. Digestive Enzyme with HCl should be taken at a dose of one to three per meal. This is one supplement that should **always be taken with food,** and you should not simply take it when it's most convenient.

### REACTIONS

Reactions to Digestive Enzyme with HCl are rare; however, if you notice stomach warmness, burning, or pain or reflux after using, simply discontinue and keep working through our Great-in-8.

## ADRENAL-SUPPORT PROTOCOL

We have established that adrenal support can help with gut healing. We have also discussed how adrenal support can help with the symptoms of adrenal fatigue (fatigue, insomnia, and depression, for example). So, using adrenal support makes sense.

When is the best time and what is the best way to use adrenal support? It's best to start now,

in step 2, the support step, and stay on adrenal support until you work your way to step 7, the weaning step. As the name implies, step 7 "Wean," is when we will wean you off everything in your program, including adrenal support. Our goal in step 7 is to determine the minimal amount of support needed.

***There are two options for your adrenal support.*** The first option, Adrenal Support Complete is a combination of adrenal adaptogenic herbs and adrenal glandular extracts. For this option, you'll take two capsules one to two times per day, with or without food.

I like this as option because the herbal and glandular extracts work differently, and combining them gives a broad spectrum of adrenal support.

The second option, Adrenal Support Herbal is a mixture of adrenal adaptogenic herbs. For those who are vegetarian, this is a good option. For this option, you'll take two capsules one to two times per day, with or without food.

Could we make your adrenal support more elaborate? Yes. Do we need to? In my opinion, no. Remember more doesn't mean better. There are no magic supplements, including adrenal supports. The magic is in the process. If you do not feel noticeable improvement from the adrenal support, simply stay on the minimal dose of either option and continue to work your way through our Great-in-8.

## VITAMIN D

You can add in vitamin D as an optional add-on. It's likely many of you have already taken vitamin D and may have levels within the normal range. Clinical trials have shown vitamin D supplementation can improve IBS and IBD.[1]

The vitamin D lab range is 30–100 ng/mL at most labs. I like to see patients in between 40 and 50 ng/mL. If they have an autoimmune condition, however, then shooting for as high as 50–60 ng/mL may be appropriate. Ideally, try to obtain vitamin D from the sun. As stated earlier, when you supplement with vitamin D, it's important to use a balance of vitamin D and vitamin $K_2$. In the clinic, I use a vitamin D supplement that is balanced with adequate vitamin D and vitamin $K_2$. I usually recommend a conservative dose of 2,000 to 4,000 IUs of vitamin D per day. If you are on a blood-thinning medication, like warfarin or Coumadin, you should consult your doctor before taking a supplement that contains vitamin K.

## ACTION-PLAN RECAP

Here is a recap of what we have done so far:
- Step 1
  - Established a healthy lifestyle plan, including exercise, time in nature, and sleep
  - Identified your ideal diet
- Step 2
  - Supported your gut and microbiota with probiotics and digestive enzymes (enzymes, acid, and bile)
  - Supported your adrenals and, indirectly, your gut, with adrenal support
  - Supported your gut and immune system with vitamin D

# STEP 2 ACTION-PLAN SUMMARY

## PROBIOTICS PROTOCOL

### Probiotics

| Name | Dose | Times/Day | w/ Food |
|------|------|-----------|---------|
| Lacto-Bifido Probiotic Blend | 1/4 tsp. | 1–2 | N |
| Saccharomyces Boulardii Probiotic | 2–4 pills | 1–2 | N |
| Soil-Based Probiotic | 1–2 pills | 1–2 | Y |

## DIGESTIVE-ENZYMES PROTOCOL

### Digestive Enzymes and Acid

| Name | Dose | Times/Day | w/ Food |
|------|------|-----------|---------|
| Lacto-Bifido Probiotic Blend | 1/4 tsp. | w/ meals | Y (always) |

## ADRENAL-SUPPORT PROTOCOL

### Adrenal-Hormone Support

| Name | Dose | Times/Day | w/ Food |
|------|------|-----------|---------|
| Adrenal Support Complete | 2 pills | 1–2 | N/A |
| Adrenal Support Herbal | 2 pills | 1–2 | N/A |

## VITAMIN D PROTOCOL

### Nutritional Support

| Name | Dose | Times/Day | w/ Food |
|------|------|-----------|---------|
| Vitamin D with $K_2$ | 2 drops | 1–2 | Y |

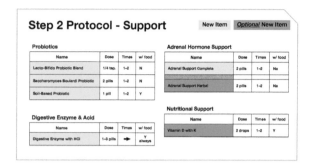

## IMPORTANT NOTES

- *All of the above should be taken during step 2. \*__If you know yourself to be sensitive or reactive__\*, you can add in one supplement at a time.*
- *Unless you've had a reaction, stay on all supplements in this step until we reach step 7.*
- *If you have a negative reaction to a supplement, simply discontinue its use.*

# REASSESSING

We have now gone through step 2. Make sure to give this step at least two to three weeks, and then evaluate how you feel. If you're feeling much better, great. Move directly to step 5. If you're only feeling slightly better or feeling no better, continue to step 3. If you're feeling somewhere in between these two, stay here on step 2 a little longer (a few more weeks) and see what happens. If you continue to improve with time and get to a satisfactory level of improvement, you can move on to step 5. However, if you don't feel much better with the additional time, continue to step 3.

*Feeling much better:*

step 1 → step 2 ⎯⎯⎯→ step 5 and on

*Not feeling better:*

step 1 → step 2 → step 3 → step 4 → step 5 and on

*What symptoms should be improving?*

Look for *any* symptomatic improvements. They might be digestive, but they might be sleep or mood or skin or mental clarity or joint pain.

Step 3 is where we remove unwanted gut bacteria or overgrowths of bacteria, fungi, and parasites. Let's head there now.

1    A. Abbasnezhad et al., "Effect of Vitamin D on Gastrointestinal Symptoms and Health-Related Quality of Life in Irritable Bowel Syndrome Patients: A Randomized Double-Blind Clinical Trial," *Neurogastroenterology and Motility: The Official Journal of the European Gastrointestinal Motility Society* 28, no. 10 (2016): 1533–44, doi:10.1111/nmo.12851; Tibor Hlavaty et al., "Vitamin D Therapy in Inflammatory Bowel Diseases: Who, in What Form, and How Much?," *Journal of Crohn's & Colitis* 9, no. 2 (2015): 198–209, doi:10.1093/ecco-jcc/jju004.

# CHAPTER 26

# STEP 3: REMOVE

## STEP 3: REMOVE/ REDUCE UNWANTED GUT BACTERIA WITH ANTIMICROBIAL HERBS

How are you feeling so far? Are you doing OK with your diet? If you are, great. However, if you're starting to feel bored, or you would love to start eating a certain food, we can make some compromises and allow you to loosen up your diet a bit. These compromises help in two ways:

1. They will keep you motivated (if diets are too restrictive, they can be hard to comply with).
2. If your health has been helped only minimally by diet up until now, diet might not be your main problem, so there is no need to follow a highly restrictive diet and you can cut yourself some slack.

Yes, you should keep your diet generally healthy, but there's no point in following a highly restrictive diet if diet isn't making a big difference. If you need some freedom, take a little, and let's see how you do with it. Start by adding back in a couple of foods that you are really craving, following

the reintroduction guidelines that we will cover in step 5. If you don't notice any regression from adding a new food into your diet, great—enjoy it.

Maybe you really miss coffee and a little cream. OK, let's give it a shot. Or maybe you cut out eggs and haven't reintroduced them yet. Or how about a responsible amount of wine? Maybe you would just like the occasional pizza and beer with friends. That's fine, try it. The only way to know what your boundaries are is to test them. With the pizza and beer, you may want to try gluten-free pizza and beer, if they are available to you. Do some checking around—you might be surprised how easy this is to obtain. Remember that this is not a license to eat unhealthy foods all the time, but it is a reminder that you don't have to be perfect all the time. So, if you're getting bored with the diet, you can open the boundaries a little to help keep you motivated. We will officially broaden your diet when we reach step 5. Your dietary reprieve is not far off.

Now that we've checked in, let's discuss the details of step 3 "Remove." You might be wondering why we didn't just start with this step if you're not feeling well. By working up to this point as we have, we've laid important groundwork to allow you to respond much better to the removal step. It's understandable for you to want the magic protocol to cure SIBO or fungus or bloating or whatever your symptoms or conditions are. Unfortunately, the search for the magic protocol usually results in going from protocol to protocol with little to no results. The reason many of these patients have been struggling is because the entire Great-in-8 *process* is what's needed, not just a protocol. Through the process we have worked through thus far, we have started to improve your internal environment. The stage is set for optimal microbiota expression. We just need to remove the bad guys that are preventing this.

Remember, there are a host of imbalances and bad guys that could be present. Here are a few examples:

- Imbalance may include SIBO, fungal overgrowth (yeast or candida), excessive inflammation, H. pylori, and biofilms.
- Bad guys might include Blastocystis hominis, giardia, amoebas, or parasitic worms.

> *Also remember everything needed for these protocols is available through www.DrRuscio.com/GutBook.*

## REMOVE PROTOCOL LEVEL 1—CLEANING OUT THE BAD BUGS

Earlier, we discussed how antimicrobial approaches, whether dietary or using herbal antimicrobials directly, can help with numerous conditions, including

- IBS and SIBO;
- weight loss and metabolism;

- thyroid autoimmunity;
- IBD (ulcerative colitis and Crohn's disease);
- celiac disease;
- blood sugar and insulin resistance;
- depression.

When we start the herbal antimicrobials, you will continue taking the items from step 2 and using whatever dietary approach you have settled in on (but with a little leeway, if you need it). This is especially important for the probiotics, because they enhance the effect of the antimicrobials. We have very high-level scientific data that has shown when probiotics are given at the same time as antibiotics, they enhance the antibiotics' ability to clear an infection or imbalance. This has been shown with H. pylori bacteria via meta-analyses and systematic reviews.[1]

We also have evidence showing that some probiotics are as effective as antifungal drugs in treating fungus.[2] And there is some documentation that probiotics are as effective as antiparasitic medications in treating parasites.[3]

The antimicrobial protocol is two months in duration. We use two antimicrobial formulations for the first month and two different formulations for the second month. These formulas can address all the imbalances we listed earlier: bacteria, SIBO, fungus, candida, yeast, H. pylori, Blastocystis hominis, giardia, protozoa, and worms.

> *This is important: before using any of these antimicrobials, you should check with your doctor.*

### Month One
During the first month, you'll take Biota-Clear 1a. Take three pills twice a day. This will require three bottles total. You will have a few extra, which you can take with the month-two protocol until the bottle is empty.

The other antimicrobial you'll take during month one is Biota-Clear 1b. Take two pills twice a day. This will require two bottles total.

**Month Two**

During this month, you'll take Biota-Clear 2a. Take two pills twice a day. This will require one bottle total.

The other antimicrobial you'll be taking is Biota-Clear 2b. Take three pills twice a day. This will require two bottles total.

These antimicrobials are best taken on an empty stomach. However, if you experience stomach upset or nausea, take them with food. If it's much easier for you to take these with food, that's fine. Do what's easiest for you. The antimicrobials can be taken at the same time as your probiotics; however, if you can leave a thirty-minute window in between, the antimicrobials may be slightly more effective. For example, you could take your probiotics first thing in the morning with a glass of water. Then take the antimicrobials a little later, before breakfast. If this feels daunting, take them all together. Keep it simple, and do what is easiest for you.

## REMOVE PROTOCOL LEVEL 1
## MONTH-ONE ANTIMICROBIALS

| Name | Dose | Times/ Day | w/ Food | Bottles Needed |
|---|---|---|---|---|
| Biota-Clear 1a | 3 pills | 2 | Best w/o | 2 |
| Biota-Clear 1b | 2 pills | 2 | Best w/o | 2 |

## REMOVE PROTOCOL LEVEL 1
## MONTH-TWO ANTIMICROBIALS

| Name | Dose | Times/ Day | w/ Food | Bottles Needed |
|---|---|---|---|---|
| Biota-Clear 2a | 2 pills | 2 | Best w/o | 2 |
| Biota-Clear 2b | 3 pills | 2 | Best w/o | 2 |

# PERSONALIZATION, OPTIONAL ADD-ON

If you are still experiencing constipation at this point in the plan, you may want to add in a magnesium supplement. Use magnesium citrate. Start with one tablespoon per day, and gradually increase by one tablespoon every few days until your bowels become more regular. If you take too much magnesium, you may experience loose stools. If this happens, simply decrease your dose.

## OPTIONAL ADD-ON

| Name | Dose | Times/ Day | w/ Food | Notes |
|---|---|---|---|---|
| Magnesium Citrate | 1 T | 1–4 | Y | Slowly increase your dose. If your stools become loose, you are taking too much and should decrease your dose. |

## IF YOU ARE SENSITIVE

If you have noticed you tend to be sensitive to supplements in general, you may want to slowly work your way into our removal protocol. Start with one formula at a time, and work up to the full recommended dose over a few days. There is no rush. Then add in the second formula, and do the same.

## REACTIONS

We introduced the concept of a die-off reaction when we discussed probiotics in step 2. As you may recall, symptoms of a die-off reaction include

- fatigue;
- irritability;
- headache;
- flu-like symptoms;
- digestive upset;
- altered stool frequency or consistency.

This is your body's reaction to the bad bugs (bacteria, fungi) dying. It's very important to note that this should last a few days, maybe a week, but no longer. If these symptoms (or any other negative symptoms that start when you begin taking antimicrobials) last more than a week, you may have an allergy to one of the compounds. The key difference that distinguishes a die-off reaction from an allergic reaction is time. Die-off reactions are temporary. Allergic reactions don't stop. So, if you do notice a prolonged reaction (more than a week), stop taking all antimicrobials for a few days and see how you feel. If you feel better, you know it was something in the antimicrobials. Once the reaction has subsided, try adding back the formulas one at a time. This will help you isolate which formula you were reacting to, and then you can simply stop using it (or use a lower dose, if tolerable).

Here is what this might look like: You start taking the Biota-Clear 1a and 1b and notice you're having diarrhea and fatigue. This lasts from Monday to Monday of the next week and doesn't seem to be getting any better. This suggests an allergy. You then stop taking both formulas and notice after three days you're back to normal. You then slowly add back in just the Biota-Clear 1a and notice no negative reaction. You slowly add back in Biota-Clear 1b and notice the diarrhea and fatigue start to return. So, you would then take only the Biota-Clear 1a at the recommended dose and for the recommended duration. You would not take Biota-Clear 1b because it's causing a negative reaction.

Here's a tip: Remember the modified fast we used earlier in step 1a? If this worked well for you, it's a great approach to revisit, should you have a reaction. Simply stay on the modified fast for two to four days to help calm things down.

GUT GEEKS

*If you have had a reaction to these herbal antimicrobial blends, you might need to try a few different formulas to find the ones you tolerate. Below are a few options to consider. It's best if you can find two formulas that work for you. If you do, you can take them for up to two months. You can find these in our clinic store:*

- *Allicin, which is contained in the product Allimax Pro 450 mg—take three capsules twice per day, with or without food*

- *Berberine, as berberine HCl 500 mg—take four capsules three times a day, with or without food*

- *Atrantil—take two to four capsules two times a day, with or without food*

GUT GEEKS

*There is also the option of pharmaceutical antimicrobial treatments, specifically antibiotics or prescription antifungals or antiprotozoals. I wouldn't recommend beginning with these, because pharmaceuticals don't have the broad action that herbs do. Remember, one herb can kill bacteria, fungi, and protozoa. You would need three different pharmaceutical prescriptions to do so. Here are a few options to consider discussing with your doctor:*

- *For SIBO, ask about rifaximin or rifaximin with neomycin.*

- *For fungus, ask about fluconazole.*

- *For protozoa, ask about Flagyl.*

Having reactions to the antimicrobials can be frustrating. This is something that is supposed to help, and it can feel defeating when it seems to make you worse. The good news is we have another approach you can try if the herbal antimicrobials don't work well for you: the elemental or semielemental diet. We will detail this a little later, but essentially this entails using hypoallergenic liquid meals to help heal the gut, reduce inflammation, and starve unwanted bacteria.

## REASSESSING

As you near the end of the two months, it's important to assess how you're doing. You will likely be in one of these three positions:

1. Feeling great—you're satisfied with your current level of improvement. This usually means you feel 70% improved or more. Note, 70% is not perfect, but people who experience this much improvement in only a few months usually go on to realize the rest of the improvement with a little time, as their bodies continue to heal.
2. Feeling OK—you feel better but not as good as you would like. This usually means you feel 30%–70% improved.
3. Feeling the same or worse—this usually happens if someone has had a reaction to the antimicrobials. If all the antimicrobials caused reactions, don't worry; we have another option.

**If you are at position 1:** move right to step 4. We have achieved our objective with the antimicrobial phase, and now it's time to move on.

**If you are at position 2:** go to "Remove Protocol Level 2," below. We've made improvements but need more work in the removal phase to achieve the desired result.

**If you are at position 3:** go to "Remove Protocol Level 3." This is a different approach to removing unwanted bacteria and rebalancing the gut. We will use a liquid-elemental/semielemental diet, which tends to work better for those who are sensitive or reactive to antimicrobials.

### What symptoms should be improving?
Look for *any* symptomatic improvement that occurs during this time. It might be digestive, but it also might be sleep, mood, skin, mental clarity, or joint pain.

## REMOVE PROTOCOL LEVEL 2—CLEANING OUT HARD-TO-KILL BAD BUGS AND REDUCING INFLAMMATION

We have given the microbiota a nudge with the previous antimicrobials, but sometimes this isn't enough to tip the balance in the favor of the good guys and reestablish a healthy equilibrium. There are three factors that often cause this resistance to rebalancing: inflammation, biofilms, and protozoa.

In "Remove Protocol Level 2," we add in natural compounds that reduce inflammation, break open the biofilms certain bugs can hide in, and kill unwanted protozoa (protozoa are like advanced bacteria).

The level 2 protocol consists of adding in artemisia, NAC (N-acetylcysteine), and InterFase Plus. These will be in addition to the level 1 herbal antimicrobials that you're already taking. You will be repeating level 1, with the addition of level 2. Here is what this looks like:

### Month One (taken again, just as before)

- Biota-Clear 1a—take three pills twice a day
- Biota-Clear 1b—take two pills twice a day

### Month Two (taken again, just as before)

- Biota-Clear 2a—take two pills twice a day
- Biota-Clear 2b—take three pills twice a day

### Plus the following during Level 2 Months One and Two

- NAC—one capsule twice per day, preferably with food; this will require two bottles total, one per month
- Biota-Dissolve—two capsules twice per day, preferably without food; this will require two bottles total, one per month

### And follow a special dosing schedule for artemisia as artemisinin

- This has a dosing schedule of one week on, followed by a two-week break, followed by one more week on. So, take Artemisinin for week one, then do not take it for weeks two and three, and then take it for one more week (week four). Then you are done for good.
- During the "on" weeks, take 600 mg in the morning and another 600 mg in the evening, preferably on an empty stomach. This will require two bottles.

### Check with your doctor before starting "Remove Protocol Level 2."

## REMOVE PROTOCOL LEVEL 2 MONTH-ONE ANTIMICROBIALS

| Name | Dose | Times/ Day | w/ Food | Bottles Needed |
|------|------|------------|---------|----------------|
| Biota-Clear 1a | 3 pills | 2 | Best w/o | 3 |
| Biota-Clear 1b | 2 pills | 2 | Best w/o | 2 |

## REMOVE PROTOCOL LEVEL 2 MONTH-TWO ANTIMICROBIALS

| Name | Dose | Times/ Day | w/ Food | Bottles Needed |
|------|------|------------|---------|----------------|
| Biota-Clear 2a | 2 pills | 2 | Best w/o | 2 |
| Biota-Clear 2b | 3 pills | 2 | Best w/o | 2 |

## REMOVE PROTOCOL LEVEL 2 ANTI-INFLAMMATORY AND ANTIBIOFILM SUPPORT (MONTHS ONE AND TWO)

| Name | Dose | Times/ Day | w/ Food | Bottles Needed |
|------|------|------------|---------|----------------|
| Artemisinin | See special dosing instructions, above | N | | 2 |
| Biota-Dissolve | 3 pills | 2 | Best w/o | 2 |
| NAC | 3 pills | 3 | Y | 2 |

## REASSESSING

At the end of Remove Protocol Level 2, most people are feeling much better. If you are, move on to Step 4 "Rebalance." If you are still not feeling better or have had reactions to all the antimicrobials, there is one more strategy we can try: an elemental or semielemental diet.

## REMOVE PROTOCOL LEVEL 3—THE ELEMENTAL AND SEMIELEMENTAL DIETS

At this point in our Great-in-8, most people will have experienced noticeable improvement. But there are some who may only feel slightly better or those who have had negative reactions to the antimicrobials. I have found using an elemental or semielemental diet to be a game changer for many of these patients. We discussed the elemental diets in chapter 18, but as a refresher, these are liquid diets that can have different forms, usually elemental or semielemental. These diets can help with IBS, intestinal inflammation, intestinal autoimmunity, celiac disease, and perhaps general autoimmunity.

This liquid-only diet can be incredibly reparative, antibacterial, and anti-inflammatory for your gut. If you have a gut "injury" and are eating three times a day, it can be hard for the gut to heal. Using a liquid diet can give your gut a break and aid in healing the same way avoiding activity can help heal a sprained ankle.

As we discussed before, I suspect that another reason an elemental diet works so well is because it has an especially favorable impact on the small intestine. The small intestine houses the majority of your immune system and is most prone to damage and leaky gut—it's a very important but underappreciated part of your digestive system.

## HOW MUCH?

Let's revisit the guidelines for the elemental and semielemental diets. You can consume as much of the liquid as you desire. If you're feeling hungry, drink some more. It's best to sip on the solution throughout the day, instead of consuming large amounts in short periods. Sipping throughout the day will help keep a steady supply of nutrients and calories in your system, which will help prevent hunger and fatigue (it will also help prevent low blood sugar, if you have this tendency). While you're on the diet, you can engage in normal activity, but you might want to avoid highly rigorous exercise. Be sure to get plenty of rest and to drink water throughout the day.

## HOW LONG?

Elemental diets can be used in one of three general ways in terms of length.

### Short term, as a reset

When used in the short-term, the elemental or semielemental diet is used exclusively (your only source of calories) for two to four days. This can be very helpful to quell a flare.

### Exclusive liquid nutrition

For one to three weeks, your only source of calories is the liquid shakes you make. This is using the elemental diet as a more formal treatment. As we saw in the research, this approach has been shown to be very helpful; however, this should be done under the supervision of a doctor.

It may sound daunting, but many patients tell me

- *they feel so good that they don't even miss food;*
- *they were not hungry and had no cravings;*
- *it was actually very convenient not to have to worry about food and to be able to simply sip on their shakes throughout the day.*

### Longer term, with intermittent/hybrid use

Elemental diets can also be used intermittently as a gut-healing tool. The intermittent or hybrid use means that you get some of your calories from an elemental/semielemental formula and the rest of your calories from normal food; it's a combination of normal food plus an elemental diet. This could be a daily use, with half food and half elemental, or it could be 70% food and 30% elemental or vice versa. If you use the hybrid approach, I recommend you experiment to find a method of incorporation that feels best to you—there is no set rule. For example, many patients like using one of these shakes as a meal replacement for breakfast, every day or most days. Some use the shakes as a meal replacement for breakfast *and* lunch and then eat a nice, big whole-foods dinner. Or some patients will do one full day of exclusive liquid nutrition per week. Others may only use elemental diets on and off, occasionally, when they feel like their guts are in need of a break. They may do anywhere from one to four days until symptoms have subsided—this is more like the reset approach.

## WHICH APPROACH IS BEST FOR YOU?

We discussed this earlier, but the points are worth repeating. Remember, it's best to use the elemental diet under a doctor's or health-care provider's supervision, but here are some guidelines to discuss with your doctor regarding an intermittent or hybrid use of the elemental diet.

A good way to start is with a two-to-four-day trial. Depending on how well you do with that, you may want to extend the diet for one to three weeks. How long you perform the diet really depends on the severity of your condition and how quickly you respond. As a general rule,

> **the greater the severity, the longer the duration.**

Listen to your body, and when you feel like you have achieved the maximum benefit, then it's a good time to transition to the hybrid approach. The longer you are on the elemental diet, the more important it is to transition to a hybrid approach.

For example, if you performed the elemental diet for two days and felt 90% improved, you could simply transition back to whole foods using the "Transitioning Back to Whole Foods" tips we cover in step 1a of the Great-in-8 plan. However, if you were on the elemental diet for two weeks, you should transition to the hybrid approach. Again, the hybrid approach is when some of your daily nutrition is from whole foods and some is from the elemental-diet shakes. For example, you could have a shake for breakfast, a shake for lunch, and then have a whole-foods dinner. Over time,

you'd gradually decrease the number of shakes while increasing the amount of whole foods you eat in a day.

Elemental/semielemental diets have been used like this in long-term studies. These studies have shown consuming as much as half your calories from a liquid solution can decrease inflammation and autoimmunity in the small intestine, and that this is safe. We will cover this information when we discuss safety.

Bear in mind that over time, you should be continually working toward the minimum use of elemental diets. While these diets are designed to be complete nutritional sources and have been shown to be safe when used long-term, it's still best to get as much of your nutrition from whole foods as possible.

## HOW TO MAKE THEM

For those of you who are wondering, here is a reminder of how to make the shakes. It's actually very simple. Just follow the instructions on the bottle. The shakes come in powder form, and you blend them with ice and water to make a shake. If the label instructs you to, you can add in a source of healthy fat. It's very easy. Mix and drink. There are only two exceptions: for the homemade elemental diet and some of the commercial semielemental diets. For the homemade elemental diet, just follow the instructions on www.DrRuscio.com/GutBook. Some of the commercial semielemental diets come premixed, in a can, similar to other diet shakes. Simply open and drink. You may want to dilute these with some water or even blend with water and ice.

Elemental Heal calls for the addition of fat. If you are highly sensitive, you may want to try it for a day or two without fat and see how you do and then gradually add in fat. Udo's Oil 3·6·9 Blend is a good option that will work well for most. An MCT oil (medium-chain triglyceride oil) can also work well, especially if you are constipated. MCT oil can have a laxative effect, so be careful with it if you are prone to diarrhea. You can also try coconut oil, olive oil, cod-liver oil, or fish oil. Follow the dosing instructions listed on the Elemental Heal bottle.

## SUPPLEMENTS AND MEDICATIONS DURING AN ELEMENTAL DIET

During the elemental diet, continue any prescribed medications. Also, make sure to speak with your doctor before performing an elemental diet to make sure it's safe for you to do so.

There are no set rules on taking supplements during the elemental diet, but here is what I would recommend: For the first few days, don't take any supplements; this will allow you to isolate for the effects of the elemental diet. Then consider adding in probiotics and antimicrobial herbs, and see if you feel even better with these. Of course, if you had a reaction to a probiotic or an antimicrobial, do not add it back in.

## REACTIONS

Reactions on an elemental diet can occur. The *best* elemental diet is usually the one that causes the *fewest* reactions. However, it's also important to give a particular formula a few days to assess how well it works for you. Some patients will notice they don't feel well until a few days in, so hang in there. If after two or three days, you're not any better, you may want to try a different version. Some common reactions that can occur are white tongue, diarrhea, bloating, gas, constipation, abdominal upset, and fatigue.

## TRANSITIONING BACK TO WHOLE FOODS

The concepts we covered in step 1A about transitioning back to solid foods after the modified fast apply to the elemental diet as well, so let's go over them again. When you start eating solid foods again, go slow: start with smaller meals rather than large ones. Opt for softer foods, like steamed veggies, rice, and soups, rather than hard foods, like raw veggies and charred meats.

A great time to listen to how your body reacts to certain foods is when you're transitioning back to solid foods. People will often notice they can pick out a specific food that doesn't agree with them after performing the elemental diet. To help make this easier, it's best to limit the number of new foods you eat at once. For example, on your first day of eating foods, try to limit yourself to one or two vegetables and one protein. Eat this food for a day or two, then move to a different vegetable and protein for another day or two. Doing this will help you isolate how you react to a certain food. There are no exact rules, but the guiding principle is to reintroduce just a couple of foods every one or two days, so that if you do have a reaction, you'll know what food you're reacting to. Don't overthink this step; just do your best. You're taking huge steps to start feeling better!

If you've been using the elemental diet for a week or longer, you may want to consider transitioning to a hybrid approach—part food and part liquid. There are no set rules on exactly what the best method is, but here is an example: For your first three days, you have only elemental-diet shakes except for one whole-foods meal. Then, for the next three days, you have half liquid diet and half whole foods. Then, for a few more days, you replace breakfast with an elemental-diet shake but all your other meals are whole foods. It's a gradual transition. This is not required, but for many this gradual transition works best.

## THREE STEPS FORWARD, ONE STEP BACK

This is a very important concept for us to cover. When you're on an elemental/semielemental diet, you may feel the best you have in a long time, which is great. However, when you transition back to whole foods, you may notice you don't feel as well as when you were on the elemental diet. You will likely feel better than you did before starting the elemental diet, but you might feel like you regressed when going back onto whole foods. Patients often think this means it didn't work or that they're "broken." This couldn't be further from the truth. This is a healing *process*. Your gut will heal gradually, and your symptoms (including food reactivity) will also diminish gradually. So, if you feel like you've taken three steps forward and one step back, remember that this is good: you're two steps more healed than you were before. Healing can take time, so be patient.

## REASSESSING

At this point, we've gone through some of the best treatments available for improving your gut health and rebalancing your microbiota. This should have you feeling noticeably better than you were before. If you don't feel 100% "fixed" yet, don't worry. Time is an important factor, meaning your body may need additional time before you realize full improvement. There are also a few more important steps to come in our Great-in-8, so stick with it. As long as we continue to make forward progress, we're doing OK.

**GUT GEEKS**

*If you have come this far and have still not noticeably improved, histamine intolerance might be a problem for you. This is particularly the case if you've been eating lots of fermented foods and historically have been using probiotics. Many "healthy" foods are high in histamines, and for those who are histamine sensitive, this can be a problem. A quick search in our website's search box or on the Internet will reveal a general list of high-histamine foods. If you're eating lots of these, consider the low-histamine diet (which most of the articles you find online will outline). The effects should be noticeable within a few days, so it's a quick and fairly easy trial to run.*

Are you feeling overwhelmed with supplements? This step in our program is the most intense in terms of the amount of supplements to take. It's important that I mention the goal is to have you on little to nothing in the long term. We are working now to correct imbalance and heal your gut so that you can maintain improvements in the long term with little to no supplementation. We will work to reduce your program to the minimum in step 7 "Wean." As you can see from the diagram, step 3 requires the most supplementation. But the good news is it gets easier from here. So hang in there!

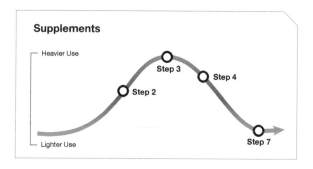

## STEP 3 ACTION-PLAN SUMMARY

- Perform the level 1 antimicrobial protocol.
- If you don't respond completely, perform the level 2 protocol.
- If you have a negative reaction to the antimicrobials or don't fully respond after performing the level 2 protocol, try the level 3 protocol—the elemental/semielemental diet.

Now that we have given the microbiota a nudge with antimicrobials and, if needed, antibiofilm and antiprotozoal agents, and maybe even an elemental diet, it can start to rebalance itself. This leads to our next step, which is designed to aid in rebalancing.

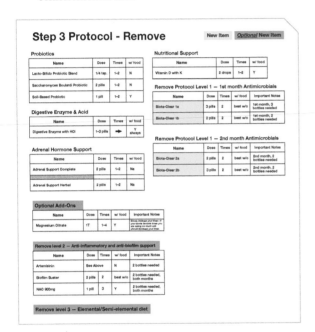

### Step 3 Protocol - Remove     New Item   *Optional* New Item

**Probiotics**

| Name | Dose | Times | w/ food |
|------|------|-------|---------|
| Lacto-Bifido Probiotic Blend | 1/4 tsp. | 1–2 | N |
| Saccharomyces Boulardi Probiotic | 2 pills | 1–2 | N |
| Soil-Based Probiotic | 1 pill | 1–2 | Y |

**Digestive Enzyme & Acid**

| Name | Dose | Times | w/ food |
|------|------|-------|---------|
| Digestive Enzyme with HCl | 1–3 pills | ➡ | Y always |

**Adrenal Hormone Support**

| Name | Dose | Times | w/ food |
|------|------|-------|---------|
| Adrenal Support Complete | 2 pills | 1–2 | Na |
| Adrenal Support Herbal | 2 pills | 1–2 | Na |

**Nutritional Support**

| Name | Dose | Times | w/ food |
|------|------|-------|---------|
| Vitamin D with K | 2 drops | 1–2 | Y |

**Remove Protocol Level 1 — 1st month Antimicrobials**

| Name | Dose | Times | w/ food | Important Notes |
|------|------|-------|---------|-----------------|
| Biota-Clear 1a | 3 pills | 2 | best w/o | 1st month, 3 bottles needed |
| Biota-Clear 1b | 2 pills | 2 | best w/o | 1st month, 2 bottles needed |

**Remove Protocol Level 1 — 2nd month Antimicrobials**

| Name | Dose | Times | w/ food | Important Notes |
|------|------|-------|---------|-----------------|
| Biota-Clear 2a | 2 pills | 2 | best w/o | 2nd month, 2 bottles needed |
| Biota-Clear 2b | 3 pills | 2 | best w/o | 2nd month, 2 bottles needed |

**Optional Add-Ons**

| Name | Dose | Times | w/ food | Important Notes |
|------|------|-------|---------|-----------------|
| Magnesium Citrate | 1T | 1–4 | Y | Slowly increase your dose—if your stools become loose you are using too much and should decrease your dose. |

**Remove level 2 — Anti-inflammatory and anti-biofilm support**

| Name | Dose | Times | w/ food | Important Notes |
|------|------|-------|---------|-----------------|
| Artemisinin | See Above | N | | 2 bottles needed |
| Biofilm Buster | 2 pills | 2 | best w/o | 2 bottles needed, both months |
| NAC 900mg | 1 pill | 3 | Y | 2 bottles needed, both months |

**Remove level 3 — Elemental/Semi-elemental diet**

1   Rong Zhu et al., "Meta-Analysis of the Efficacy of Probiotics in Helicobacter Pylori Eradication Therapy," *World Journal of Gastroenterology* 20, no. 47 (2014): 18013–21, doi:10.3748/wjg.v20.i47.18013; Min-Min Zhang et al., "Probiotics in Helicobacter Pylori Eradication Therapy: A Systematic Review and Meta-Analysis," *World Journal of Gastroenterology: WJG* 21, no. 14 (2015): 4345–57, doi:10.3748/wjg.v21.i14.4345; Ener Cagri Dinleyici et al., "Saccharomyces Boulardii CNCM I-745 in Different Clinical Conditions," *Expert Opinion on Biological Therapy* July (2014): 1–17, doi:10.1517/14712598.2014.937419; H. Szajewska et al., "Systematic Review with Meta-Analysis: Saccharomyces Boulardii Supplementation and Eradication of Helicobacter Pylori Infection," *Alimentary Pharmacology & Therapeutics* 41, no. 12 (2015): 1237–45, doi:10.1111/apt.13214.

2   Gamze Demirel et al., "Prophylactic Saccharomyces Boulardii versus Nystatin for the Prevention of Fungal Colonization and Invasive Fungal Infection in Premature Infants," *European Journal of Pediatrics* 172, no. 10 (2013): 1321–26, doi:10.1007/s00431-013-2041-4.

3   Ener Cagri Dinleyici et al., "Clinical Efficacy of Saccharomyces Boulardii or Metronidazole in Symptomatic Children with Blastocystis Hominis Infection," *Parasitology Research* 108, no. 3 (2011): 541–45, doi:10.1007/s00436-010-2095-4; Bulent Besirbellioglu et al., "Saccharomyces Boulardii and Infection Due to Giardia Lamblia," *Scandinavian Journal of Infectious Diseases* 38, no. 6–7 (2006): 479–81, doi:10.1080/00365540600561769.

# CHAPTER 27

# STEP 4: REBALANCE

## STEP 4: REBALANCE GUT BACTERIA AFTER TREATMENT WITH ANTIMICROBIAL HERBS

Once we have removed/reduced bacteria and fungi that shouldn't be there, the ecosystem of your gut will start to rebalance all on its own. However, there are a couple of things we can do now to gently aid in this rebalancing. You will notice the steps from here on tend to be easier than our first three steps. This is because we have gone through most of the major interventions, and now we just focus on fine-tuning and personalization.

## TRANSITIONING TO STEP 4

At this point you should be done with the two-month (or more) antimicrobial program from step 3. When starting step 4, maintain the same diet and lifestyle you've already established. Don't forget that *you* create the internal environment that influences the balance of your microbiota. Continue with level 2's supports (adrenal support, digestive enzymes/acid, probiotics). Remember that probiotics will help the microbiota return more quickly into balance after the nudge we gave it with the antimicrobials.[1] In step 3, *if* you performed the elemental/semielemental diet and responded well, you may have also transitioned to a hybrid approach. If so, continue the hybrid diet during step 4.

Now, we will add an agent that helps your gut bacteria return to optimum balance—a prokinetic. What is a prokinetic? Prokinetics are agents that support healthy motility in your stomach and intestines. Motility just means that food moves through your intestinal tract at the right pace. When food moves through at the appropriate pace, it keeps your bacteria in balance. However, if food is moving too slowly, it can cause bacteria to overgrow. We want to make sure things are flowing through your intestinal tract and not stagnant to prevent bacterial or fungal overgrowths.

# PROKINETICS PROTOCOL

### OPTION ONE—MOTILPRO

MotilPro can be dosed one of two ways. You can take four to six capsules before bed, or you can take two capsules three times a day in between meals. Either method works; choose one based upon your personal preference.

MotilPro contains a fair amount of ginger, and this can sometimes cause a reaction known as ginger burn. This typically manifests as indigestion, stomach burning, or a general feeling of digestive irritation. If you notice this reaction, MotilPro is probably not a good choice for you.

*Prokinetics Option One*

| Name | Dose | Times/Day | w/Food | Notes |
|------|------|-----------|--------|-------|
| MotilPro | 4–6 capsules | Once before bed | N | You can also dose as 2 capsules 3x/day between meals |

### OPTION TWO—IBEROGAST

Iberogast has limited availability in the United States. It can be dosed one of two ways: you can take sixty drops before bed, or you can take twenty drops three times a day, in between meals. Either method works; choose based upon your personal preference.

*Prokinetics Option Two*

| Name | Dose | Times/Day | w/Food | Notes |
|------|------|-----------|--------|-------|
| Iberogast | 60 drops | Once before bed | N | You can also dose as 20 drops 3x/day between meals |

### OPTION THREE—PRESCRIPTION ALTERNATIVE

Low-dose erythromycin or low-dose naltrexone are two prescription prokinetics that can be used.

We discussed low-dose erythromycin in chapter 19, but we haven't discussed low-dose naltrexone. You can think of low-dose erythromycin or low-dose naltrexone as a milder replacement for the tegaserod we discussed in chapter 19. You will need to check in with your doctor for specifics on these and to determine if either of these are right for you. Low-dose erythromycin is usually given at a dose between 50 mg and 62.5 mg one to two times per day. Low-dose naltrexone is usually given at a dose starting at 1 mg and slowly built to as much as 4.5 mg per day. Low-dose Resolor (prucalopride) can also be used at 0.5 mg to 1.0 mg per day. This drug is more difficult to obtain because it is not available in the United States. If you live in the United States, your doctor would be required to write a prescription, and then you would obtain it through a pharmacy outside the United States.

### HOW DO YOU KNOW IF A PROKINETIC IS WORKING?

Since prokinetics are a preventive measure, they don't cause much of a symptomatic change in most. So, most people don't feel much different while on them. However, if you don't take a prokinetic, there is an increased chance that weeks or months later you will notice your symptoms returning. However, some *do* notice their digestion improves. If people are constipated, they may notice improved bowel frequency. Sometimes people report feeling like "things are moving" better in their digestive tracts or that their symptoms of indigestion are improved. Whether you feel improvements or not, stay on the prokinetic until we wean you off it in step 7 "Wean."

# REASSESSING— IMPORTANT

We've just added a prokinetic to aid with intestinal motility. This is a key moment in our process. This is when we're hoping that your gut ecosystem returns to a healthy balance after a little nudge from the antimicrobial step. Time is an important factor in determining this. For many, as the weeks go by, they will maintain their improvements or even continue to improve. This means the ecosystem has achieved a healthy balance.

However, there are some people who will regress during step 4. They go from feeling well to slowly returning to feeling how they did before. For these people, the ecosystem hasn't achieved a healthy balance and has likely slipped back into an unhealthy state. If you're one of these people, don't worry—it's OK. This just means that your microbiota may need a little more attention to get back to balance. If you notice that you regress during step 4, here are a few things to ask yourself:

- Have I drifted back to old eating habits?
  - » Sometimes when people are feeling better, they get careless with their diet. You may have started to eat more unhealthy foods than your gut is ready to tolerate and need to return to a stricter diet for a short time.
- Have I drifted back to poor lifestyle habits?
  - » When you start feeling better, it's easy to begin doing more, sleeping less, skipping exercise, or not taking your walks in nature. You may need to return to healthier lifestyle practices again.

If you answered yes to the above and are experiencing a regression, don't be discouraged. You might have simply done too much too soon. It doesn't mean anything is wrong or broken but just that you need to revisit some of these healthy diet and lifestyle principles for a while. You'll get a chance to try relaxing the boundaries on diet and lifestyle later.

***What if you have kept your diet and lifestyle somewhat constant and still appear to be regressing during step 4?***
This is also OK and doesn't necessarily mean anything is wrong. This usually indicates we need to revisit the antimicrobial step, step 3. More specifically, this usually means one of two things:

1. You may need to revisit the antimicrobial approach of step 3 again and give your gut microbiota another nudge. You can perform the two-month antimicrobial program from step 3 up to three times. Sometimes the microbiota just needs a little more nudging to rebalance.
2. You may also need to advance one level in the three available protocol levels of step three. For example, add in level 2's supports if you have not done them yet, or you may need to go to level 3 and incorporate the elemental-diet approach if you did not perform it yet.

## FOR THE MOST STUBBORN CASES
After some time and observation, you may notice you always feel better when you're on antimicrobials in step 3 and then *repeatedly* regress in step 4. If this is you, you may need low-dose cyclical antimicrobial therapy.

## LOW-DOSE CYCLICAL ANTIMICROBIAL THERAPY
If you notice that you feel best when you're *on* antimicrobials and not as well when you come *off* them, you may wonder whether you can just take antimicrobials indefinitely. For some patients a modified version of the antimicrobials in the longer term may be necessary. This is known as low-dose cyclical antimicrobial therapy and might look like someone performing the following:

*Low-Dose Cyclical Antimicrobials*

| Name | Dose | Times/Day | w/Food | Notes |
|------|------|-----------|--------|-------|
| Biota-Clear 1a | 2–3 pills | 1 | best w/o | For 1 month only, then switch |
| Biota-Clear 1b | 2–3 pills | 1 | best w/o | For 1 month only, then switch |
| Biota-Clear 2a | 2–3 pills | 1 | best w/o | For 1 month only, then switch |
| Biota-Clear 2b | 2–3 pills | 1 | best w/o | For 1 month only, then repeat from first month |

In low-dose cyclical antimicrobial therapy, you take a low dose of one antimicrobial formula at a time and rotate the antimicrobial formula from month to month. After you've done this for several months, try to slowly wean yourself off them and see how you do. Remember, you should always be working toward the *minimal* amount of supplements needed. Please note you only take one antimicrobial formula at a time. Don't look at the antimicrobials as an easy way to alleviate symptoms, one that allows you to disregard healthy diet and lifestyle. It may be possible to develop resistance to antimicrobials, so we do not want to rely on them exclusively.[2]

## HOW DO YOU KNOW IF YOU SHOULD REVISIT STEP 3 OR PRESS FORWARD TO STEP 5?

First, remember that if you are merely reading this and not performing the steps, it will be much harder to gauge. Most of these decisions will be apparent as you actually go through the process. So, if during your first read it doesn't seem clear, don't worry. Here are some additional guidelines:

- If during step 4 you have experienced a minor regression, say roughly by 30%, give yourself some time, and stay in step 4 for a few more weeks. It's possible your body needs more time to adjust, and you will be better in a few weeks. It's also possible

that you will achieve the lost 30% of improvement as you continue through the rest of our steps.

- If during step 4 you are experiencing a major regression, over 50%, then revisiting step 3, as we just outlined, makes sense.

## WHEN IS THE IDEAL TIME TO TRANSITION TO STEP 5?

Step 5 is where you start eating a less restrictive diet. We remove dietary restrictions and determine where your dietary boundaries are. Staying in step 4 longer is the more conservative approach.

It's best to stay in step 4 for at least four weeks, but you can stay here for up to four months. How quickly you move through this step depends on you:

- If you have been battling somewhat severe symptoms for a while, you may not want to rock the boat. It's a good idea to stay in step 4 for a while, letting your gut heal and enjoying the relief from your symptoms.
- If you had only minor symptoms to begin with, you may want to move on to step 5 more quickly (after one month) to see what additional benefits you can obtain from our subsequent steps and to be able to eat some foods that you're missing.

## IN SUMMARY

- If you have a significant relapse during step 4, evaluate if you have drifted back to poor dietary or lifestyle habits. If you have, try revisiting a stricter dietary and lifestyle plan.
- If you are still following a good diet and lifestyle plan, you may want to revisit aspects of step 3 as we outlined above.
- Move to step 5 after spending anywhere from one to four months in step 4.

# STEP 4 ACTION-PLAN SUMMARY

- Maintain the same diet and lifestyle we have already established. Continue with step 2's program: adrenal support, digestive support, and probiotics.
- If in step 3 you performed the elemental/semielemental diet and responded well, you may want to consider transitioning to a hybrid approach during step 4.
- Take a prokinetic.
- Consider revisiting aspects of step 3 if you regress in step 4.
- Move to step 5 after spending anywhere from one to four months in step 4.

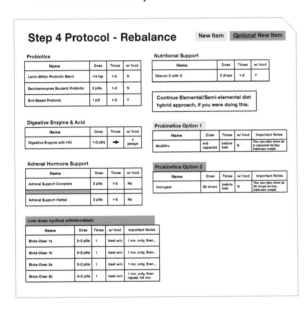

**Step 4 Protocol - Rebalance**  New Item  *Optional* New Item

**Probiotics**

| Name | Dose | Times | w/ food |
|---|---|---|---|
| Lacto-Bifido Probiotic Blend | 1/4 tsp. | 1-2 | N |
| Saccharomyces Boulardi Probiotic | 2 pills | 1-2 | N |
| Soil-Based Probiotic | 1 pill | 1-2 | Y |

**Nutritional Support**

| Name | Dose | Times | w/ food |
|---|---|---|---|
| Vitamin D with K | 2 drops | 1-2 | Y |

Continue Elemental/Semi-elemental diet hybrid approach, if you were doing this.

**Digestive Enzyme & Acid**

| Name | Dose | Times | w/ food |
|---|---|---|---|
| Digestive Enzyme with HCl | 1-3 pills | ➡ | Y always |

**Prokinetics Option 1**

| Name | Dose | Times | w/ food | Important Notes |
|---|---|---|---|---|
| MotilPro | 4-6 capsules | before bed | N | You can also dose as 2 capsules 3x/day between meals |

**Adrenal Hormone Support**

| Name | Dose | Times | w/ food |
|---|---|---|---|
| Adrenal Support Complete | 2 pills | 1-2 | No |
| Adrenal Support Herbal | 2 pills | 1-2 | No |

**Prokinetics Option 2**

| Name | Dose | Times | w/ food | Important Notes |
|---|---|---|---|---|
| Iberogast | 60 drops | before bed | N | You can also dose as 20 drops 3x/day between meals |

**Low-dose cyclical antimicrobials**

| Name | Dose | Times | w/ food | Important Notes |
|---|---|---|---|---|
| Biota-Clear 1a | 2-3 pills | 1 | best w/o | 1 mo. only, then... |
| Biota-Clear 1b | 2-3 pills | 1 | best w/o | 1 mo. only, then... |
| Biota-Clear 2a | 2-3 pills | 1 | best w/o | 1 mo. only, then... |
| Biota-Clear 2b | 2-3 pills | 1 | best w/o | 1 mo. only, then repeat 1st mo. |

1    Mary Ellen Sanders, "Impact of Probiotics on Colonizing Microbiota of the Gut," *Journal of Clinical Gastroenterology* 45 Suppl., no. December (2011): S115–9, doi:10.1097/MCG.0b013e318227414a.

2    Kisaburo Nagamune et al., "Artemisinin-Resistant Mutants of Toxoplasma Gondii Have Altered Calcium Homeostasis," *Antimicrobial Agents and Chemotherapy* 51, no. 11 (2007): 3816–23, doi:10.1128/AAC.00582-07.

# CHAPTER 28

# STEP 5: REINTRODUCE

## STEP 5: REINTRODUCE FOODS YOU REMOVED IN STEP 3

### ORIENTATION TO STEP 5

Welcome to step 5. Let's all get on the same page, because there are three different groups of people who will be arriving at step 5:

- Those coming from step 1 (who skipped steps 2–4)
- Those coming from step 2 (who skipped steps 3–4)
- Those who did not skip any steps and are coming from step 4

Regardless of which step you've just completed, you should perform this reintroduction step. It's important to mention that those of you who went through more steps have a higher chance of reaction and should be more cautious with your reintroduction step. Whichever steps have led you to this one, stay on the program that we have established through our previous steps. Here is what this should look like:

- Those coming from step 1 on their personalized diets after completing step 1
- Those coming from step 2 on the step 2 protocol plus their personalized diets
- Those who did not skip any steps and from step 4 on the step 4 protocol plus their personalized diets

Now that we have worked to rebalance and heal your gut, there is an excellent chance you will be able to tolerate foods you were not able to tolerate before. This is a great time to perform a reintroduction to discover any newly found food freedom. Almost everyone will notice an increased ability to tolerate foods that were previously problematic, *but* you will also likely notice a handful of foods don't work for you. Let's cover the specifics of the reintroduction.

# REINTRODUCTION GUIDELINES AND ENJOYING NEW FOOD FREEDOM

Once you're feeling better and feel somewhat stable in that improvement, it's a good time to reintroduce. How long should you feel improved and stable before proceeding? This could be anywhere from a couple of weeks to a couple of months. This partially depends on how severe your symptoms were—generally speaking, the worse your symptoms were, the longer you should wait to perform the reintroduction. It also depends on where you are mentally. For example, if you really miss certain foods, you may want to perform the reintroduction sooner rather than later. When you feel the urge to move on, go ahead. It's important to wait to reintroduce until you're somewhat stable, because we will monitor to see if a new food causes a fluctuation in how you feel. So, we need a somewhat stable baseline to compare against. The principle of eliminating foods and then later reintroducing them can be applied to the main aspects of our dietary plan:

- Allergens (which we removed with the Paleo and autoimmune-Paleo diets)
- Foods that feed bacteria (which we addressed with the low-FODMAP diet)
- Carb intake

The overarching principles of eliminating problematic foods and then reintroducing them are as follows:

1. Remove something for about two to four weeks and then see how you feel (in my experience people usually feel at least 30% better after eliminating problematic foods).
2. Gradually reintroduce what you cut out, and see if you notice regression in any of the improvements you were experiencing.

You may be reintroducing non-Paleo foods, like dairy. Or you may reintroduce high-FODMAP foods, like cauliflower. The negative reactions or regressions can apply to any symptom. The specific symptom is not important. What is important is that you notice if a symptom reappears after reintroducing a certain food.

How exactly should you reintroduce? Again, the rules here are not rigid, so don't stress yourself in attempts to be perfect. There are, however, a few principles that you should adhere to.

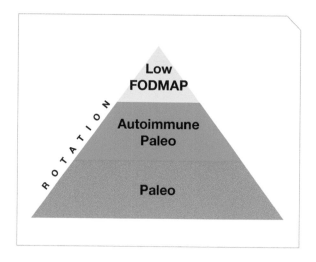

*The first principle is to reintroduce the most restrictive foods first.* Looking at our pyramid helps visualize this. You eliminate from the base up and then reintroduce from the top down. So, wherever you are on the pyramid, you reintroduce from that position down. For example, reintroduce FODMAPs *before* reintroducing non-Paleo foods. Also, try to reintroduce the least problematic foods first, as depicted in this diagram.

*The next principle is to try to reintroduce foods one at a time.* If you reintroduce many foods at once, like dairy, soy, gluten—you won't be able to pinpoint what is causing a reaction. For example, if you're trying to determine if you have a problem with dairy, pizza is not a good reintroduction test food, because you're getting dairy and gluten.

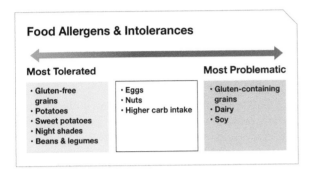

**Food Allergens & Intolerances**

| Most Tolerated | | Most Problematic |
|---|---|---|
| • Gluten-free grains<br>• Potatoes<br>• Sweet potatoes<br>• Night shades<br>• Beans & legumes | • Eggs<br>• Nuts<br>• Higher carb intake | • Gluten-containing grains<br>• Dairy<br>• Soy |

*The next principle is to try to have a few servings a day, for a few days.* You need to have enough of a food to see if it causes a reaction. By "enough," I mean you need to have an adequate amount (dose) and number of servings (number of doses). For example, having a spoonful of dairy might not be enough to cause a reaction. Also, having only one serving might not be enough—you might only notice a reaction after your third serving. I can have one serving of espresso a day, three or four times a week, with no problems. But if I have it more often than this or if I have more than one serving in a day, I start to feel bloated and tired.

This bring us to an important concept. Are food allergies all or nothing? In my opinion, no. There tends to be variability: some people can tolerate more or less of a certain food than others. With time and observation, you will home in on what your problem foods are, how much of them you can have, and how often. Again, don't over-think this. Just start to broaden your diet when performing your reintroduction and observe how you feel—with time and observation you will settle into the ideal diet for you. Trust your gut here—pun intended.

*Another principle to remember is the more severe your intolerance, the more obvious it will be upon reintroduction.* Sometimes, patients become overly analytical and painstakingly analyze if they may or may not have had a food reaction. Do not do this—it creates unneeded stress. If you have a severe allergy, it will be more important to avoid a food. Fortunately, a more severe allergy means you also have a more severe reaction. Conversely, if it's a minor allergy, it's less important to avoid and reactions are usually less strong. Gluten, dairy, and soy are good examples of this. Some patients do fine with these foods. But some have severe and very clear reactions. So, I advise my patients to practice avoidance that corresponds with their level of reaction. The worse the reaction, the more you should avoid it. Simple and practical, right?

*The final principle is you should periodically revisit your reintroduction.* With time, and as your gut heals, you will likely have fewer allergies, so you should periodically revisit the reintroduction. After eating healthy for one year, you will likely be able to tolerate more foods than after eating healthy for one month. Again, this is because your gut, your microbiota, and your immune system will have had longer to heal and balance.

Does this seem like a lot? This aspect of diet can be the most overwhelming for people. Your outlook on this is important. Here are a few things I have found helpful. First, remember to take this one step at a time—change can be a gradual process. Initially, some of this may seem hard or foreign, but with a little practice and planning, I think you'll be surprised by how quickly eating this way becomes second nature. Try to look at this as a chance to see how great you can feel and as an opportunity to load your body with healthy food and nutrients. Focus on this and not on what you can't eat. Remember—it's not all or nothing. If you miss a meal here or there, it's OK. You won't ruin the diet if you do. I tell my patients,

> *"If you are 100% compliant, you can reap 100% of the rewards. If you are 80% compliant, you can reap 80% of the rewards, and 80% is still pretty darn good."*

As long as it's done within reason (not excessively), eating off plan is a good chance to test your boundaries and should not be looked at like failure. Enjoy it! Finally, remember we are all human, and sometimes life gets in the way. Do your best, and if you have a setback, turn your gaze forward, and don't beat yourself up.

## WHERE DO CARBS FIT INTO THE REINTRODUCTION?

As we touched on earlier, you'll naturally start to reintroduce carbs as you work through the reintroduction we discussed above. This is because as you work up the pyramid, there tend to be fewer carbs allowed; and, of course, when you work down the pyramid (that is, you reintroduce foods) there are more carbs allowed. However, just because there are more carbs allowed on the diet doesn't mean you should eat more carbs. Listening to your body will help you determine what "more carbs" should mean for you. Let's revisit the guidelines from chapter 8 for predicting if you will do better on a higher- or lower-carb diet:

**You may do better on a lower-carb diet (100 grams/day or less) if**
- you have tried a lower-carb diet and felt good;
- you have a family history of diabetes;
- you have diabetes or prediabetes (type 2);
- you are overweight;
- you crave carbs or can't stop eating carbs/sugar once you start eating them;

- you are of a more northern descent than equatorial descent (Irish versus Venezuelan, for example).

**You may do better on a moderate-carb diet (100–175 grams/day or more) if**
- you have tried a higher-carb diet and felt good;
- you are an athlete or highly active;
- you need to gain weight;
- you are of a more equatorial descent than northern descent (Venezuelan versus Irish, for example).

**How to know if you aren't eating enough carbs:**
If you have been eating a lower-carb diet for a while and feel like your health is regressing, you may want to try increasing your carbs. Common symptoms of not eating enough carbs include fatigue, insomnia, irritability, carb cravings, brain fog, feeling cold, and digestive upset. If you increase your carbs and feel better, you have confirmation that your diet was too low carb. If you increase your carbs but don't notice any change, carbs are probably not the issue.

How, specifically, should you reintroduce carbs? Good news! This fits in nicely with our reintroduction step. First, we need to determine if you tolerate sources of carbs (like rice or potatoes). You'll be testing this during your reintroduction. Then, once you know what carb sources you're OK with, you can experiment with upping your overall carb intake and seeing how you feel. Here is what this might look like:

You went on the autoimmune-Paleo diet and felt better. Now, you will be reintroducing foods that were not allowed on the autoimmune-Paleo diet, like potatoes and sweet potatoes. You do this, and they seem fine. You then move on to foods not allowed on the Paleo diet, like rice. Rice was also OK.

Now we know you can tolerate these foods, but the question is, will you feel better when you eat these carb-dense foods regularly, which will increase your daily carb intake?

You now add a small serving of rice, potato, or sweet potato to each meal for a couple of days, and see how you feel. You could count your carb grams if you'd like, but you don't need to. The reason you don't need to is because you're not shooting for a given number or level but rather paying attention to see when your body feels best.

When people increase their carbs, they notice one of two things: they feel better, or they feel worse. Of course, if you feel worse, reduce your carbs. If you feel better, continue with the carbs. With time and observation, you should settle into the right level of carb intake for you. If you don't notice any difference when eating more or fewer carbs—congratulations. You have a versatile ecosystem that can thrive on either.

## SAFE CARB SOURCES

If you notice you feel better with a moderate to higher carb intake, here is a list of higher-carb foods that tend to work well for most:

- White rice
- White potato
- Sweet potato
- Gluten-free bread products
- Oats
- Plantains
- Cassava, taro, yucca
- Rutabaga
- Corn (non-GMO)

## REINTRODUCTION RECAP

Keep these things in mind as you reintroduce foods:

- Reintroduce from the top of our pyramid down.
- Start your reintroduction with "safer" foods first.
- Try to reintroduce foods one at a time.
  - » This helps isolate which foods are problematic. If you reintroduce five foods at the same time and have a reaction, it's hard to say which food caused it.
- For a given food, try to have a few servings a day for a few days.
  - » It's not all or none. Some people can tolerate small amounts of trigger foods, so having a few servings will help you identify if you have a certain threshold.
- The more severe your intolerance, the more obvious it will be upon reintroduction—meaning the more severe your reaction will be.
- Increasing your carb intake is part of the reintroduction. Listen to your body as you reintroduce foods that are carb dense, and adjust accordingly.
- Don't drive yourself crazy with details.
  - » Think big picture and about what you do most of the time. Don't fret over minute dietary details or about an occasional off-plan meal.
- Periodically revisit your reintroduction.
  - » This is what we are doing now :)

## HERE ARE A FEW ADDITIONAL POINTS WORTH EMPHASIZING

### Be confident

You need to find the right diet *for you*. You have taken enormous steps to heal your gut so that you can tolerate the broadest range of foods possible, and now we will determine what that range is in our reintroduction step. Wherever you end up, be confident in your diet. Don't give in to pressure from stuff you read on the Internet. If you settle into a low-carb approach, you may read that low carb is bad because it "starves your gut bugs." We've already debunked this concept, so have confidence that if this is what feels best for you, *it is* the best for you. Or, if you have settled into a higher-carb approach, you may read that higher-carb diets can cause weight gain and diabetes. But we've already talked about how some people will actually do better with their weight and blood sugar on a higher-carb diet. So, be confident that the diet you feel best on is the best diet for you and for your unique ecosystem.

Don't compare yourself to anyone else. If your friend does great on lots of fiber and high-FODMAP foods—good for her. That type of diet may decimate others. So be OK with the diet *you* feel best on—honor your unique ecosystem. And, yes, even if your friend has great digestion, it doesn't mean you should follow her diet. Some people have it easy, and they will have great digestion no matter what they eat, just like some people will stay thin no matter what they eat. This doesn't mean you should look to these people for dietary advice. Just because some people have been dealt a fortunate genetic hand does not mean they have any clue what they are doing. Trust our Great-in-8 process, and continue to work through it. This will get you to the best and broadest diet for you.

### It is not all or none

There tend to be levels of food tolerance. For example, some people can eat dairy in any quantity with absolutely no problem. Others can't have any without feeling lousy. And right in the middle of these people, are those who can have *some* dairy, but if they have *too* much, they don't feel well. Just because you don't do well with large quantities of a certain food doesn't mean you need to avoid it 100%. Keep this in mind, because it can help make your diet less restrictive.

For example, I mentioned my limitations with espresso earlier. I can do one espresso drink (usually two to three shots), but if I do more than this, my gut is not happy. I also don't seem to digest Brussels sprouts well. I can eat small quantities, but larger servings don't sit well with me. I have

no problem with gluten or dairy, but I still don't make gluten a dietary staple.

It's probably not a good idea to consume any of the foods you notice a reaction to every day. For example, I don't have espresso every day. If I do, after a while I notice my digestion starts to regress. But this doesn't mean that I can't have one or two espresso drinks in a given week if I'm in the mood, or if I'm traveling and the coffee available looks delicious, that I can't have an espresso drink every day while traveling and then return to my occasional consumption when I get home. Does this make sense? Be flexible with your avoidance of trigger foods, because it will make your life a lot easier, more enjoyable, and tastier.

### Diets are tools, not religions

The diets we have covered (Paleo, low FODMAP, lower carb, and the others) are tools to help you more quickly identify foods that might be problematic. Most people end up with a unique blend of helpful observations taken from these diets. Don't worry if you don't follow *all* the rules for a given diet religiously. Our ultimate goal is to get you to the *broadest* possible diet. Everyone is different in terms of what their dietary boundaries will be, but everyone has to go through the process of testing these boundaries to see where they are.

### Do not fear food

Again, it's important to mention that people will often notice a dramatically increased ability to eat foods that used to bother them after they have worked up to step 5. It's important that we establish this, because some patients get scared into thinking they can never again have a bite of gluten, dairy, high-FODMAP foods, non-Paleo foods, or [insert food here]. This is not true, and this belief is not healthy. Yes, you will likely notice there are some foods you can't eat or can only have in small quantities. But do you remember how powerful placebos are? If you have the belief that you will get sick from a certain food, there is a strong chance you will "placebo" this into being. One of the most freeing and beneficial moments I witness in the clinic is when I tell a patient, "It's OK to test your food boundaries, and I anticipate you will be able to eat many of your 'problem' foods with no problem at all. Enjoy them."

### Setbacks are OK

Patients are often afraid of "making a mistake" after working hard to heal their guts. They tend to think that months of work can be undone by a couple of bad meals. This is not true. Remember how important the environment you create for your microbiota is? If you're eating and living healthily most of the time, you will create an environment that fosters a healthy microbiota. Most of the time means it's OK to have occasional deviations. If the police in your city took three afternoons off over the course of a month, would your city suddenly be overrun with crime? No, of course not. Your gut is the same way. It's what you do *most* of the time that's important, so don't beat yourself up or be fearful that an occasional off-plan meal will be a deal breaker.

## BUT WHAT IF YOU HAVE A REACTION?

If you have a reaction, does this mean you're doing damage and that bacterial or fungal imbalances have returned? No. Reactions are part of the process of determining what your dietary boundaries are. The only way to know where your boundaries are is to test them. A single reaction or even a few reactions due to eating foods that aren't right for you are not enough to cause irreparable harm. Yes, it might be an unpleasant few hours or days, but this is not enough to undo months of healing.

It's also important to realize that bacterial and fungal imbalances do not occur from a few bad meals. It takes weeks of constant feeding to allow a bacterial or fungal colony to substantially grow. Think about it this way: If you left a piece of white bread out on the counter, would mold be growing on it the next day, or would you slowly and gradually see mold appear over a couple of weeks? The same thing happens in the gut. It takes weeks of eating the wrong stuff all the time for you to substantially refeed bad bugs. Don't freak out about a few off-plan meals or about experimenting with former trigger foods. You may still have a reaction, but a reaction doesn't mean that months of our rebalancing work is now undone. It just means your gut didn't like what you ate, and your reaction is a temporary irritation response. Learn from this, but don't be fearful that a major imbalance has occurred because of it.

## HOW LONG SHOULD YOU REINTRODUCE?

There is no specific answer to this question, but there are a few guidelines. I think of reintroduction as a gradual process. First, we go on a somewhat restrictive diet (such as Paleo or low FODMAP) and then, after a number of weeks on this more restrictive diet, we test the boundaries with a reintroduction. At the start of a reintroduction, it's good to be methodical and follow the rules we have already covered. Over the course of a few weeks, you should be able to test most of the foods you're eager to bring back into your diet. Once you've done this, you should have a general sense of what works and what doesn't work. Here is what this might look like:

- You can do cheeses and butter just fine, but regular milk doesn't agree with you.
- You can have gluten on occasion, but if you have it more than that, you feel tired.

- You can eat most of the high-FODMAP foods, except cauliflower, which seems to bloat you.
- Rice feels good to you, but potatoes don't.

Once you have established some of these big-picture boundaries, you can start to run periodic mini tests to see how you do. Maybe you noticed bloating after eating gluten-free bread. But then when you read the ingredients, you realized that it has a lot of potato starch in it, and maybe it's the *potato* that is bloating you. So, you try a gluten-free bread made mostly with rice flour, and you're fine.

Sometimes life will present you with an opportunity to retest something. Maybe you are at your cousin's for brunch, and she has made lattes that are outstanding. Maybe you decide to have one or two, even though this is more milk than you usually have, because these lattes are just so good. OK, this is a life-induced test of your dairy tolerance.

In the long term, you should view the reintroduction as a gradual process of eating and observing how your body responds. Learn and adjust from your observations, but also remember not to overthink things.

## REASSESSING

At this point, you are likely feeling much better than when you started the Great-in-8. You are likely able to eat more foods than you were before but also have discovered what foods do not work for you. There have probably been a few setbacks along the way, which is OK. Remember to periodically test the boundaries of your diet so you're always working toward the broadest diet possible. Listen to your body, and you will gradually settle into the diet that is perfect for you.

If you notice that you are starting to drift back to not feeling well, here are a few thoughts:

- Try revisiting a stricter diet and lifestyle—if this resolves the problem, great.
- If this does not help, you may want to revisit step 3 and consider going through more of the optional add-ons. Make sure you move to step 4 after step 3 and work step by step from there.

You should be feeling better and have noticed that, as promised, our steps are becoming easier: there's less stuff to do, and your diet is becoming broader. If you're feeling well right now, stay with your current plan for a while. There's no need to rush to step 6 (staying with step 5 anywhere from two weeks to two months is fine).

Part of the reason for not rushing is because there is a potential for reactions in step 6. As a general rule, the more severe your symptoms were at the start of the Great-in-8, the more careful you should be with step 6 "Feed." Feeding can help some but also make others worse. Let's wade into this slowly and cautiously, so if you turn out to be one whose symptoms will be made worse, we'll minimize any type of reaction. We're almost done with our Great-in-8! When you feel ready, let's continue on to step 6.

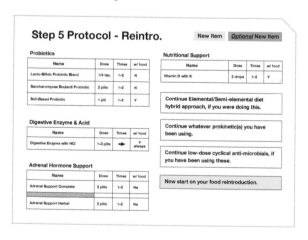

# STEP 5 ACTION-PLAN SUMMARY

- Now that we have worked to heal and balance your gut, you should be able to tolerate more foods, so we will perform a reintroduction to determine any new food freedom.
- Don't fret if you experience setbacks here; this is part of determining what your dietary boundaries are.
- Don't fear food or be religious about your diet.
- Be confident in the dietary plan you are now settling into.
- Things should be getting easier; you should be feeling better and also eating a broader diet.
- Our goal is to get you on the broadest diet possible, gradually, with time and observation.

# CHAPTER 29

# STEP 6: FEED

## STEP 6: FEED THE GOOD BACTERIA

### ORIENTATION TO STEP 6

Welcome to step 6, where we will focus on feeding your microbiota. First, stay on the supplement program that you have previously established. Continue to eat whatever diet you have now settled into. As we transition into step 6, we'll take steps to feed your gut bugs. We've already been feeding them as we've gone through our reintroduction and broadened your diet. But we can take this a step further by adding in specific items that feed the microbiota, like fiber and prebiotics. However, remember that this feeding isn't good for everyone, so be cautious during this step. *The more severe your symptoms were, the more careful you should be here.* This doesn't mean if you have severe symptoms, you shouldn't try the feeding step. Just be on the lookout for reactions, because they're more likely to happen in those who previously had more severe symptoms. For example, those who only needed to do step 1 or step 2 and then skipped to step 5 usually do better with adding in our feeding supplements. Those who needed to

go through steps 3 and 4 have a higher likelihood of negatively reacting to our feeding supplements. Again, this doesn't mean the latter group shouldn't give this a try; just be a little more cautious.

If feeding can cause reactions, why even bother at all? There are two reasons: feeding may cause improvements, and now is the ideal time to experiment with feeding. The steps we've worked through up to this point have helped to balance your microbiota, thus ensuring you'll have the best possible outcome from feeding your microbiota. There are three aids that can be useful in feeding the microbiota: fiber, prebiotics, and resistant starch. We have already discussed the impact of fiber and prebiotics on your health in previous chapters. Let's now discuss how to use them.

## STEP 6: FEED—PROTOCOL

As we established in previous chapters, the belief that you must feed your gut bacteria copious amounts of fiber is an exaggeration. But you still might benefit from upping your fiber and prebiotic intake, so it's worth some experimentation. As a reminder, we have already worked to increase your fiber, carb, and prebiotic intake in our reintroduction in step 5. Remember, fiber, carbs, and prebiotics tend to be found together in a lot of the same foods, so when you reduce one of these, you tend to reduce them all, or if you increase one, you tend to increase them all. We will now take this one step further and experiment with supplemental fiber, prebiotics, and resistant starch.

Resistant starch is added last because it's the most fermentable and strongest prebiotic,[1] which means it also carries the highest risk of causing a reaction.

## FIBER

There are two items to balance when choosing a supplemental fiber: solubility and fermentability. Solubility refers to the fiber's ability to dissolve in water; fermentability refers to how much it will feed your gut bacteria. Soluble fiber is usually soft, whereas insoluble fiber is hard. Since insoluble fiber doesn't dissolve, it is also much harder for your gut bacteria to eat. If your gut bacteria can't eat it, it can't be fermented. So, insoluble fiber is less able to feed your gut bugs; therefore, it's less fermentable. Here is a quick summary of solubility and fermentability as they relate to the two different fiber types:

Insoluble fiber
- tends to be rougher, which increases the chances it will irritate your intestines;
- will not dissolve in water;
- is less fermentable (less prone to cause gas and bloating).

Soluble fiber
- tends to be softer, which decreases the chances it will irritate your intestines;
- is more fermentable (more prone to cause gas and bloating).

Which one is best? The majority of the studies point to *soluble* fiber being the most beneficial and well tolerated. But no one fiber will be right for all people, so let's go through a few options you can experiment with. Keep in mind the overall benefit of supplemental fiber is minimal, so if you try one or two different fibers and experience no benefit, simply move on to our next step.

If supplementing with soluble fiber tends to work better than supplementing with insoluble fiber, does this mean you should strive for a diet higher in soluble fiber and lower in insoluble fiber? Not exactly. Trying to organize your diet around solubility can be tricky, and I wouldn't recommend it. However, as we discussed earlier, I would first start with avoiding hard sources of fiber, like raw veggies or the skins of fruits and vegetables, and opting for peeled, steamed, or sautéed sources, which will be softer. Then, as your gut heals, incorporate more of the harder fiber sources, and see how you do.

For all the fibers listed below, use the following dosing:

- Use one to two tablespoons, one to two times per day; slowly build to full dose.
- Take with water or juice.
- Take on an empty stomach or with food.
- Take with or without supplements.

### Fiber #1—general fiber, a good all-around support
Biota-Fiber contains 3 g soluble and 1 g insoluble fiber derived from natural sources—mostly fruits and vegetables. I have found this fiber works best for a variety of conditions, and it is the first fiber you should try.

If you have tried the Biota-Fiber and did not tolerate it, try Fiber #2.

### Fiber #2—low fermentability and low FODMAP, mostly soluble
If you've noticed that you experience gas or bloat easily, or are very FODMAP sensitive, either of

these fibers might be a good fiber for you. Only try these if you don't react well to the Biota-Fiber.

- Heather's Tummy Fiber is a natural fiber made from acacia that contains only soluble fiber and is low FODMAP.
- Citrucel is a synthetic fiber that contains only soluble fiber and is not fermentable. It comes in both pill and powder form. Citrucel powder does contain artificial sweeteners; the capsules do not.

If you have tried Fibers #1 and #2 and did not tolerate them, try Fiber #3.

### Fiber #3—low fermentability and low FODMAP, partially soluble

There is one final fiber that is worth trying should the other fiber types not work: psyllium.

- Psyllium husk has a two to one ratio of soluble to insoluble fiber. Most grocery and health-food stores have a psyllium-husk fiber in stock, so this should be easy to obtain locally. If you try a psyllium fiber, make sure psyllium is the only ingredient (avoid fiber blends).

### GUT GEEKS

Here are some fiber sources that are high in FODMAPs—these are more prone to cause bloating and/or gas reactions if you are very sensitive:

- Inulin—mostly obtained from chicory root or Jerusalem artichoke
- Beet fiber, corn fiber, soy fiber, citrus fiber
- Carrageenan is a water-soluble fiber found in certain types of seaweed
- Guar gum

Remember that most people will tolerate FODMAPs after healing their guts by going through our Great-in-8 steps.

### Follow these guidelines for the fiber supplementation

Experiment with a few of the fibers we've just discussed following our guidelines:

- Slowly build up to the recommended dose over one to two weeks.
  - » You may notice you're fine with a lower dose but don't do well with the full recommended dose. If this is the case, use the dose that works for you.
- Wait a few more days to gauge your response: improved, no change, or worse.
- If you have a reaction to one fiber, discontinue it and move on to the next fiber.
- Try to find one fiber that works for you, and then move on to the prebiotic supplementation. If you can't find a fiber that you can tolerate, move on to the prebiotic supplementation.
- You only need to find one fiber.
  - » If you tried the first fiber and had a reaction, move to the second fiber option. If the second fiber option works well for you, you are ready to move from fiber to the prebiotic supplements.

### Fiber Supplements*

| Name | Dose | Times/Day | w/ Food | Notes |
|------|------|-----------|---------|-------|
| Biota-Fiber | 1–2 T | 1–2 | N | See below |
| Heather's Tummy Fiber or Citrucel | 1–2 T | 1–2 | N | See below |
| Psyllium | 1–2 T | 1–2 | N | See below |

*Take only one of these—not all three.
Note: Slowly build to full dose over 1–2 weeks. May cause gas/bloating/pain for a few days, which should then subside.

## PREBIOTICS

After some fiber experimentation, we now add in prebiotics. A Biota-Boost Prebiotic contains a mixture of natural prebiotics that support the growth of healthy bacteria.

### Follow these guidelines for the prebiotic supplementation

The guidelines for prebiotics are very similar to the ones you used for fiber:

- Take one to three capsules, one to two times per day.
- Take with water.
- Slowly build up to the recommended dose over one to two weeks.
  - » You may also notice you are fine with a lower dose of prebiotics but do not do well with the full recommended dose. If this is the case, use the dose that works for you.
- Wait a few more days to gauge your response: improved, no change, or worse.
- As long as you are not feeling worse, you can move on to the resistant starch.
- If you have a reaction, discontinue and move on to the next step.
  - » If you have had a negative reaction to the prebiotic, you should be very careful with the resistant starch, because you have a higher chance of negatively reacting to it.
- Take with or without food or supplements. As we discussed earlier, a dose of 3.5–5 grams (3,500 to 5,000 milligrams) per day might be ideal, causing improvement to digestive function but also having a minimal risk for negative reactions. Two capsules contain 1,500 mg. So, if you take
  - » two capsules once per day, you'll be taking 1,500 mg;
  - » two capsules twice per day, you'll be taking 3,000 mg;
  - » three capsules twice per day, you'll be taking 4,500 mg.

**Prebiotic Supplement**

| Name | Dose | Times/Day | w/ Food | Notes |
|------|------|-----------|---------|-------|
| Biota-Boost Prebiotic | 2–3 | 1 to 2 | either | Slowly build to top dose over 2 weeks. May cause gas/bloating/pain for a few days, which should then subside |

## RESISTANT STARCH

Resistant starch is the final feeding strategy we will experiment with. There are many sources of resistant starch, but I recommend experimenting with supplemental tapioca. If you don't tolerate tapioca, you can try green banana, potato, or corn starch. Resistant starch comes in powder form and should be taken just like fiber or prebiotics. A good brand is Bob's Red Mill Tapioca Starch.

### Follow these guidelines for resistant starch

Follow the guidelines below when you start taking resistant starch:

- The dose is one teaspoon, one to two times per day, taken with water and with or without food or supplements.
- Slowly build up to the recommended dose over one to two weeks.
  - » You may notice you are fine with a lower dose but do not do well with the full recommended dose. If this is the case, use the dose that works for you.
- Wait a few more days to gauge your response: improved, no change, or worse.
- As long as you are not feeling worse, you can move on to the step 7.
- If you have a reaction to one, discontinue and move on to step 7.

## Resistant Starch Supplement

| Name | Dose | Times/Day | w/ Food | Notes |
|------|------|-----------|---------|-------|
| Unmodified Tapioca Starch | 1 t | 1–2 | N | Slowly build to top dose over 2 weeks. May cause gas/bloating/pain for a few days, which should then subside |

## Morning smoothies

A morning smoothie can be made that combines many of the items from your current program:

- A protein powder
  - » Whey or pea protein or vegetable protein
- Water or milk
  - » Coconut milk, rice milk, dairy milk
- Fresh or frozen berries
  - » A mixture combining strawberries, blueberries, and raspberries; berries are low in sugar but high in antioxidants
- A fiber supplement
  - » Select from above
- Prebiotics capsules
  - » From above
- A resistant starch powder
  - » From above
- A greens powder

### RECIPE ONE
- ½ cup unsweetened almond milk
- 1 cup frozen blueberries
- 1 ripe frozen banana
- 2 tablespoons pea protein
- 1 tablespoon greens powder
- 1 teaspoon chia seeds
- ¼ teaspoon (to start) of resistant starch
- 1 tablespoon of fiber supplement
- pinch of cinnamon
- 1 prebiotic capsule

Combine almond milk, blueberries, banana, pea protein, greens powder, chia seeds, resistant starch, fiber supplement, and cinnamon into a blender and mix on high until smooth. Open prebiotics capsule, and add contents to blender. Mix on low for a few seconds. Pour into glass and enjoy!

### RECIPE TWO
- 1 cup unsweetened vanilla almond milk or vanilla rice milk (you can use plain almond or rice milk; just add a touch of vanilla bean powder or extract)
- 1 cup mixed frozen berries
- 1 large frozen banana
- 1 tablespoon pea protein
- 1 tablespoon greens powder
- 1 tablespoon of flaxseed
- 1–2 tablespoons of almond butter (substitute sun butter if avoiding nuts)
- ¼ teaspoon (to start) of resistant starch
- 1 tablespoon of fiber supplement
- 1 prebiotics capsule

Combine milk, berries, banana, pea protein, greens powder, flaxseed, almond butter, resistant starch, and fiber supplement into a blender and mix on high until smooth. Open prebiotics capsule, and add contents to blender. Mix on low for a few seconds. Pour and serve!

## REACTIONS

The same rules regarding reactions that we discussed in step 5 also apply here. Remember, a reaction is not necessarily a bad thing; it's part of the process of determining where your boundaries are.

## WHO MIGHT DO BEST WITH "FEEDING," AND WHO IS AT RISK FOR REACTIONS?

Those who had severe symptoms initially have a higher likelihood of reactions when going through step 6. We can break this down into three risk groups:

- Lowest chance of negative reaction in step 6
  » Those who skipped steps 2 through 4
- Moderate/small chance of a negative reaction in step 6
  » Those who skipped steps 3 and 4
- Highest chance of negative reaction in step 6
  » Those who did not skip any steps

This doesn't mean step 6 is a bad idea for those with the highest chance of a reaction, but it's important that you have an idea of what to expect. This is especially important to prevent you from repeatedly trying to force prebiotics and fibers upon your microbiota because you've been led to believe you should. There is no right or wrong here; the best approach is learning to listen to your body and being confident with the dietary and supplemental plan you end up on.

## STEP 6 ACTION-PLAN SUMMARY

Experiment with fibers, prebiotics, and resistant starches as we have just discussed following our guidelines:

- Slowly build up to the recommended dose over one to two weeks.
- Wait a few more days to gauge your response: improved, no change, or worse.
- If you have a reaction to one fiber, discontinue it and move on to the next item.

## REASSESSING

The main item to reassess here is if you experienced improvement from any type of feeding: fiber, prebiotics, or resistant starch. If you did, great—continue using. If you didn't, simply do not use these. From here, everyone will move to step 7 as we round the final corner in our Great-in-8 plan.

In case you're wondering, "Will I be on all of this stuff forever?" the answer is no. We want to find the minimal dose and number of supports needed in the long term. In our next step (step 7 "Wean"), we will start the process of finding the *minimal* program needed.

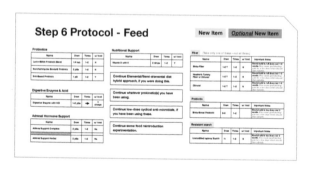

1    Alan W. Walker and Trevor D. Lawley, "Therapeutic Modulation of Intestinal Dysbiosis," *Pharmacological Research*, 2013, doi:10.1016/j.phrs.2012.09.008.

# CHAPTER 30

# STEP 7: WEAN

## STEP 7: WEAN YOURSELF OFF THE SUPPLEMENTS IN YOUR PLAN

### ORIENTATION TO STEP 7

In step 7, we will work to find the minimal program needed to maintain your improvements. Our goal is to get you on little to nothing in the long term. We will take steps to identify the supports that are most helpful and continue only those. This coincides with the changes we made earlier with your diet: we worked to reduce the amount of dietary restrictions you were following so as to find the broadest diet possible. Now we will work to reduce the amount of supplements and other supports you need.

When is the best time to start step 7? It's best to be stable in your improvement for at least two to three months before starting to curtail your supplement program. The reason for this is because we want to give your body time to heal before we start curtailing. Think of it like wearing a knee brace while recovering from a knee injury. The brace is helpful, and eventually it won't be needed,

but if you stop using the brace too soon, your knee won't be ready and you could reinjure yourself.

Why is it important to curtail the program? Curtailing the program is important because of what I call supplement creep. This is where more and more supplements slowly creep into your regimen over time. As different supplements come into vogue, they're added, then more are added, then later even more are added. If you never take time to assess if a particular supplement actually helps you, you end up on too many over time. It's important to periodically assess if you still need a supplement by discontinuing it and seeing how you respond.

This is also performed with drug therapy. It's known as a "drug holiday," which simply means patients discontinue a drug that was previously helpful to see if they can maintain their improvements without it.[1] I noticed this in myself also. After years of enjoying recovered gut health, I started to have bloating, loose stool, and insomnia. When I took stock of my diet and program, I found I was eating *lots* of high-FODMAP foods (which I used to feel great on) and taking a fairly high dose of probiotics. After a while, this ended up being too much for my gut. I reduced the FODMAPs and decreased my probiotic dose.

Within a few days I was improving, and within a few weeks I was back to normal.

# STEP 7: WEAN PROTOCOL

How exactly do you wean yourself off the supports in your program to determine what is and what is not needed? There are no set rules for this, but there are some questions to consider. These come from my observations in the clinic:

1. Which supplements should you try coming off first?
2. Should you come off a particular supplement all at once or gradually?
3. How long should you wait in between the supplements you discontinue?
4. How do you know if you need something? What are the signs to look for?
5. Should you periodically retest your dietary boundaries?

## 1. WHICH SUPPLEMENTS SHOULD YOU TRY COMING OFF FIRST?

Start by coming off those supplements that you feel have been the least helpful. Most people tend to have a sense of what these are.

If you're not sure, you can work through coming off your program in the order below. You may not be using all the supplements listed below; if you're not using one, just skip ahead to the next.

1. Adrenal support
2. The prokinetic from step 4 (either Iberogast or MotilPro)
3. Low-dose cyclical antimicrobial therapy
4. Resistant starch, prebiotics, and fiber—in this order
5. Hybrid use of the elemental/semielemental diet
6. Digestive acid and/or enzymes
7. Probiotics

## 2. SHOULD YOU COME OFF A PARTICULAR SUPPLEMENT ALL AT ONCE OR GRADUALLY?

There is no set rule here, and I really don't think it matters. Choose whatever method appeals to you. If you choose to wean off gradually, doing so over a week is a good interval to shoot for.

## 3. HOW LONG SHOULD YOU WAIT IN BETWEEN THE SUPPLEMENTS YOU DISCONTINUE?

Again, there is no set rule. We want to leave enough time to allow you to gauge how you are doing being off a supplement, but we don't want to wait so long that this whole process feels like it takes forever. Anywhere from one to three weeks between supplements works.

## 4. HOW DO YOU KNOW IF YOU NEED SOMETHING—WHAT ARE THE SIGNS TO LOOK FOR?

Do you notice any of your improvements regress shortly after you discontinue a supplement? Feeling slightly different for a few days is normal. Wait a few days, and see if you return to normal; your body may just need a few days to adjust. If you do not return to normal after a few days, go back on and see if you return to normal. If you return to normal, this suggests the supplement was helping.

I recommend repeating this process one or two more times to make sure this wasn't a coincidence. The symptoms that can return after discontinuing a given supplement will not be the same for everyone, so remember to be on the lookout for *any* regression that starts after discontinuing something. Also, remember not to overthink this. If something is helping or not helping, it should be apparent. You are looking for noticeable shifts, not for extremely subtle variations in how you feel. It's normal to feel a little better or worse from day to day; we're humans not robots. Don't micromonitor yourself. To provide you with a little more guidance, let's look at adrenal support as an example.

What should you expect when coming off adrenal support? At this point in our process, most people will notice little to nothing when coming off adrenal support—meaning they will maintain their improvements. There may be a few days at first where they don't feel quite the same pep, but then a few days later, their bodies adjust, and they feel just as good as when they were on adrenal support. This is similar to coming off caffeine. Our goal is for you to come off adrenal support and still feel great, and this is what will likely happen.

A small number of people, maybe 15%, notice they don't feel as well when they come off adrenal support. If this is you, go back on adrenal support for a few more months, and then try coming off again several months later. If you try again and notice you just can't seem to come off adrenal support without feeling like you regress, check in with a well-trained functional-medicine doctor who can help determine if there might be a lingering problem that's preventing your adrenals from recovering. The same logic for the adrenal support should be applied to all your other supplements.

## 5. SHOULD YOU PERIODICALLY RETEST YOUR DIETARY BOUNDARIES?

Here are a few notes and reminders about diet:

- With time, you should be able to eat more foods and have fewer dietary restrictions.
- Some people do better on a low-carb diet for a while but several months later notice it doesn't seem to be working. If this is you, you might need to up your carbs.
- If you have a setback, you may need to return to a stricter diet for a period.
- If you are under a lot of stress, you might notice you have to be stricter with your diet until things settle down. You may also want to bring back in some of the supplements you were previously able to cut out. For example, adrenal support and probiotics can help buffer some of the negative effects of stress on the gut. You can also use the modified fast or revisit two to four days on an elemental/semielemental diet to quell a flare.

## REASSESSING

After some time, tinkering, and observation, you should be able to reduce some of the supplements in your program. This could include both the number of and/or the dose of any of your supplements. This will not be the same for everyone, and it depends on how your body reacts to coming off certain supplements. Some people will be on nothing right now and feel fine. Others may have only been able to come off one supplement. There is no right or wrong here. If you were only able to come off one supplement, remember that your body may simply need more time to heal before you're able to curtail your program further. Wait a little while, and try again.

## STEP 7 ACTION-PLAN SUMMARY

In this step, we work to find the minimum number and lowest dose of supplements you need to maintain your improvements. This step can be performed quickly or slowly. For those who feel they are sensitive or want to be cautious, proceed slowly. For those who just want to get on with it, proceed more quickly. Remember, we always want to be working toward the lowest amount of supplements and the broadest array of foods. If you aren't able to come off a supplement now, wait a few months and try again.

Along with weaning you off your supplements and dietary restrictions, we are trying to wean your focus off health and increase your focus on other fun stuff in your life. This is a good transition to step 8, where we work on maintenance and fun.

1   Robert H. Howland, "Medication Holidays," *Journal of Psychosocial Nursing and Mental Health Services* 47, no. 9 (2009): 15–18, doi:10.3928/02793695-20090804-01.

# CHAPTER 31

# STEP 8: MAINTENANCE AND FUN

## STEP 8: MAINTAIN YOUR IMPROVEMENTS, AND ENJOY YOUR NEWFOUND HEALTH

Welcome to the final step in our Great-in-8, where we will briefly cover maintenance and fun. After reading this book and then going through our steps, you will have given your health quite a bit of attention, time, and energy. This is a good thing, because it has allowed you to improve your health. But there comes a point when it's helpful to shift your focus back to your *life*, to the things you enjoy, to fun.

There is also the issue of maintenance, or how to maintain your improvements. We have already discussed tips and tricks for what to do if you have a setback, but now is a good time to review this and also add a few additional pointers. For those who haven't achieved the desired level of improvement, we will cover how to find a good health-care provider and also provide you with a list of things to discuss with them. There are different types of providers (doctors, nutritionists, and health coaches, to name a few), and our discussion will provide you with tools that can help you find the health-care professional that is the best fit for you. Let's first discuss fun.

## THE IMPORTANCE OF FUN

Why is the *fun* aspect so important? We've discussed this a few times throughout this book, but to put it simply: because it's the next step in the healing and recovery process. When you aren't feeling well, it's understandable that you will dedicate more time to your health and health research. But once you're improving, it's important to get back to the other things in your life that may have suffered during your health-focused period—things like social outings, hobbies, perhaps staying up a little too late and enjoying wine, an occasional dessert with friends, music, and so on.

There are three reasons why getting back to your life is so critical: First, having enjoyment in your life has been shown to help you heal faster.

Remember earlier we discussed how social stress delays wound-healing time? Second, from a psychological or spiritual perspective, maintaining these activities provides a balanced life and should translate to you feeling happier. Remember Dan Buettner's findings from his book *Thrive: Finding Happiness the Blue Zones Way* that we discussed earlier? Those with less money or power who had time with friends and community were happier than the wealthier and more powerful. Third, if you don't replace your health/research-focused time with other activities, you can easily fall into a black hole of chronically overobsessing about your health, even though your health has improved. This can lead to a syndrome where people are never happy with their health, which makes them feel stressed out and depressed, which is *then* usually followed by more elaborate diets and supplement programs that don't work. This is often accompanied by *more* time spent on the Internet researching, and this increased Internet use has been shown to increase depression and anxiety. This is then followed by even *more* elaborate diet and supplement programs. All the while, the missing ingredient of "getting back to their life" is being neglected. Please don't let this become you.

In case this *is* you, here is one additional thought. Even the best doctors and health gurus, many of whom are my good friends, deal with health issues from time to time. So even the best are not perfect. If *they* aren't perfect, how reasonable is it for *you* to expect to be perfect? As long as you're feeling well most of the time, don't sweat the small stuff. No one is perfect, and no one is invincible. Minor setbacks and flares are going to happen from time to time.

# MAINTENANCE PROGRAM

What does an ideal maintenance program look like? It really depends on what *you* notice after you go through step 7. I would emphasize that you should listen to *your body* and not allow yourself to be influenced by whatever the hot supplement of the moment is.

Here is one variation of a sample maintenance program:

- Vitamin D, 2,000 IUs per day during the fall and winter months (because you're outside getting sunshine during the spring and summer)
- Probiotics
  - » One teaspoon of Lacto-Bifido Probiotic Blend most mornings
  - » One capsule of Saccharomyces Boulardii Probiotic most mornings
  - » One capsule of Soil-Based Probiotic most mornings
- One heaping scoop of Biota-Fiber most mornings
- One to two capsules of Digestive Enzymes with HCl with *larger* meals only
- Occasional performance of one to two days of the modified fast or an elemental diet when your gut doesn't feel happy
- Occasional use of an adrenal support if you're dealing with abnormally high amounts of stress
- A moderate-carb Paleo diet most of the time, but periodic indulgences in gluten or dairy or whatever, as long as you don't notice very strong negative reactions

Here is a variation of a sample maintenance program for someone with more sensitive digestion:

- Vitamin D, 2,000 IUs per day during the fall and winter months
- Probiotics
  - » One teaspoon of Lacto-Bifido Probiotic Blend most mornings
  - » One capsule of Saccharomyces Boulardii Probiotic most mornings

- » One capsule of Soil-Based Probiotic most mornings
- One to two capsules of Digestive Enzyme with HCl with *most* meals
- Occasional use of adrenal support if you are dealing with abnormally high amounts of stress
- Fasting and liquid dieting
  - » On most days, you practice intermittent fasting (you skip breakfast but eat a slightly larger lunch and dinner).
  - » Every Sunday you perform the modified fast for one full day.
  - » Once every couple of months you perform four full days on the elemental diet using Elemental Heal.
- Low-dose cyclical antimicrobial therapy
  - » You notice you feel best when taking
    - two pills per day of Biota-Clear 1a for one month, then switching to a different antimicrobial;
    - two pills per day of Biota-Clear 1b for a month, and so on as the protocol indicates.
- Generally eat according to the Paleo low-FODMAP diet but enjoy periodic indulgences:
  - » You do not tolerate gluten, so you make sure any indulgences are gluten-free.
  - » You can tolerate a small amount of dairy.

# HANDLING INEVITABLE SETBACKS

Setbacks are going to happen. Knowing this is normal can prevent you from feeling defeated or overly worried when they do occur. A simple principle regarding handling setbacks is to revisit what has worked well for you. For some, this might be as simple as briefly revisiting a stricter diet and lifestyle, as we've already discussed. Perhaps you were feeling great when

- eating less carbs;
- getting one more hour of sleep a night;
- exercising one day less per week.

But after a while you started

- having more carbs;
- sleeping a little less;
- exercising more.

Then you gradually noticed you were not sleeping as well, were tired during the day, and were a bit bloated. Let's have you revert to what previously worked well. Once things settle down, you may want to play with each one of these variables to determine if your regression came from the carbs, the sleep, or the exercise. With time and observation, you will learn what works best for you.

The simplest strategy is to revisit what has worked for you from a diet and lifestyle perspective. However, there will be those of you for whom the diet and lifestyle changes didn't make a large difference. You may have noticed the most difference when on the probiotics and adrenal support. If that's the case, return to those. Or you might not have noticeably improved until you performed the antimicrobials or one of the elemental/semielemental diets. If so, return to this. Once you have gone through the Great-in-8, you should have a good sense of the aspects that were the most helpful for you. If you have a regression, you can briefly return to these aspects of the plan for a few weeks.

Remember, you can use a short-term liquid fast as a quick and easy reset. Either the modified fast (the lemonade or broth we discussed earlier) or one of the elemental diets can be used for two to four days as a reset. Then, after this, you can incorporate the other aspects of the Great-in-8 you found to be helpful, if you need additional improvements.

Here is one additional thought for those of us who are type A personalities. I'm sure we've all heard the expression that too much of a good thing can become a bad thing. This can hold true for your diet and for supplements in your program. Sometimes, the best thing for a person is to stop everything. While something like a probiotic, adrenal support, or digestive enzyme can be helpful, sometimes everything together is too much for your body and ends up having the opposite of the desired effect. If you have been struggling, you may simply want to stop everything and see how you do. This also applies to diet, meaning take a break from worrying about food. You should have already been moving in this direction when we performed step 5 "Reintroduce" and during step 7 "Wean." However, sometimes it can be helpful to reframe this and completely go off any diet or supplements—it's a mental break, and for some this is the best medicine.

Depending on how often you're having setbacks, you may want to consider bringing in a professional. Here's a simple rule: if you feel like you are spending more time having setbacks than feeling well, it's time to seek professional guidance. I realize saying "see a doctor" is too vague to be helpful, so let's cover some specifics to help you find the right health-care provider, should you need one.

# CHAPTER 32

# IF YOU NEED MORE HELP— FINDING A GOOD DOCTOR

I should mention first that my office offers visits at our physical office in Walnut Creek, California, and via phone or Skype for those who aren't in our area. We can help. All the information you need can be found here: https://drruscio.com/gethelp/.

## HOW TO FIND A GOOD DOC

A term you may not have known until you read this book is "functional medicine." If this is a new term to you, let's cover a few common questions.

### WHAT IS FUNCTIONAL MEDICINE?

This is how I define functional medicine: functional medicine is a health-care practice that attempts to treat the underlying cause of disease and illness, usually doing so as naturally as possible and emphasizing dietary and lifestyle changes, nutritional supplements, and herbal medicines. Lab testing is used to guide treatment and determine what an underlying cause of illness might be. The goal of functional medicine should be to reestablish a healthy equilibrium in the body so that you can maintain well-being by adhering to healthy diet and lifestyle practices.

### HOW DOES A FUNCTIONAL-MEDICINE DOCTOR DIFFER FROM A CONVENTIONAL DOCTOR?

Functional medicine is not a replacement for conventional medicine. This is a key point. A functional-medicine clinician and a conventional clinician will have areas of overlap but also key differences. Let's use hypothyroidism for example. Functional-medicine doctors are very good at treating the underlying cause of hypothyroidism (which is thyroid autoimmunity) with diet, supplements, and improving gut health. But those with thyroid autoimmunity are at increased risk for thyroid cancer, which most functional-medicine clinicians will not be screening for. So, you should see your functional-medicine provider and continue to follow up with whatever screening your conventional doctor has recommended.

## WHY WOULD YOU SEE A FUNCTIONAL-MEDICINE PROVIDER?

Here are a few examples:

- You have symptoms (fatigue, weight gain, depression . . .), but your conventional doctor says everything is normal.
- You have chronic constipation, bloating, or abdominal discomfort. Your conventional doctor prescribed a laxative, but you feel like this hasn't *fixed* the problem.
- You have chronic heartburn or reflux, and your regular doctor prescribed an acid blocker. You read up on it and are uncomfortable with the long-term risks and side effects of this medication.
- You have been diagnosed with hypothyroidism and told you need medication, but you would like a second opinion before starting to see if there is anything that can be done to reduce or eliminate your need for medication.

A good functional-medicine doc can also help you prioritize information you read about and think might be important: testing, supplements, or dietary modifications, for example. A good provider will *save you* time and money, because he or she can help guide you to what's needed instead of you doing it on your own via trial and error.

## WHO CAN PRACTICE FUNCTIONAL MEDICINE?

Unfortunately, there are currently no regulations—beware not all providers are created equal. Even someone with good academic credentials is not guaranteed to be a good clinician, so do your research. Let's discuss some specifics to help you with this.

## WHAT TYPE OF FUNCTIONAL-MEDICINE PROVIDER MIGHT BE BEST FOR YOU?

You can visualize a spectrum of functional-medicine providers. At one end there are health coaches, and at the other end there are doctors.

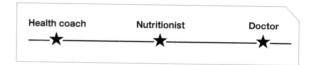

If you only have mild symptoms, then anyone can likely help: a health coach, nutritionist, or doctor. If you have more severe symptoms, are highly sensitive, or have a disease diagnosis, you could still start with the health coach or nutritionist, but it might be best to find a licensed doctor (ND, DC, MD, DO) who specializes in what you need.

## ARE THERE SPECIALTIES WITHIN FUNCTIONAL MEDICINE?

There are not formal specialties within functional medicine. However, as much as functional medicine claims to not specialize but instead be holistic and treat the underlying cause of disease, the underlying cause may emanate from different systems of the body. So, finding a provider whose area of specialty or focus aligns with your needs is a good idea. For example, some functional-medicine providers focus on digestive health. Others focus on women's health. Some may focus on thyroid health, and others may focus on Lyme disease. If someone claims to specialize in several things, it likely means they don't specialize in one area but are a generalist in all. This is not a bad thing, but it's something to be aware of. A generalist is fine if you don't have a specific condition or area you need help in. However, if you have chronic IBS, you may do best with a functional-medicine provider who focuses on digestive conditions.

Who you work with is a calculated decision. Here is a breakdown on this:

The health coach/nutritionist
- Pro—will likely cost less, be more accessible, and may know more about diet
- Con—may have less clinical expertise

The doctor (ND, DC, MD/DO)
- Con—will likely cost more, be less accessible, and may know less about diet
- Pro—more clinical expertise

Please keep in mind these are merely generalizations to help guide you. There will be exceptions to these rules. This doesn't mean one clinician is better or worse; it just depends on what you need. If you are someone who hasn't changed your diet, you should probably start with a health coach or nutritionist. However, if you have changed your diet or are trying to manage a diagnosed condition, you may want to see a doctor. You have to find the right balance for you, depending on if you have changed your diet, the severity of your illness, your motivation, and your financial situation.

When I fell ill in my twenties, I already had a very healthy diet and lifestyle, so working with a health coach or nutritionist didn't make sense. I saw a few conventional doctors, and they were no help either. I needed to see a DC (doctor of chiropractic) practicing functional medicine and specializing in digestive conditions to diagnose and treat my intestinal parasite.

## RED FLAGS

There are some red flags that indicate a particular provider may not be a good fit. Before we go through these points, remember there are exceptions to every rule. So, these points may indicate the provider is one to avoid, but they do not guarantee it.

### When a provider requires you to purchase a costly package to receive care

This could be something like requiring you to sign up for a six-month plan that costs $5,000 and includes all testing, treatment, and office visits. A shorter-term and less expensive package might be OK, especially if it includes nutritional coaching, as this provides structure. However, when lab testing and treatment are all bundled into a package, I would be a little cautious. Again, it is not a set rule but something to be aware of.

### If they appear hard-driving, overly opinionated, or don't listen

Do you get the sense they're not listening to you? Do they seem unwilling to think outside their box? Do they make strong claims and seem overly opinionated? You want a provider who will look at you as a teammate rather than a subordinate.

### If they require excessive testing out of the gate

For example, if the provider requires you perform $3,500 of testing before getting started, this is likely a red flag. There may be an exception here if the provider sees chronically ill patients and knows these patients need this thorough testing. Outside of this exception, be wary. In my opinion, a good clinician should recommend only a few tests that are most appropriate (personalized) for the person sitting in front of them—this keeps the testing fee more reasonable.

Functional medicine is a wonderful field that helps a lot of people. However, sometimes it's too excessive and patients end up footing a rather large bill, unnecessarily. Things are starting to change, and functional-medicine care is becoming more cost-effective. Be on the lookout for some of these red flags to help prevent you from spending way more than you need to. When done the right way, functional medicine should ultimately be a cost savings because a good clinician will help you get well as efficiently as possible.

# THINGS TO DISCUSS WITH YOUR DOCTOR

We have discussed many of these throughout the book, but they're worth repeating. It's also important to remember that nondigestive symptoms, like fatigue, weight gain, depression, insomnia, joint pain, and skin problems, could all be coming from an undetected digestive issue. So, even if you don't have overt digestive symptoms, like gas, bloating, and constipation, you should consider having a digestive evaluation—if the Great-in-8 hasn't resolved your symptoms.

# CONDITIONS AND TESTING TO CONSIDER

## SIBO (SMALL-INTESTINAL BACTERIAL OVERGROWTH)

This is the most common imbalance I find in the clinic. We have already discussed the most common symptoms of SIBO: gas, bloating, constipation, diarrhea, abdominal pain, and reflux. The Great-in-8 works fantastically well for most cases of SIBO, so if you have it, you should have seen at least some improvement. But you may have a challenging case that needs to be quantified and tracked with testing. SIBO is tested using a breath test that should measure both hydrogen and methane gas over the course of three hours. Glucose or lactulose are given in the drink used as part of this test. This test usually costs about $200 and is often covered by insurance.

## DYSBIOSIS AND DIGESTIVE-TRACT INFECTIONS: PARASITES, FUNGI, BACTERIA, AMOEBAS, PROTOZOA

Dysbiosis refers to imbalances in the bacteria or fungi that naturally occur in the digestive tract.

How exactly we define dysbiosis is a bit vague, so you will have to work with a good clinician on this.

Infections are a bit more clear-cut. It's not practical to list all the possible infections, but here are a few more common ones: H. pylori, Yersinia enterocolitis, Toxoplasmosis gondii, Blastocystis hominis, and Entamoeba histolytica. To test for both dysbiosis and infections, a doctor can perform a panel that tests stool and may also test breath, blood, saliva, and urine. Many good tests are available through insurance, so you might not need to pay out of pocket.

## GUT-MOTILITY AUTOIMMUNITY

Autoimmunity can occur against the part of the intestines that regulates motility. If this happens it can make SIBO more likely to recur. There are two companies that currently offer a test for this: IBS Check by Common Wealth Diagnostics and IBSDetex by Quest Diagnostics. They both assess antibodies against what's known as vinculin and CdtB. If this test is positive, it may indicate the prokinetics medications we discussed earlier would be an important part of treatment. It's also important to note that this does not appear to apply to those who are predominantly constipated.[1]

This test appears most useful in determining if IBS is the cause of your diarrhea, which would make further testing for celiac disease or inflammatory bowel disease unnecessary.

## TESTING THE MICROBIOTA

We have already discussed that specific microbiota tests can be used for research purposes only and have no true clinical meaning at this time. It's important you understand this so as to not get sucked into speculative testing and treatment programs. The most advanced microbiota testing to date (in mid-2017, the time I'm writing this book) currently offers two tests that are nearing clinical application. Things in this field are changing rapidly, so depending on when you read this, it may be more or less relevant.

The first test uses a special microbiota analysis that can screen for IBD.[2] This test is not yet available for doctors, but the researchers hope to be offering clinical training for doctors on how to use this test as a screening tool soon.

The second test recently became available in clinical practice. The initial research regarding this test was able to show dysbiosis (imbalances) in the microbiota that correlated with IBS and IBD.[3] Over 70% of those with either IBS or IBD displayed dysbiosis via this test, whereas only 16% of healthy controls had dysbiosis. However, whether this test can improve *treatment* has yet to be established. At the time of this writing, we are working on collaborating with this lab and research group to see if this test might be able to improve the treatment of IBS or IBD.

## HYPOTHYROIDISM

Sometimes it's important to also look outside the digestive tract. A screening for hypothyroidism can be very helpful here. This is a blood test that measures two things: TSH and T4. Here is the approach I would recommend regarding thyroid health. Start with this simple TSH and T4 evaluation for hypothyroidism. If you are truly hypothyroid, you will need to be on thyroid-hormone medication. If you are not truly hypothyroid, but your values look slightly off, work to improve your gut health, and you will likely see this imbalance improve. True hypothyroidism means your TSH is high *and* your T4 is low, according to the conventional ranges. True hypothyroidism usually requires medication. Most thyroid problems are driven by either inflammation and/or autoimmunity; both of which can be remedied by improving the health of your gut. It's not a guarantee, but start with the gut, and then reevaluate. There is

a good chance that fixing your gut will improve your thyroid.

## FEMALE HORMONE IMBALANCES

Sometimes women will notice they feel worse during different parts of their cycle. If you notice symptoms that coincide with your cycle, your female hormones (estrogen and progesterone) might be imbalanced. If you noticed certain symptoms started around the time of menopause, you may also have a hormonal imbalance. Female hormones do affect your gut and vice versa. If, after working to improve your gut health, you still have some lingering symptoms, you might need support specific to your hormones. Some typical symptoms are

- bloating or cramping;
- constipation;
- hot flashes;
- insomnia;
- irritability;
- depression;
- cravings;
- vaginal dryness;
- altered cycle length;
- altered menstrual flow.

There are herbal medicines available that help to balance female hormones, whether they are high or low. Because these herbs act in a corrective way, testing is not needed. A few examples are black cohosh and dong quai, which work to balance estrogen, and chaste tree, which works to balance progesterone.

If you are cycling, you can try the compound Estro-Harmony at two capsules one to two times per day and Progest-Harmony at one to two capsules two times per day. Both are made by Functional Medicine Formulations, and both can be taken with or without food. Start at the lower dose, give it a few weeks, and then move to the higher dose if your symptoms have only partially responded. If you are not cycling (meaning you are menopausal or postmenopausal), you can try Estro-Harmony alone at the same dose. You can locate both of these through www.DrRuscio.com /GutBook.

## ANEMIA

In anemia, certain nutrient deficiencies (iron and B vitamins) alter red blood cell production. This can cause fatigue and other symptoms. Those with lots of digestive symptoms, those with an autoimmune condition, and especially those who are underweight are at risk for anemia. To detect anemia, you can perform a test called a CBC (complete blood count) with differential.

## IBD (INFLAMMATORY BOWEL DISEASE)

IBD is usually diagnosed as Crohn's disease or ulcerative colitis, but there are a few less common types. As we have discussed, this is an autoimmune condition directed against your gut bacteria and/ or intestinal tissue. Some common symptoms are diarrhea, bloating, abdominal pain, and frequent stools. Here are some tests to discuss with your doctor:

- C-reactive protein
- Erythrocyte sedimentation rate (ESR)
- Lactoferrin
- Calprotectin
- A series of antibodies that can detect the underlying autoimmunity, which are abbreviated as ACCA, ALCA, AMCA, gASCA, pANCA
- Physical exam
- Colonoscopy and endoscopy/capsule endoscopy

## ABDOMINAL AND/OR PELVIC ADHESIONS

Abdominal and/or pelvic adhesions are essentially scar tissue that can form in your abdomen and/or pelvis. They can occur secondary to trauma, like a C-section, a hysterectomy, or impact trauma. They can also occur due to inflammation. When they occur, it can be like stepping on a garden hose and obstructing its flow—the scar tissue is like your foot putting pressure on and obstructing the hose that is your intestine. Some people will not see complete resolution of their symptoms until this scar tissue is addressed. Fortunately, certain types of manual therapy, very similar to massage, can be used to break down this scar tissue. You can see more on this here: http://goo.gl/4jeSlM.

## STRUCTURAL ABNORMALITIES OF THE DIGESTIVE TRACT

There are other structural abnormalities that thwart improvements. Having an evaluation with a well-trained gastroenterologist can help you assess if any of these are present. These are rare, but if nothing else is working for you, an evaluation is worth considering.

## DIGESTIVE-TRACT MOTILITY

IBD, adhesions, structural abnormalities, and/or autoimmunity can interfere with proper intestinal motility. "Motility" just means movement. It's important that food moves through your intestinal tract at the appropriate pace. Motility studies can be performed to assess this. If a motility problem is found, it can often be treated with a motility agent, as we discussed earlier, using Iberogast, MotilPro, low-dose erythromycin, or Resolor.

Additionally, if constipation is your main complaint, asking your gastroenterologist for a referral to a motility specialist can be helpful to rule out a motility problem. This could include slow-transit constipation, constipation due to pelvic-floor imbalance, or what's known as dyssynergic constipation.

## AN IMPORTANT NOTE REGARDING TESTING

When you're not feeling well, the idea of a test that will tell you what is wrong with you is very appealing. Testing can be very helpful in making a diagnosis and getting you to the corresponding treatment. However, there is another side to the testing issue. Testing is only helpful if it demonstrably changes the way in which you will be treated. There are many new tests in functional medicine that are more academic than clinical. What I mean is there are tests that show interesting information, but we have no idea what it means or how to treat it. We touched on some tests like this throughout this book. As a health-care consumer, it's difficult to know all the good tests versus nonuseful tests, so this is where finding a *good* doctor whom you trust is important. If you understand the concept of "more testing does not mean better results" and search for a health-care provider who seems conservative and reasonable, you will most likely end up with the appropriate amount of testing. But be cautious. Not all doctors get this, and it can result in you spending way more than you need to on lab testing.

Another challenge with tests that are more academic than clinical is what they do to your psyche. If you see a "positive" or "high" for one of your test results, it can be disconcerting. However, this positive or high result could be for a marker that is *meaningless*; however, if you didn't know that, you might be quite worried. Also, there are times when someone has a positive or high result, and then when this marker is retested just a few weeks later, it's normal again, all on its own. I offer this in the hope you will understand that just because there is a marker that is out of range, it doesn't mean you should be alarmed. A good health-care provider will be able to help you interpret your labs practically and guide you to the appropriate course of action.

Here is a simple example. Rob came in with gas, bloating, constipation, and fatigue. We ran some testing and found SIBO. We treated Rob for his SIBO, and within a few weeks his gas, bloating, constipation, and fatigue improved remarkably, and he was thrilled. When we retested his SIBO, the labs were improved, but he was still positive for SIBO. When Rob saw his results were still positive, he was crushed. He felt like a failure.

This is where having a good clinician is key. I reassured Rob that if his symptoms were gone, I wasn't concerned about his labs, because the labs and the patient don't always match. I told Rob he hadn't done anything wrong and to enjoy his newfound health. I also recommended we follow up again in two to three months just to keep tabs on him. Guess what? When I saw him at his follow-up, Rob was still doing great! Now, what if I had framed this differently? Rob could have felt like a failure, been nervous about his SIBO, and been subjected to another round of unneeded SIBO treatment. He may have needlessly gone home and spent hours on the Internet searching about SIBO rather than playing with his kids or spending time with his wife. Instances like this are why I emphasize finding a good provider.

## PERIODIC CHECKUPS

I would recommend you find a doctor who is highly skilled in digestive health to perform a periodic gut checkup. The time interval between checkups really depends on you, so follow your doctor's lead here. If you need help with this, feel free to contact our office. We have been working hard to find ways to make this care available to more people through my office. We offer phone visits for those who are at a distance, and I have been training another doctor in order to increase our accessibility.

1   Ali Rezaie et al., "Assessment of Anti-Vinculin and Anti-Cytolethal Distending Toxin B Antibodies in Subtypes of Irritable Bowel Syndrome," *Digestive Diseases and Sciences* 62, no. 6 (2017): 1480–85, doi:10.1007/s10620-017-4585-z.

2   William A. Walters et al., "Meta-Analyses of Human Gut Microbes Associated with Obesity and IBD," *FEBS Letters* 588, no. 22 (2014): 4223–33, doi:10.1016/j.febslet.2014.09.039.

3   C. Casén et al., "Deviations in Human Gut Microbiota: A Novel Diagnostic Test for Determining Dysbiosis in Patients with IBS or IBD," *Alimentary Pharmacology and Therapeutics* 42, no. 1 (2015): 71–83, doi:10.1111/apt.13236.

# CHAPTER 33

# CLOSING THOUGHTS

In this book, we've covered a lot. In part 1, we discussed how crucially important your gut health is and how the health of your gut affects your entire body, either positively or negatively. We detailed how problems in the gut can cause almost any symptom, from depression to insomnia, and how fixing a problem in the gut can often remedy these symptoms.

We have learned about this world of bacteria in your gut called the microbiota and covered some important misconceptions. We have learned that every ecosystem is different and how important it is we find and create the environmental factors that will allow your unique gut ecosystem to thrive. We have also detailed the importance of your small intestine, which is often left out of the conversation. Then we discussed the importance of early life factors and how pivotal these are in the formation of your microbiota and your immune system. We touched on how to use science the right way, rather than as a marketing tool.

In part 2, we covered dietary factors that are important for your gut and overall health. Much of

what we learned here built upon the concept that different gut ecosystems require different diets, just like different geographic ecosystems require different amounts of rain. Some people will do better on fewer carbs, while others will do better on more carbs. Some feel best on two meals per day, while others feel best on three or more meals per day. We established the important concept of eating to create a healthy internal environment, which then fosters healthy bacteria, which is the key to creating a healthy microbiota.

In part 3, we discussed key external environmental factors (like time in nature and sun exposure) and how these can create a healthy internal environment. We provided an accurate recommendation regarding sun exposure and updated the antiquated, skin-cancer-centric recommendations that have predominated the discussion. We also discussed exercise and stress and how they impact your gut. We closed this section with a reminder of how important friends and social time are for healing and happiness.

In part 4, we detailed the available gut-treatment options like probiotics, enzymes, antimicrobial herbs, and supplemental fiber and prebiotics. We gained a healthy understanding of how these different treatment options can help us and when a particular treatment is not a good fit. This hopefully provided valuable information to refer back to when you're confused or unsure about claims you read on the Internet.

Finally, in part 5, we translated all this information into a clinical approach, codified in our Great-in-8. We started by helping you discover the right diet for your gut ecosystem. This wasn't about finding the "one best diet" but rather navigating the available diets to find what was best for you. We then continued with our Great-in-8, which organized the available gut treatments into a logical sequence of personalized steps. In doing this, we worked together to create a healthy internal environment so your gut and microbiota can rebalance and achieve a healthy equilibrium. There were likely some ups and downs along the way, but just as a good gardener tends his garden, we listened to and tended your responses to help you end up in a far better position at the end than when you started.

We worked to find the minimal kinds and dosages of supplements and the broadest diet possible, and we did this with the goal of not making you feel dependent upon a restrictive diet and an excessive supplement plan. Finally, we covered a few strategies for handling setbacks, tips for finding a doctor, and things to discuss with him or her, should you need more help.

I hope you've learned a lot from this book. I mean that in the deepest sense. I hope you feel you've grown as a health-care consumer. Today's health-care consumers deserve better than they've been getting, from both conventional and natural medicine. This book was written to empower you, not only by helping you get well but by giving you the tools you need to understand *why* you got well. You're smarter and more capable than you think. If you apply a little logic and learn to listen to your body, you don't need to be dependent upon doctors or health gurus.

This book has been a labor of love. I love this work and love witnessing how dramatically it improves the lives of my patients. I look forward to hearing how this book has improved *your* life and welcome feedback and communication. If you visit www.DrRuscio.com/GutBook, you'll see a number of resources to help you as you work through this process. There are message boards where you can communicate with others who are going through the steps of the Great-in-8, and all the supplements needed for the Great-in-8 can also be found there.

I also invite you to connect with me by following my podcast, weekly articles, and weekly videos at www.DrRuscio.com. If you're a doctor or health-care provider, you can follow our health-care-practitioner newsletter at www.drruscio.com/review.

## If this book has helped you, please share it so this message can reach and help more people.

Thank you for taking the time to read this book. I sincerely hope you found it worthwhile and that it will help you vastly improve your health.

In health,
Dr. Michael Ruscio

# ABOUT THE AUTHOR

Dr. Michael Ruscio is a functional-medicine practitioner, clinical researcher, and international lecturer. He is a leader in the movement to make integrative medicine and natural health solutions more accepted and accessible. His clinical practice is located in Northern California.

CPSIA information can be obtained
at www.ICGtesting.com
Printed in the USA
BVHW050814180219
540527BV00032B/4751

9 780999 766804